A LANGE medical book

LANGE
SMART CHARTS

D1469571

PHYSIOLOGY

Shauna Lyn, MD

LANGE MEDICAL BOOKS / McGRAW-HILL
Medical Publishing Division

New York   Chicago   San Francisco   Lisbon   London   Madrid   Mexico City
Milan   New Delhi   San Juan   Seoul   Singapore
Sydney   Toronto

Lange Smart Charts: Physiology

Copyright © 2004 by the **McGraw-Hill Companies**, Inc. All rights reserved.
Printed in the United States of America. Except as permitted under the United States
Copyright Act of 1976, no part of this publication may be reproduced or distributed
in any form or by any means, or stored in a data base or retrieval system, without the
prior written permission of the publisher.

1 2 3 4 5 6 7 8 9 0 QPD/QPD 0 9 8 7 6 5 4

ISBN 0-07-139507-5
ISSN 1547-4100

This book was set in Goudy by Joanne Morbit and Deirdre Sheean of McGraw-Hill Professional's
Hightstown, N.J. composition unit.
The editors were Janet Foltin, Harriet Lebowitz, and Mary E. Bele.
The production supervisor was Phil Galea.
The art manager was Charissa Baker.
The cover designer was Mary McKeon.
The index was prepared by Nancy Newman.
Quebecor World Dubuque was printer and binder.

This book is printed on acid-free paper.

NOTICE

CONTENTS

PREFACE

Lange Smart Charts: Physiology is written specifically for students in the field of medicine. The book not only highlights the information that students need to learn for course examinations and for the physiology component of the USMLE Step I boards, but also makes it easier to study and remember this material.

The unique approach of this book is immediately apparent. **Tables and diagrams** are used exclusively to present well-selected information clearly and concisely. This chart method gives an instant picture of how the various facts are connected, thereby making study time productive and successful. The special feature **Terms to Learn** introduces each chapter and provides the reader with a quick understanding of certain high-yield facts—the information most often targeted on examinations and boards. **Mnemonics** are also included throughout the book to make immediate recall easier.

The material presented in *Smart Charts* is detailed enough for review in physiology courses, yet concise enough for board review. The selection and organization of information is designed to promote efficient use of study time by reducing the amount of re-reading required to master this subject area.

I would like to thank my husband, Tom Savel, for his inspiration and tireless assistance during the writing of this book. I also want to thank my parents, Eleanor and Lowell Lyn, and my sister Cerise for always supporting me.

HOW TO USE THIS BOOK

Layout of the book	The book is composed entirely of tables and diagrams to clarify relationships and interactions among the various elements of the organ systems of the body.
Using *Lange Smart Charts: Physiology* in conjunction with your physiology course	For optimal benefit, start using this book early in the year to follow along with the content of your physiology course. *Lange Smart Charts: Physiology* is designed to make the most of your studying time. Each chapter is introduced by an **outline** of the physiologic processes that are the focus of study. This is followed by **Terms to Learn**, which provides a basic review of expressions needed for the comprehension of physiologic concepts. **Diagrams** of mechanisms and pathways allow quick memorization and **illustrations** clarify difficult concepts. **Tables** make it easy to associate the functions and clinical significance of components of each of the organ systems. **Mnemonics** and other learning aids in each chapter promote quick recall of details.
Using *Lange Smart Charts: Physiology* as a physiology review for the USMLE Step 1.	Begin by reviewing each of the chapter outlines and the Terms to Learn. Use the tables and diagrams to fill in the details. Learn the mnemonics to improve your recall. Find your weaknesses by using a physiology question book and then review these topics in the relevant chapters. With this approach, you should be able to review physiology in a matter of days.

CHAPTER 1
BASIC CONCEPTS OF PHYSIOLOGY

I. GENERAL CELL PHYSIOLOGY

Cell Structure and Function

Cellular Organelles

Intercellular Junctions

Intercellular Junctions in the Mucosa of the Small Intestine

Intercellular Communication

Intercellular Communication by Chemical Mediators

Process of Intracellular Communication

Intracellular Mediators

II. PHYSIOLOGY OF SPECIALIZED CELLS: NERVE CELLS

Structure and Function of Nerve Cells

Components of a Motor Neuron

Action Potential

Action Potential in a Neuron

Events Occurring at Chemical Synapses

Biochemical Process at Cholinergic Endings

Presynaptic and Postsynaptic Responses

Specific Neurotransmitters

Disorders Involving the Neuromuscular Junction

Motor Neuron Diseases

III. PHYSIOLOGY OF SPECIALIZED CELLS: MUSCLE CELLS

Organization of Skeletal Muscle Fiber

Components of the Sarcomere

Actin and Myosin in Skeletal Muscle

Events in the Contraction and Relaxation of Skeletal and Smooth Muscle

Initiation of Muscle Contraction by Ca^{2+}

Comparison of Skeletal, Smooth, and Cardiac Muscle

Responses of Skeletal Muscle to a Repeated Stimulus

Muscular Dystrophies

IV. BODY FLUIDS

Body Fluid Compartments

Differences in Terms Related to Osmotic Pressure and Osmolality of Solutions

Transport Across Cell Membranes

Equations Relating to the Transport of Ions and Fluids

ABBREVIATIONS

ACh = acetylcholine

AMPA = a-amino-3-hydroxy-5-methyl-4-isoxazoleproprionate

ANS = autonomic nervous system

ATP = adenosine triphosphate

cAMP = cyclic adenosine monophosphate

cGMP = cyclic guanosine monophosphate

CNS = central nervous system

DAG = diacylglycerol

DNA = deoxyribonucleic acid

ECF = extracellular fluid

ECM = extracellular matrix

GABA = γ-aminobutyric acid

GI = gastrointestinal

GDP = guanosine diphosphate

GTP = guanosine triphosphate

5-HIAA = 5-hydroxyindoleacetic acid

ICF = intracellular fluid

IP$_3$ = inositol triphosphate

mRNA = messenger RNA

NMDA = N-methyl-D-aspartate

PNS = peripheral nervous system

RER = rough endoplasmic reticulum

RNA = ribonucleic acid

SER = smooth endoplasmic reticulum

SR = sarcoplasmic reticulum

TBW = total body water

Acetylcholinesterase	Enzyme that inactivates the neurotransmitter acetylcholine by catalyzing its hydrolysis into choline and acetate in the synaptic cleft.
"All-Or-None" Law	Under a given set of conditions, an action potential occurs with a constant amplitude and form regardless of the strength of the stimulus if the stimulus is at or above threshold intensity; it fails to occur if the stimulus is subthreshold.
Apoptosis	Programmed cell death.
Choline Acetyltransferase	Enzyme that catalyzes the condensation of acetyl coenzyme A and choline to produce acetylcholine; located in the motor nerve terminal.
Depolarization	*Decrease* in the potential difference, or polarization across a membrane (eg, -90 mV $\rightarrow -70$ mV).
Hyperpolarization	*Increase* in the potential difference, or polarization across a membrane (eg, -90 mV $\rightarrow -100$ mV).
Meiosis	"Reduction division"; two-stage type of cell division that results in four daughter cells, each having half the number of chromosomes (*haploid number*) of the original cell.
Membrane Potential	Electrical energy difference between the inside and outside of a cell, produced by separation of charge and measured in millivolts.
Mitosis	One-stage type of cell division in which the chromosomes duplicate and then divide, resulting in two daughter cells, each having the same, full complement of chromosomes (*diploid number*) as the original cell.
Na$^+$-K$^+$-ATPase (also known as Na$^+$-K$^+$ pump)	Enzyme that catalyzes the hydrolysis of ATP; it acts as a carrier molecule in active transport by pumping Na$^+$ out and K$^+$ into cells, preventing those ions from reaching equilibrium and maintaining the resting membrane potential.
Osmolality	Number of osmoles per kilogram of solvent; not affected by volume of solutes or temperature.
Osmolarity	Number of osmoles per liter of solution; not affected by volume of solutes or temperature.
Osmole	One osmole equals the gram-molecular weight of a substance, which equals the number of freely moving particles each molecule liberates in solution.
Summation of Contractions	Repeated stimulation of a muscle before relaxation occurs, producing additional contractions that are added to the one already present. This produces a tension greater than that developed during a single muscle twitch; *not the same as tetanus*.

Continued

Syncytium	Mass of protoplasm that contains several nuclei; the actions of both cardiac and smooth muscle cells are so interconnected that these cell types are described as "syncytiums."
Tetanus	*Fusion* of rapidly repeated contractions into one that is greater and prolonged. *Complete* tetanus has no relaxation between stimuli, and *incomplete* tetanus has periods of incomplete relaxation between stimuli; *not to be confused with summation.*
Tetany	Spasm and twitching of muscles, especially of the face, hands, and feet. Low concentration of extracellular Ca^{2+} increases excitability of nerves and muscles; seen in alkalosis, hypoparathyroidism, and rickets.
Tone (tonus)	State of partial contraction maintained by visceral smooth muscle and characterized by continuous, irregular contractions that are independent of neural stimulation.
Tonicity	Osmolality of a solution relative to plasma.
Wallerian Degeneration	Orthograde degeneration of a nerve; if an axon is the predominant input, the postsynaptic cell may also undergo degeneration or death. *Regeneration of neurons can occur in the PNS but is inadequate in the CNS.*

I. General Cell Physiology

CELL STRUCTURE AND FUNCTION

Structure	Description	Function	Clinical Significance
Cell (plasma) Membrane	• *Semipermeable* membrane made up of proteins floating in fluid *phospholipid bilayer*. • Contains ion channels and transport proteins that regulate crossing substances. • Polar (hydrophilic) heads of phospholipids are exposed to aqueous exterior of cell and its aqueous interior cytoplasm. • Nonpolar (hydrophobic) tails meet in nonaqueous interior of membrane.	• Regulates all substances entering and leaving cell. • Cell membrane proteins variably serve as carriers in facilitated diffusion; cell adhesion molecules; enzymes; ion channels; ion pumps; and receptors for antigens, hormones, and neurotransmitters.	Human immunodeficiency virus must attach to cholesterol-rich regions of cell membrane before it can replicate and infect other cells.
Nucleus	• Contains DNA in form of *chromatin* (complex of DNA and proteins), which forms *chromosomes* during cell division. • Contains *nucleolus*. • Surrounded by double membrane called *nuclear envelope*.	• Control center of cell. • Site of DNA and RNA synthesis. • Transcription: DNA → mRNA in nucleus. • Translation: RNA → protein in cytoplasm. • Nucleolus contains RNA and is site of ribosome synthesis.	Abnormalities in cell's ability to transport substances between nucleus and cytoplasm may cause disease (eg, Huntington disease).
Centrosome or Centromere	• Located near nucleus. • Made up of two centrioles that form poles of mitotic spindle.	Anchors and organizes microtubules during cell division.	

Continued

CELL STRUCTURE AND FUNCTION (Continued)

Structure	Description	Function	Clinical Significance
Mitochondria	• Organelle with double membrane. • Outer membrane contains enzymes involved in oxidation. • Inner membrane is folded to form shelves (cristae) and contains enzymes that convert products of metabolism into CO_2 and H_2O.	• "Powerhouse" of cell. • Chemical energy within nutrients is trapped and stored through formation of ATP. • Site of most cellular respiration.	Patients with disorders such as lupus, rheumatoid arthritis, and primary biliary cirrhosis often test positive for antimitochondrial antibodies.
Endoplasmic Reticulum	System of membranes in cell cytoplasm.		• SR (SER of muscle cells) actively pumps Ca^{2+} from sarcoplasm and stores it in terminal cisterns. • Ca^{2+} is released when there is an action potential.
	RER has ribosomes attached to cytoplasmic side of membrane.	• Site of protein synthesis. • Passes vesicles of newly synthesized proteins to Golgi apparatus for packaging.	
	SER does not have ribosomes attached to cytoplasmic side of membrane.	• Different functions in different cell types. • Works with mitochondria to produce steroid hormones and contains enzymes needed to detoxify drugs.	
Golgi Apparatus	• Group of stacked membrane-enclosed sacs (cisterns). • Located near nucleus.	• Processing and packaging of proteins and lipids. • *Cis* side receives vesicles of newly synthesized proteins from RER that are passed to *trans* side, where they are transferred to lysosomes and exterior of cell by exocytosis.	Defective proteins are detected and degraded, allowing for normal body function.
Lysosomes	Membrane-enclosed structures in cell cytoplasm that contain acidic enzymes.	Cellular digestive system.	Tay-Sachs disease and iron storage diseases are caused by congenital absence of lysosomal enzymes.

Peroxisomes	Structures similar to lysosomes, except they contain peroxisome-specific proteins.	Peroxisome-specific proteins carry substances into and out of peroxisome matrix to catalyze anabolic and catabolic reactions.	X-linked adrenoleukodystrophy and Zellweger syndrome are fatal childhood diseases caused by defects in peroxisomal membrane transport.
Cytoskeleton	System of fibers (microtubules, intermediate filaments, and microfilaments) and proteins that secure them together.	• Maintains cell structure. • Permits movement of cell as a whole as well as movement of its internal organelles and proteins.	• Hereditary elliptocytosis is disorder of red blood cells caused by genetic mutation that causes disruption of red blood cell cytoskeletons. • This disorder may result in hemolytic anemia.
Microtubules	• Long, hollow, cylinder-like structures. • 15 nm in diameter. • Composed of two protein subunits, α and β. • Assembly of microtubules is facilitated by warmth and inhibited by cold.	• Provide tracks for transport of vesicles and organelles from one part of cell to another. • Form spindle apparatus to move chromosomes during mitosis.	• Microtubules form *cilia*, tiny hair-like organelles that project from surface of epithelial cells. • Cilia protect bronchioles from mucus and foreign bodies. • Anticancer drug paclitaxel (Taxol) binds microtubules, restricting movement of the cell and its organelles. As a result, mitotic spindles cannot form and cells die.
Intermediate Filaments	• Fibers 8–14 nm in diameter. • Composed of various subunits.	Form a flexible scaffolding for cell, which helps resist external pressure.	Abnormal intermediate filaments cause cells to rupture more easily (eg, skin blistering).
Microfilaments	• Long, solid fibers 4–6 nm in diameter. • Have contractile properties. • Composed of actin, the most abundant protein in mammalian cells.	Aids in cell crawling, phagocytosis, and muscle contraction.	• Actin interacts with myosin to allow muscle contraction. • Actin supports microvilli on epithelial cells in small intestine.

CELLULAR ORGANELLES

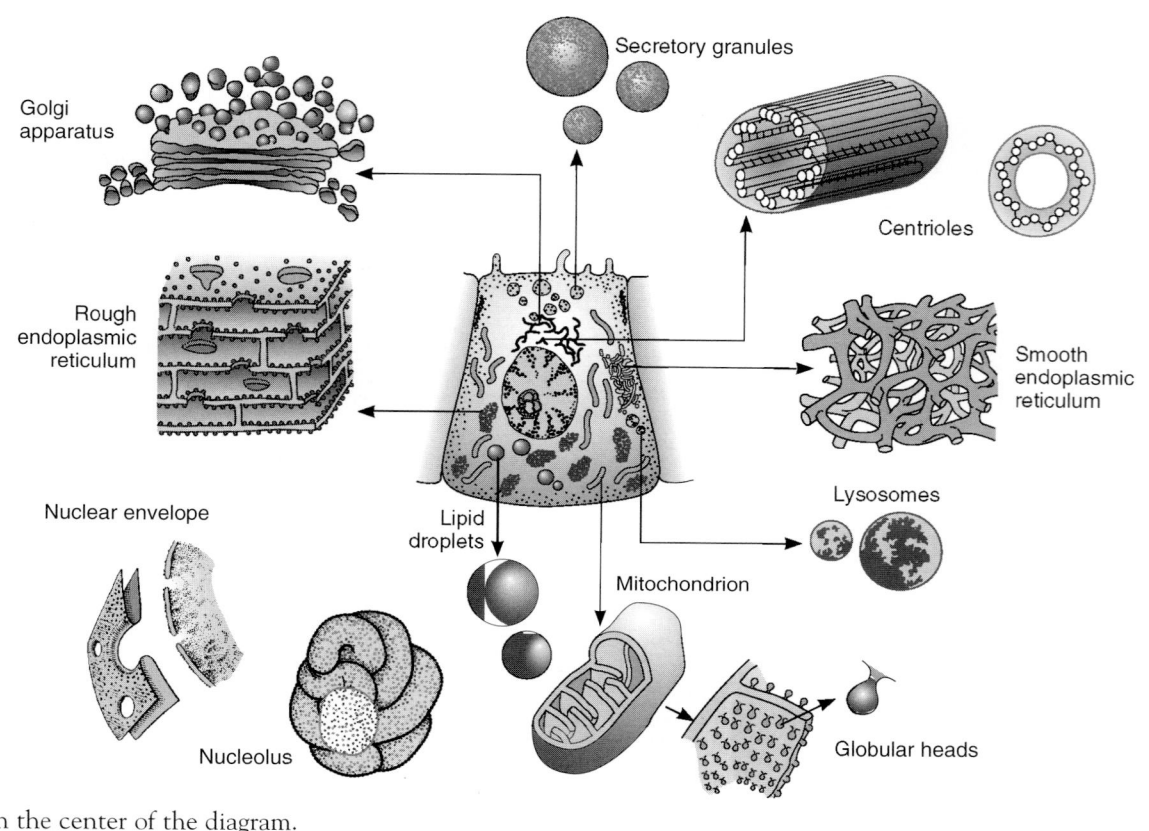

A hypothetical cell is seen in the center of the diagram.

Reproduced, with permission, from Junqueira LC, Carneiro J, Kelley RO: *Basic Histology*, 9th ed. McGraw-Hill, 1998.

INTERCELLULAR JUNCTIONS

Type	Description	Transmembrane-Linking Protein	Function	Examples
Tight Junctions (Zonula Occludens)	• Membranes of two adjacent cells fit against each other snugly, essentially sealing cells together and *preventing flow of fluid and ions between cells*. • Located near apical surface of cell.	Cadherin.	• Ties cytoskeleton of adjacent cells together, providing strength and stability. • Helps establish apical polarity of cell.	Epithelia such as intestinal mucosa, renal tubules, and choroid plexus.
Zonula Adherens	• Belt-like structure that encircles apical cell, beneath zonula occludens. • Major site of attachment for intracellular microfilaments, including actin and myosin.	Cadherin.	• Ties cytoskeleton of adjacent cells together. • Helps establish apical polarity of cell.	Epithelial cells.
Desmosomes (Macula Adherens)	Spot-like regions of tight adhesion scattered throughout the cell, below zonula adherens.	Cadherin.	• Ties cytoskeleton of adjacent cells together. • Apposed patches of thickened areas of membranes of two adjacent cells are attachment sites for intermediate filaments.	Epithelia such as skin and smooth muscle.
Hemidesmosome	• Half of a desmosome. • Located at cell base. • Connected intracellularly to intermediate filaments.	Integrin.	Ties cytoskeleton of cell to basal lamina and ECM.	Epithelial cells.

Continued

INTERCELLULAR JUNCTIONS (Continued)

Type	Description	Transmembrane-Linking Protein	Function	Examples
Focal Adhesions	Protein complexes associated with intracellular structure and signaling as well as microfilaments (actin) and cell movement.	Integrin.	• Tie cytoskeleton of cell to basal lamina and ECM. • Serve as points of traction with surface over which cell pulls itself.	Epithelial cells.
Gap Junctions	Hexagonal arrangement of connexin (called connexon) forms channels that permit transfer of molecules between adjacent cells.	Connexin.	Allows direct passage of small molecules and ions between adjoining cells.	Myocardial cells, hepatocytes, intestinal smooth muscle cells.

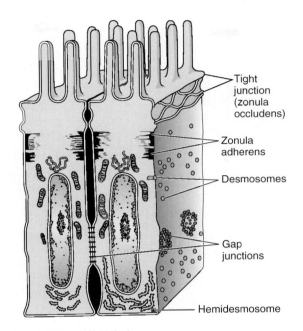

Reproduced, with permission, from Ganong WF: *Review of Medical Physiology*, 21st ed. McGraw-Hill, 2003:16.

INTERCELLULAR COMMUNICATION

Type	Description	Means of Message Transmission	Local or General	Examples
Autocrine	Process by which cell produces substance that regulates that cell or neighboring cells of same type.	By diffusion in interstitial fluid.	Locally diffuse.	• Prostaglandins released by uterine tissue induce contractions of uterine smooth muscle. • Prostaglandins released by bronchiolar smooth muscle induce vasodilation.
Endocrine	Process by which cell secretes regulatory substance directly into bloodstream, which affects cells that may be some distance away.	By circulating blood.	General.	• Anterior pituitary secretes prolactin, which travels via bloodstream to mammary glands to stimulate milk synthesis. • Pancreatic cells in islets of Langerhans secrete glucagon, insulin, somatostatin, and pancreatic polypeptide (pancreas has both exocrine and endocrine function).
Exocrine	Process by which cell delivers regulatory substances to an epithelial surface.	Usually via a duct.	Local.	• Pancreatic acinar cells secrete digestive enzymes (eg, carboxypeptidase, pancreatic lipase, ribonuclease, trypsin) into pancreatic duct of Wirsung, which joins common bile duct to form ampulla of Vater. • Ducts of sweat and salivary glands.
Neural (Synaptic)	Process by which neurons release neurotransmitters across synaptic cleft to postsynaptic cells.	Across synaptic cleft.	Local.	• At neuromuscular junction, motor nerve releases ACh, which increases Na^+ and K^+ conductance of muscle membrane. • This action causes influx of Na^+ and produces depolarizing potential.

Neurocrine	Process by which neuron releases regulatory substances into bloodstream to affect distant cells.	Axonal transport to bloodstream.	General.	• Hypothalamus releases antidiuretic hormone into bloodstream. • Antidiuretic hormone acts on distal tubule and collecting duct of kidney to increase NaCl reabsorption and H_2O retention.
Paracrine	Process by which cell secretes regulatory substance that diffuses into ECF to affect nearby cells that are different from itself.	By diffusion in interstitial fluid.	Locally diffuse.	Histamine released from cells in wall of stomach stimulates HCl secretion by parietal cells of gastric gland.

INTERCELLULAR COMMUNICATION BY CHEMICAL MEDIATORS

	GAP JUNCTIONS	SYNAPTIC	PARACRINE AND AUTOCRINE	ENDOCRINE
Message transmission	Directly from cell to cell	Across synaptic cleft	By diffusion in interstitial fluid	By circulating body fluids
Local or general	Local	Local	Locally diffuse	General
Specificity depends on	Anatomic location	Anatomic location and receptors	Receptors	Receptors

A = autocrine; P = paracrine.

PROCESS OF INTRACELLULAR COMMUNICATION

Sequence	Action
1	Agonist binds membrane receptor.
2	• G protein is activated by binding GTP. • Amplification allows one agonist–receptor complex to activate hundreds of effectors.
3	• Activated G protein interacts with effector proteins to alter their activities. • Effectors include enzymes, ion channels, and phospholipases.
4	Effector proteins affect activities of second messengers (cAMP, cGMP, DAG, IP_3).
5	Activity of second messenger alters activity of second messenger–dependent protein kinases (cAMP-dependent protein kinases, cGMP-dependent protein kinases, protein kinase C, calmodulin-dependent protein kinase) or ion channels.
6	Level of phosphorylation of enzyme or ion channel is altered.
7	Final cellular response.

☞ AGE SPLuRge—Agonist, G protein, Effector proteins, Second messengers, Protein kinases, Level of phosphorylation, Response

INTRACELLULAR MEDIATORS

Type	Description/Example
Second Messengers	
Cyclic Nucleotides (cAMP, cGMP)	• Vision depends on cGMP-gated Na^+ channels present in plasma membranes of rods. • When rhodopsin (receptor) is activated by light (stimulus), rhodopsin interacts with the G protein transducin. • Activated transducin interacts with cGMP phosphodiesterase, which increases cGMP and causes closing of cGMP-activated Na^+ channels and hyperpolarization of photoreceptor cell.
IP_3 and DAG	• G protein activates agonist-receptor complex, which then cleaves phosphatidylinositol 4,5-bisphosphate into IP_3 and DAG. • IP_3 binds receptors on endoplasmic reticulum, leading to release of Ca^{2+} into cytosol, which triggers cellular response. • Immunosuppressant drug cyclosporine helps prevent transplant rejection by blocking this pathway.
Ca^{2+}	Ca^{2+}-calmodulin complex activates myosin light-chain kinase (a calmodulin-dependent protein kinase), which phosphorylates myosin, resulting in smooth muscle contraction.
Protein Kinases	
Protein Kinase	• Enzyme activated by second messengers that phosphorylates proteins on serine or threonine residues (protein phosphatase is enzyme that dephosphorylates proteins). • cAMP-dependent protein kinase phosphorylates rate-determining enzymes in glycogen metabolism. • Ca^{2+} stimulates *protein kinase* C, which stimulates cell division and is involved in growth of tumor cells.
Protein Tyrosine Kinase	• Membrane receptors that are themselves protein kinases. • When agonist binds receptor, protein tyrosine kinase phosphorylates protein substrates on tyrosine residues. • Receptors for insulin and those for growth factors (epidermal growth factor, colony-stimulating factor, fibroblast growth factor) are protein tyrosine kinases. • Uncontrolled protein-tyrosine kinases play major role in cell transformation and malignancy.

G Proteins	
Heterotrimeric	• Nucleotide regulatory protein that aids in translation of signals between cells and helps modulate intracellular concentrations of second messengers. • In active state, acts as GTPase, hydrolyzing GTP to GDP. • Adenylyl cyclase (enzyme that aids synthesis of cAMP) and cGMP phosphodiesterase (enzyme that breaks down cGMP) are modulated by G proteins. • Activation of phospholipase A_2 by G protein leads to production of arachidonic acid.
Monomeric	• Small G proteins involved in protein synthesis, cell proliferation, neoplastic cell transformation, and vesicle transport. • Ras-like G proteins regulate cell growth and differentiation. • Rab-like G proteins help target vesicles to membranes.

II. Physiology of Specialized Cells: Nerve Cells

STRUCTURE AND FUNCTION OF NERVE CELLS

Structure	Important Features
Soma (cell body)	Contains nucleus as well as other structures (RER, ribosomes, Golgi bodies) and substances necessary for specialized functions of nerve cell.
Nissl Bodies	RER of nerve cell.
Neurofilaments	Thin, rod-like structures of nerve cell cytoskeleton.
Lipofuscin	Pigment formed from incompletely degraded membrane components that accumulates in some nerve cells.
Dendrites	• Multiple extensions of soma that may be up to 1 mm long. • Dendrites near soma contain Nissl bodies and Golgi bodies, and those further away contain elements of cytoskeleton.
Dendritic Spines	Knobby projections on dendrites.
Axon Hillock	• Thickened area of soma from which axon originates. • Lacks RER, ribosomes, and Golgi bodies.
Initial Segment	• Unmyelinated part of axon located at and just beyond axon hillock. • Part of nerve cell with lowest threshold for an action potential and where action potentials are initiated in motor neurons.
Axon (also known as nerve fiber)	• Single process extending from soma. • Lacks RER, ribosomes, and Golgi bodies but contains SER and cytoskeleton. • Transmits impulses from cell to cell.
Axon Terminal	End of presynaptic neuron that contains synaptic vesicles.
Active Zones	Portion of axon terminal of the presynaptic cell that contain rows of Ca^{2+} channels and from where synaptic vesicles are released.
Synaptic Knobs	Terminal branches of axons that contain vesicles in which neurotransmitters are stored.

Synapse	Anatomic site where electrical impulse is transmitted from one cell to another.
Synaptic Cleft	Area between pre- and postsynaptic cells that contains acetylcholinesterase.
Myelin	• Protein-lipid complex that is wrapped around axon and speeds conduction of nerve impulses by altering electrical properties of nerve fiber. • Demyelination in PNS is seen in Guillain Barré syndrome. • Demyelination in CNS is seen in multiple sclerosis.
Schwann Cell	Myelin-producing cell in PNS that wraps around axon of single neuron.
Internodes	Length of axon covered by myelin sheath.
Nodes of Ranvier	• Unmyelinated gaps that occur at regular intervals along myelin sheath of nerve cells (between Schwann cells). • Contains high concentrations of Na^+ channels. • Sites to which nerve impulses jump during *salutatory conduction*.
Golgi Type I Neurons	Short axons that terminate near soma.
Golgi Type II Neurons	Long axons that may extend > 1 m.
Glia (neuroglia)	• "Nerve glue"; specialized supporting cells of nervous system. • 10–50 times as many glial cells as neurons. • There are four main types. Astrocytes: • Star-shaped cells present in CNS. • Component of blood-brain barrier. • Fibrous astrocytes are primarily white matter. • Protoplasmic astrocytes are primarily gray matter. Ependymal cells: • Form epithelium that separates CNS from ventricles.

Continued

STRUCTURE AND FUNCTION OF NERVE CELLS (Continued)

Structure	Important Features
	Microglia: • Scavenger cells similar to macrophages that remove products of cellular damage from the CNS. • They are thought to originate in bone marrow.
	Oligodendrocytes: • Myelin-producing cells in CNS that wrap around axons. • Have multiple processes that form myelin on many neighboring axons.

COMPONENTS OF A MOTOR NEURON

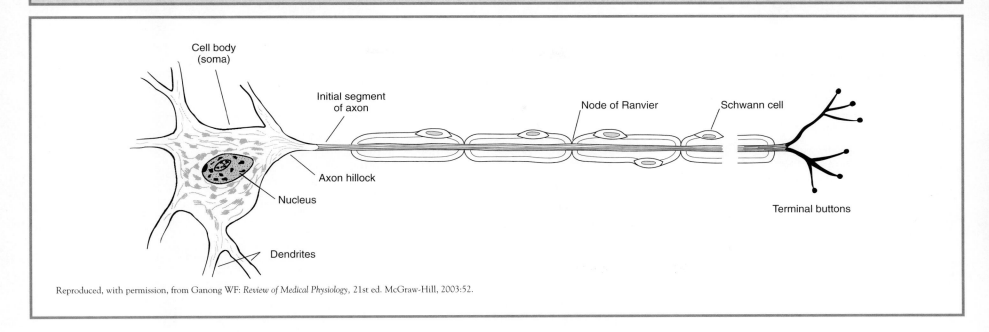

Reproduced, with permission, from Ganong WF: *Review of Medical Physiology*, 21st ed. McGraw-Hill, 2003:52.

ACTION POTENTIAL

Phase	Tracing	Description	Major Changes in Ion Conductance
Latent Period	Prior to upstroke.	• Interval at resting membrane potential. • Ends when threshold is reached and action potential begins.	Magnitude of resting potential determined mainly by extracellular K^+ concentration (Na^+ channels are closed and K^+ channels are open).
Depolarization	Firing level.	• Threshold-critical membrane potential at which excitable cells undergo rapid depolarization, resulting in action potential. • Action potential fails to occur if stimulus is sub-threshold. • Absolute refractory period begins at firing level and extends into downstroke, and *neuron is resistant to all stimulation during this time*.	Na^+ and K^+ conductance increases, resulting in movement of Na^+ into cell and K^+ out of cell.
	Upstroke.	• Decrease in magnitude of potential difference across membrane. • Potential rises toward zero. • Action potential is produced if threshold is reached.	• Fast Na^+ channels open first, causing rapid increase in conductance of Na^+. • Slow K^+ channels open later.
	Overshoot.	Portion of action potential during which membrane potential is positive.	• Conductance of Na^+ peaks at approximately same time as action potential. • Slow K^+ channels continue to open.
Repolarization	Downstroke.	• Membrane potential returns toward resting state (ie, becomes more negative). • Relative refractory period begins at end of absolute refractory period, and only stronger-than-normal stimulus can cause excitation of neuron.	• Slow Na^+ channels close. • Slow K^+ channels continue to open. • Conductance of K^+ peaks at midrepolarization.

After-depolarization	More gradual part of downstroke.	• Occurs after spike potential and after repolarization is approximately 70% complete. • Rate of repolarization is decreased.	• Conductance of K^+ decreases. • Conductance of Na^+ continues to decrease.
Hyperpolarization (hyperpolarizing after-potential)	Undershoot.	• Occurs at end of action potential, following after-polarization. • Polarization of membrane increases, and its potential becomes more negative than resting membrane potential.	• Conductance of Na^+ returns to resting level. • Conductance of K^+ remains elevated above resting level.

☞ Lazy Dogs Really Aren't Hyper—-Latent period, Depolarization, Repolarization, After-depolarization, Hyperpolarization

ACTION POTENTIAL IN A NEURON

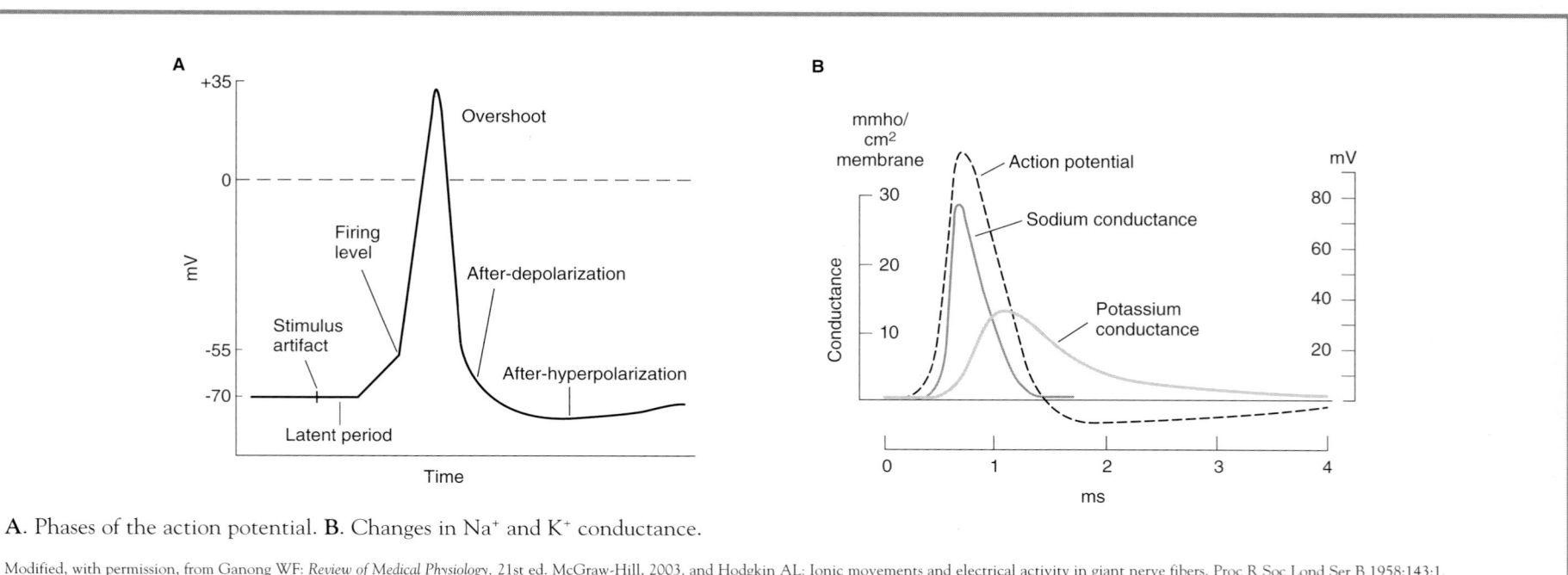

A. Phases of the action potential. **B.** Changes in Na$^+$ and K$^+$ conductance.

Modified, with permission, from Ganong WF: *Review of Medical Physiology*, 21st ed. McGraw-Hill, 2003, and Hodgkin AL: Ionic movements and electrical activity in giant nerve fibers. Proc R Soc Lond Ser B 1958;143:1.

EVENTS OCCURRING AT CHEMICAL SYNAPSES

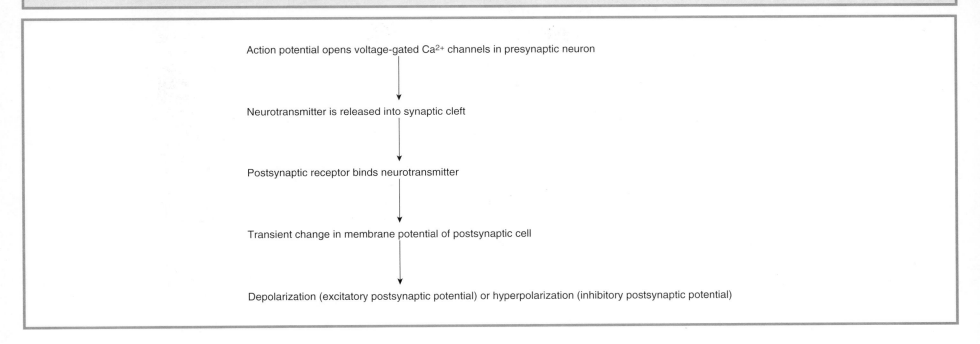

Action potential opens voltage-gated Ca^{2+} channels in presynaptic neuron

↓

Neurotransmitter is released into synaptic cleft

↓

Postsynaptic receptor binds neurotransmitter

↓

Transient change in membrane potential of postsynaptic cell

↓

Depolarization (excitatory postsynaptic potential) or hyperpolarization (inhibitory postsynaptic potential)

BIOCHEMICAL PROCESS AT CHOLINERGIC ENDINGS

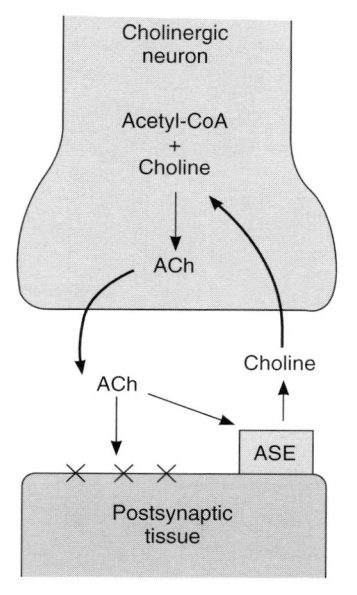

Active uptake of choline takes place via a transporter into cholinergic neurons.
ASE = acetylcholinesterase; X = receptor.

Reproduced, with permission, from Ganong WF: *Review of Medical Physiology*, 21st ed. McGraw-Hill, 2003:101.

PRESYNAPTIC AND POSTSYNAPTIC RESPONSES

Response	Description
Presynaptic Responses	
Facilitation	• Neurotransmitter (eg, serotonin) released by modulatory neuron onto affected axon decreases K^+ conductance in its nerve terminal.
	• This action prolongs action potential and causes greater influx of Ca^{2+} into nerve terminal, leading to greater release of neurotransmitter from modulated neuron and allowing it to increase its affect to postsynaptic cell.
	• Response of postsynaptic cell grows with each stimulation but dies rapidly after stimulation stops.
Inhibition	• Neurotransmitter released by modulatory neuron onto affected axon increases Cl^- conductance (eg, $GABA_A$) or increases K^+ conductance (eg, $GABA_B$) in its nerve terminal.
	• This action decreases action potential and decreases influx of Ca^{2+} into nerve terminal, leading to decreased release of neurotransmitter from modulated neuron.
	• Term also refers to direct inhibition of presynaptic neurotransmitter release independent of Ca^{2+} influx into nerve terminal.
Summation	• Integration of many excitatory and inhibitory synapses that converge on single neuron.
	• Spatial summation occurs when several inputs arrive almost simultaneously; inputs are added, resulting in larger depolarization of postsynaptic membrane than either input alone.
	• Temporal summation occurs if another action potential enters nerve terminal before first one has disappeared; two action potentials combined produce larger response.
Synaptic Fatigue	Presynaptic defect in which long-term, repeated stimulation of synapse eventually leads to point at which each successive presynaptic stimulus elicits smaller postsynaptic response.
Tetanic Stimulation	• High-frequency stimulation of presynaptic cell results in accumulation of Ca^{2+} in presynaptic nerve terminal and prolonged enhancement of postsynaptic response (posttetanic potentiation).
	• Lasts tens of seconds to minutes after stimulation has stopped.
	• Longer than facilitation.

Continued

PRESYNAPTIC AND POSTSYNAPTIC RESPONSES (Continued)

Response	Description
Postsynaptic Responses	
Accommodation	• Slow depolarization of nerve or muscle cells allows cells to adapt to stimulus and pass normal threshold without firing an action potential. • Prolonged depolarization allows open Na^+ channels to close and closed K^+ channels to open—all before threshold is reached.
Excitatory Response	Action potential increases activity of postsynaptic cell (eg, muscle contracts and gland secretes).
Habituation	Disappearance of response to repeated, benign stimulus caused by decrease in intracellular Ca^{2+} and neurotransmitter release.
Inhibitory Response	Action potential decreases or completely blocks activity of postsynaptic cell.
Local Circuit Currents and Local Responses	• Potential differences between adjacent cells travel by *electrotonic conduction*. • Result is depolarization of membrane adjacent to initial site of depolarization. • *These potential changes are not propagated but decrease in size with distance.*
Long-term Depression	Repetitive low-frequency synaptic stimulation decreases efficacy of transmission at that synapse for days to weeks.
Long-term Potentiation	• Repetitive high-frequency synaptic stimulation increases efficacy of transmission at that synapse for days to weeks. • Believed to be involved in learning and memory.
Propagation	Action potential generated at one location of axon acts as stimulus for production of action potential in adjacent region of axon *without change in magnitude of action potential.*

SPECIFIC NEUROTRANSMITTERS

Substance	Location	Important Points
ACh	ANS, brain, GI tract, neuromuscular junction, retina, sweat glands.	• Transmitter used by all motor axons that arise from spinal cord, all autonomic preganglionic neurons, and all postganglionic sympathetic fibers. • Nicotinic ACh receptors are present at neuromuscular junctions. • Muscarinic ACh receptors are present in brain and in heart and smooth muscle.
Excitatory Amino Acids		
Aspartate	Brain, spinal cord.	Believed to function primarily in visual cortex.
Glutamate	Cerebral cortex, brainstem.	• Most common excitatory neurotransmitter in brain. • Metabotropic receptors are coupled to G proteins and increase IP_3 and DAG and decrease cAMP. • Three types of ionotropic receptors that are ligand-gated ion channels: kainate, AMPA, and NMDA.
Inhibitory Amino Acids		
GABA	Brain, retina.	• $GABA_A$ and $GABA_B$ receptors are in CNS, and $GABA_C$ receptors are in retina. • $GABA_A$ and $GABA_C$ receptors mediate Cl^- influx, leading to hyperpolarization and inhibition of neurons. • GABA receptors are coupled to G proteins; they stimulate conductance of K^+ and inhibit Ca^{2+} influx and adenyl cyclase. • Benzodiazepines and barbiturates bind $GABA_A$ receptors and enhance opening of Cl^- channels.
Glycine	Brain, spinal cord, retina.	Most glycine receptors mediate Cl^- influx, leading to hyperpolarization and inhibition of neurons.

Continued

SPECIFIC NEUROTRANSMITTERS (Continued)

Substance	Location	Important Points
Amines		
Dopamine	Brain, retina, sympathetic ganglia.	• Degeneration of dopaminergic synapses from substantia nigra to corpus striatum occurs in Parkinson disease. • Acts as positive inotropic via β_1 receptors, causing increased systolic blood pressure (no effect on diastolic blood pressure). • Injection causes renal and mesenteric vasodilation, but vasoconstriction elsewhere.
Epinephrine	Brain, spinal cord.	• Has greater affinity for β receptors than α receptors. • *Not mediator at postganglionic sympathetic endings like norepinephrine.*
Norepinephrine	Brain, spinal cord, GI tract, sympathetic endings.	Has greater affinity for α receptors than β receptors.
Histamine	Brain, GI tract.	Three types of receptors: • H_1 receptors activate phospholipase C. • H_2 receptors increase cAMP. • H_3 receptors (mostly presynaptic) mediate release of histamine and other neurotransmitters via G protein. Also released from mast cells during anaphylactic reactions and in allergic conditions.
Serotonin	Brain, spinal cord, GI tract, retina.	• Reuptake of serotonin from synaptic cleft is inactivated by monoamine oxidase to form 5-HIAA. • Urinary output of 5-HIAA is used to monitor serotonin metabolism. • Involved in temperature regulation, sleep, mood, and sensory perception.
Gas		
Nitric oxide	Brain, spinal cord, GI tract.	• Functions as CNS neurotransmitter and neuromodulator in CNS. • Mediates transmission between inhibitory motor neurons of enteric nervous system and GI smooth muscle.

- Increased cytosolic Ca^{2+} stimulates nitric oxide synthase, which catalyzes nitric oxide production.
- Influences cellular processes via cGMP.

Polypeptides

Angiotensin II	Brain, spinal cord.	Also functions as adrenal hormone that stimulates renal reabsorption of Na^+ and H_2O.
Atrial Natriuretic Peptide	Brain.	Also functions as hormone in heart that increases in response to increased Na^+ intake and ECF expansion.
Cholecystokinin	Brain, retina.	Also functions as GI tract hormone that aids in gallbladder contraction.
β-Endorphin	Brain, GI tract, retina.	<ul><li>Endogenous opioid.</li><li>Modulates pain pathways.</li></ul>
Enkephalin	Brain, GI tract, retina.	<ul><li>Endogenous opioid.</li><li>Modulates pain pathways.</li></ul>
Endothelin	Brain, pituitary gland.	Also has other functions, including vasoconstriction, positive inotropy and chronotropy, increased bronchoconstriction, decreased glomerular filtration, increased gluconeogenesis.
Gastrin	Brain.	Also functions as GI tract hormone.
Inhibin	Brain.	Also functions in reproductive tract by inhibiting follicle-stimulating hormone secretion.
Motilin	Brain, pituitary gland.	Also functions as hormone by stimulating contraction of smooth muscle in GI tract.
Neuropeptide Y	Brain, ANS.	<ul><li>Augments vasoconstriction effects of norepinephrine.</li><li>Mediates appetite.</li><li>Levels increase with exercise.</li></ul>
Neurotensin	Brain, retina.	Also functions as hormone by inhibiting motility in GI tract.
Oxytocin	Brain, spinal cord, posterior pituitary.	Also functions as hormone to stimulate uterine contractions and milk secretion in pregnancy.

Continued

SPECIFIC NEUROTRANSMITTERS (Continued)

Substance	Location	Important Points
Secretin	Brain.	Also functions as GI tract hormone.
Somatostatin	Brain, GI tract, retina.	• Also secreted from hypothalamus and functions as growth hormone–inhibiting hormone. • Inhibits secretion of insulin and GI tract hormones.
Substance P	Brain, retina, endings of primary afferent pain fibers.	Inhibited by enkephalins.
Vasoactive intestinal polypeptide	ANS, brain, spinal cord, GI tract, retina.	• Functions as GI tract hormone and neuropeptide. • Inhibits smooth muscle cells, leading to vasodilation. • Excites glandular epithelial cells.
Vasopressin	Brain, spinal cord, posterior pituitary.	Also functions as adrenal hormone that increases renal reabsorption of Na^+ and H_2O.
Purines		
Adenosine	Brain.	• Neuromodulator that acts as CNS depressant. • Also acts as cardiac vasodilator.
ATP	Autonomic ganglia, brain.	• Mediates rapid synaptic responses in ANS. • May play role in sensory transmission.

DISORDERS INVOLVING THE NEUROMUSCULAR JUNCTION

Disorder/Causal Agent	Etiology	Clinical Presentation
Genetic Disorders		
Lambert-Eaton Myasthenic Syndrome	Autoimmune disorder involving production of antibodies to presynaptic Ca^{2+} channels, leading to decreased presynaptic release of ACh.	• Proximal muscle weakness of limbs that worsens with exertion, absent tendon reflexes, and paresthesias. • Two thirds of cases occur in patients with small cell lung cancer.
Myasthenia Gravis	Autoimmune disorder involving production of antibodies to nicotinic ACh receptors.	• Progressive muscle weakness and fatigability (ocular muscles are commonly affected, and weakness improves with Tensilon). • Symptoms relieved by anticholinesterases such as neostigmine. • Immunosuppressive drugs, plasmapheresis, and thymectomy help reduce antibodies.
Drug Exposure		
α-Toxin	• Binds α-subunits of ACh receptor, preventing ACh from functioning. • Found in cobra venom, curare (plant extract), and succinylcholine (paralytic drug). • Aminoglycoside antibiotics, antiarrhythmics, β-blockers, lithium, phenothiazines, and tetracyclines may also interfere with neuromuscular transmission.	Dyspnea, paresthesias, fasciculations, and limb paralysis may progress to nausea, vomiting, fever, abdominal pain, and shock.
Strychnine	Functions as competitive antagonist to glycine (inhibitory) receptors.	• Characterized by severe contractions of facial muscles ("fixed grin" or risus sardonicus). • Overdose leads to painful convulsions. • Respiratory muscle paralysis may lead to death.

Continued

DISORDERS INVOLVING THE NEUROMUSCULAR JUNCTION (Continued)

Disorder/Causal Agent	Etiology	Clinical Presentation
Infectious Disorders		
Botulism	Ingestion of endotoxin of *Clostridium botulinum* from improperly cooked foods blocks presynaptic ACh release at neuromuscular junction, causing paralysis.	• Flaccid paralysis of skeletal muscle. • Severe disease may result in cardiac or respiratory failure.
Tetanus	Skin exposure to exotoxin of *Clostridium tetani* blocks presynaptic release of ACh, causing spasmodic muscle contraction.	• Spastic paralysis of skeletal muscle • Often manifests first in jaw and neck (lockjaw) and may cause opisthotonos (whole body spasm). • May affect respiratory muscles leading to death by asphyxia.
Environmental Causes		
Black Widow Spider Bite	Neurotoxin releases significant amounts of ACh at neuromuscular junction and blocks its reuptake.	• Tingling, rash, nausea, rigid abdominal muscles, chest tightness, shortness of breath. • May also cause local damage at site of bite.
Scorpion Sting	• Venom contains neurotoxin that affects Na^+, K^+, and Ca^{2+} channels. • Potency varies depending on species.	Symptoms range from mild flu to death within 1 hour (caused by cardiovascular collapse).
Tick Paralysis	Neurotoxin blocks presynaptic release of ACh.	• Paresthesias and progressive muscle weakness. • Flaccid paralysis may result. • Symptoms subside after parasite is removed.
Organophosphate Pesticide Exposure	Pesticides irreversibly inactivate acetylcholinesterase in synaptic cleft, resulting in excess ACh.	• ☞ Remember SLUDGE, which stands for *Salivation, Lacrimation, Urination, Defecation, GI upset, (pulmonary) Edema.* • Other symptoms include bradycardia, bronchoconstriction, and pupil constriction. • Atropine and pralidoxime reverse symptoms.

MOTOR NEURON DISEASES

Disease	Description	Symptoms
Amyotrophic Lateral Sclerosis (Lou Gehrig disease)	• Progressive disease of unknown etiology. • Results in degeneration and loss of upper and lower motor neurons, destroying innervation to skeletal muscle.	• Progressive weakness, slurred speech, difficulty swallowing, shortness of breath. • *Progressive muscular atrophy*, often beginning with hands. • *Fasciculations* caused by dying α-motor neurons at all levels of spinal cord and brainstem.
Poliomyelitis	• Acquired viral disease with acute onset. • Results in destruction of lower motor neurons (anterior horn cells of spinal cord). • Reinnervation from collateral sprouts of axons of surviving α-motor neurons may occur.	• Acute symptoms include fever and lethargy. • Progressive *flaccid paralysis* (usually asymmetric) and atrophy of denervated muscles.
Spinal Muscular Atrophy	• Inherited (autosomal recessive) disorder. • Slowly progressive disease in which degeneration of anterior horn cells results in muscle weakness. • Three forms (I, II, III).	• Flaccid muscles with fasciculations. • Lower limbs more affected than upper limbs, and proximal lower limbs more affected than distal lower limbs. • Symptoms range from breathing disorders and death in young children (< 2 years of age) to proximal weakness and abnormal gait in adults.
Guillain-Barré Disease	Acute inflammatory demyelinating disease (polyradiculopathy) of unclear etiology (frequently postviral).	• Begins with paresthesias in distal extremities, resulting in rapidly developing ascending weakness with risk of respiratory failure. • Difficulty swallowing. • Bowel and bladder function preserved.

III. Physiology of Specialized Cells: Muscle Cells

ORGANIZATION OF SKELETAL MUSCLE FIBER

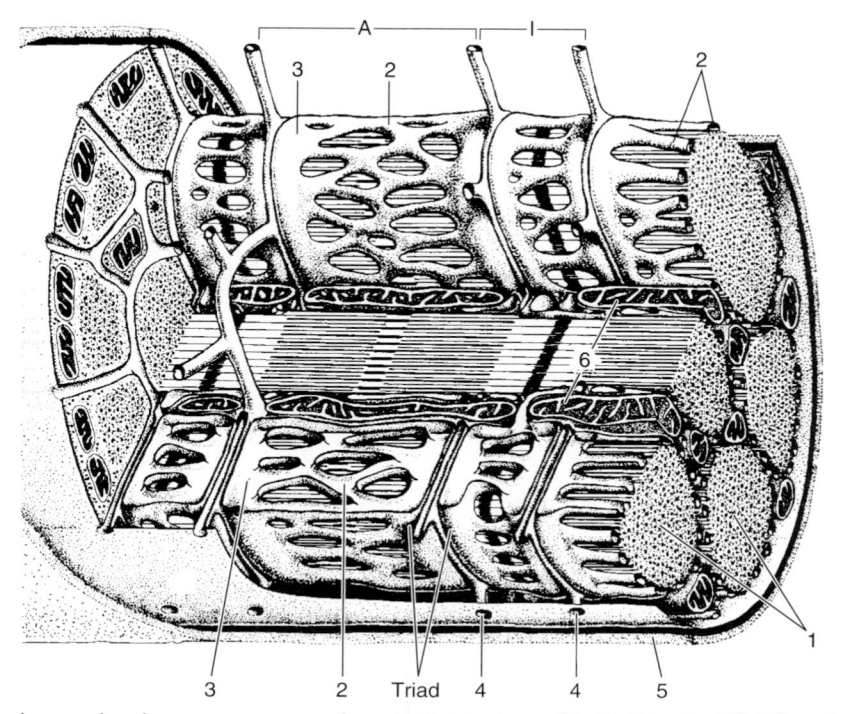

A single muscle fiber surrounded by its sarcolemma has been cut away to show individual myofibrils (1). the SR (2) with its terminal cisterns (3) surround each myofibril. The T system of tubules (4) contacts the myofibrils between the A and I bands two times in every sarcomere. The T system and the adjacent cisterns of the SR constitute a triad. A basal lamina (5) surrounds the sarcolemma. Several mitochondria (6) are apparent.

Modified, with permission, from Krstic RV: *Ultrastructure of the Mammalian Cell.* Springer, 1979.

COMPONENTS OF THE SARCOMERE

Component	Description
A Bands	<ul><li>Area of sarcomere formed by parallel myosin (thick) filaments.</li><li>*When muscle contracts, width of A bands remains constant.*</li></ul>
Actin	Contractile proteins that, along with tropomyosin and troponin, make up *thin filaments* and *I bands* of muscle fibers.
Calmodulin	Ca^{2+}-binding protein that, once Ca^{2+} is bound, activates myosin light-chain kinase, leading to contraction of smooth muscle.
Dense Bodies	Structures bound to actin in smooth muscle in absence of Z lines.
Dystrophin-Glycoprotein Complex	Proteins that provide structural support and strength to muscle fibrils.
H Bands	Regions in center of A bands where, when muscle is relaxed, thin and thick filaments do not overlap.
I Bands	Area of sarcomere formed by parallel thin filaments.
Intercalated Disks	Series of folds that form junctions at the ends of cardiac muscle fibers.
M Line	<ul><li>Area that divides H band.</li><li>Area on either side of M line is "pseudo–H zone."</li></ul>
Myosin	Contractile proteins that make up *thick filaments* and *A bands* of muscle fibers.
Sarcolemma	Cell membrane of muscle cell.
Sarcomere	Area between two adjacent Z lines that is contractile unit of striated muscle.
SR	SER of muscle cells.
Sarcotubular System	T tubules together with SR.

Continued

COMPONENTS OF THE SARCOMERE (Continued)

Component	Description
T Tubules	• Grid-like system of transverse tubules that is continuous with sarcolemma. • Aids in rapid transmission of action potential to other muscle fibrils.
Tropomyosin	• Regulatory protein that, when bound to troponin, inhibits muscle contraction by covering the sites where myosin binds to actin. • Part of *thin filaments*.
Troponin	• Ca^{2+}-binding protein made of three subunits (C, I, and T); it inhibits muscle contraction when bound to tropomyosin. • When it binds Ca2+, muscle contraction begins; part of *thin filaments*.
Z Line	• Divides I band and connects thin filaments. • Provides boundaries for sarcomere. • *When muscle contracts, Z lines move closer together*; when muscle relaxes, they move farther apart.

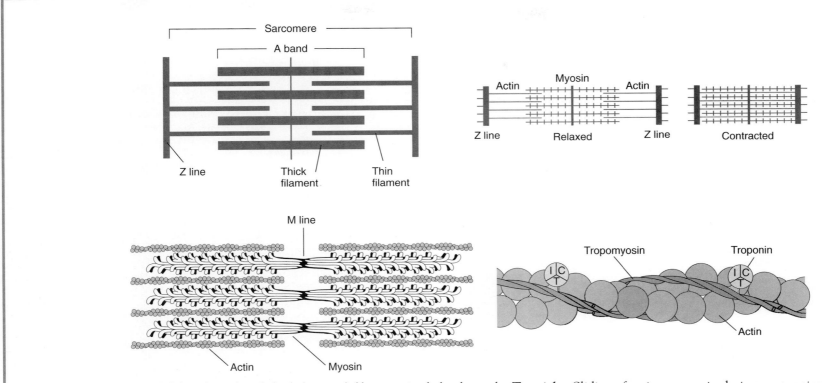

Top left: Arrangement of thin (actin) and thick (myosin) filaments in skeletal muscle. **Top right:** Sliding of actin on myosin during contraction; Z lines move closer together. **Bottom left:** Relation of myosin to actin. Note that myosin thick filaments reverse polarity at the M line in the middle of the sarcomere. **Bottom right:** Diagrammatic representation of the arrangement of actin, tropomyosin, and the three subunits of troponin.

Reproduced, with permission, from Ganong WF: *Review of Medical Physiology,* 21st ed. McGraw-Hill, 2003:67.

EVENTS IN THE CONTRACTION AND RELAXATION OF SKELETAL AND SMOOTH MUSCLE

Step	Contraction	Relaxation
Skeletal Muscle		
1	Discharge of motor neuron.	Ca^{2+} pumped backed into SR.
2	Release of ACh at motor end plate.	Release of Ca^{2+} from troponin.
3	Binding of ACh to nicotinic ACh receptors.	Cessation of interaction between actin and myosin.
4	Increased Na^+ and K^+ conductance in end-plate membrane.	
5	Generation of end-plate potential.	
6	Generation of action potential in muscle fibers.	
7	Inward spread of depolarization along T tubules.	
8	Release of Ca^{2+} from terminal cisterns of SR and diffusion to thick and thin filaments.	
9	Binding of Ca^{2+} to troponin C, uncovering myosin-binding sites on actin.	
10	Formation of cross-linkages between actin and myosin and sliding of thin on thick filaments, producing shortening.	
Smooth Muscle		
1	Binding of ACh to muscarinic receptors.	Dephosphorylation of myosin by myosin light chain phosphatase.
2	Increased influx of Ca2+ into cell.	Relaxation or sustained contraction due to latch bridge mechanisms.
3	Activation of calmodulin-dependent myosin light chain kinase.	
4	Phosphorylation of myosin.	
5	Increased myosin ATPase activity and binding of myosin to actin.	
6	Contraction.	

Modified, with permission, from Ganong WF: *Review of Medical Physiology*, 21st ed. McGraw-Hill, 2003.

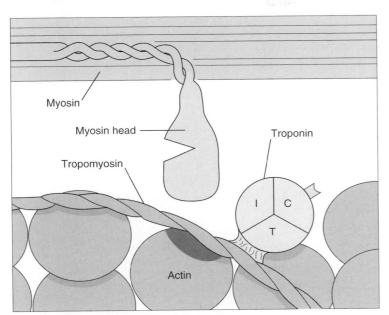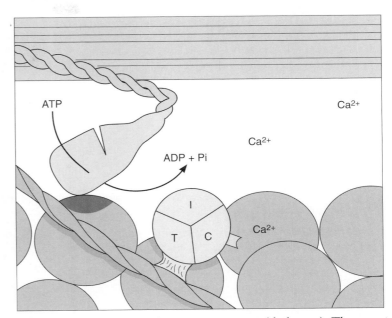

The binding of Ca^{2+} to troponin C causes lateral displacement of tropomyosin. This exposes the binding site for myosin on actin (dark area). The myosin head then binds, ATP is hydrolyzed, and the configuration of the myosin head and neck changes. (Only one of the two heads of the myosin-II head is shown.)

Reproduced, with permission, from Ganong WF: *Review of Medical Physiology*, 21st ed. McGraw-Hill, 2003:71.

COMPARISON OF SKELETAL, SMOOTH, AND CARDIAC MUSCLE

Characteristic	Type I (Slow or Red) Skeletal Muscle	Type II (Fast or White) Skeletal Muscle	Visceral (Single-Unit) Smooth Muscle	Cardiac Muscle
Location	Attached to bones and tendons.	Attached to bones and tendons.	Walls of hollow organs (eg, intestines, uterus, blood vessels).	Heart.
Structure	• Large, cylindrical, *multinucleated* cells arranged in parallel bundles. • Smaller than type II, with greater density of capillaries and mitochondria.	• Large, cylindrical, *multinucleated* cells arranged in parallel bundles. • Larger than type I.	• Small, spindle-shaped cells joined by *gap junctions* form large sheets. • Functional units are bundles or layers of cells.	• Short cells with blunt, branched, interwoven ends. • Joined by *intercalated disks and gap junctions*.
	• Uniform arrangement of sarcomere and sarcotubular system. • Troponin-based regulation. • T system is at A-I junction.	• Uniform arrangement of sarcomere and sarcotubular system. • Troponin-based regulation. • T system is at A-I junction.	• Unorganized arrangement, *no sarcomere, transverse tubule, or troponin*. • Rudimentary SR (obtain Ca^{2+} mainly from ECF). • *Dense bodies* instead of Z lines.	• Uniform arrangement of sarcomere and sarcotubular system. • Troponin-based regulation. • T system is at Z lines.
	Striated.	Striated.	Not striated.	Striated.
Function	• Strong, gross, sustained movement. • Endurance. • Recruited first. • Involved in all skeletal muscle activity (eg, long muscles of back).	• Fine, rapid, precise movement. • Recruited to increase force and power for brief periods (eg, extraocular muscles).	• Depends on location. • Functions as syncytium.	• To pump blood throughout body. • Functions as syncytium.
Primary ATP Production	Oxidative phosphorylation.	Anaerobic glycolysis.	Oxidative phosphorylation and glycolysis (variable).	Oxidative phosphorylation.

Mechanical Properties	• Increases force of contraction by increasing recruitment of motor units. • Tension developed depends on initial length of muscle fiber.	• Increases force of contraction by increasing recruitment of motor units. • Tension developed depends on initial length of muscle fiber.	• Increases force of contraction by recruiting more cross-bridges in cells. • Sustained contraction due to *latch-bridge mechanism*: myosin cross-bridges remain attached to actin for a time after intracellular Ca^{2+} concentration falls. • Tension varies for given length of muscle fiber (*plasticity*).	• Increases force of contraction by increasing free intracellular Ca^{2+}. • Tension developed depends on initial length of muscle fiber.
Source of Ca^{2+}	SR.	SR.	SR and ECF.	SR and ECF.
Mechanism of Ca^{2+} Mobilization	T tubule depolarization opens SR channels, allowing release of Ca^{2+} into myoplasm.	T tubule depolarization opens SR channels, allowing release of Ca^{2+} into myoplasm.	• IP_3 increases Ca^{2+} release. • Protein kinase A increases Ca^{2+} uptake by SR.	ECF Ca^{2+} triggers release of Ca^{2+} from SR.
Role of Ca^{2+}	Initiates contraction by binding to troponin.	Initiates contraction by binding to troponin.	Activates calmodulin, which activates myosin light chain kinase.	Initiates contraction by binding to troponin.
Electrical Properties	Resting membrane potential: −90 mV.	Resting membrane potential: −90 mV.	• No true resting membrane potential (−50 mV when quiescent). • May demonstrate prolonged plateau.	• Resting membrane potential: −90 mV. • *Prolonged plateau because of slow Ca^{2+} channels.*

RESPONSES OF SKELETAL MUSCLE TO A REPEATED STIMULUS

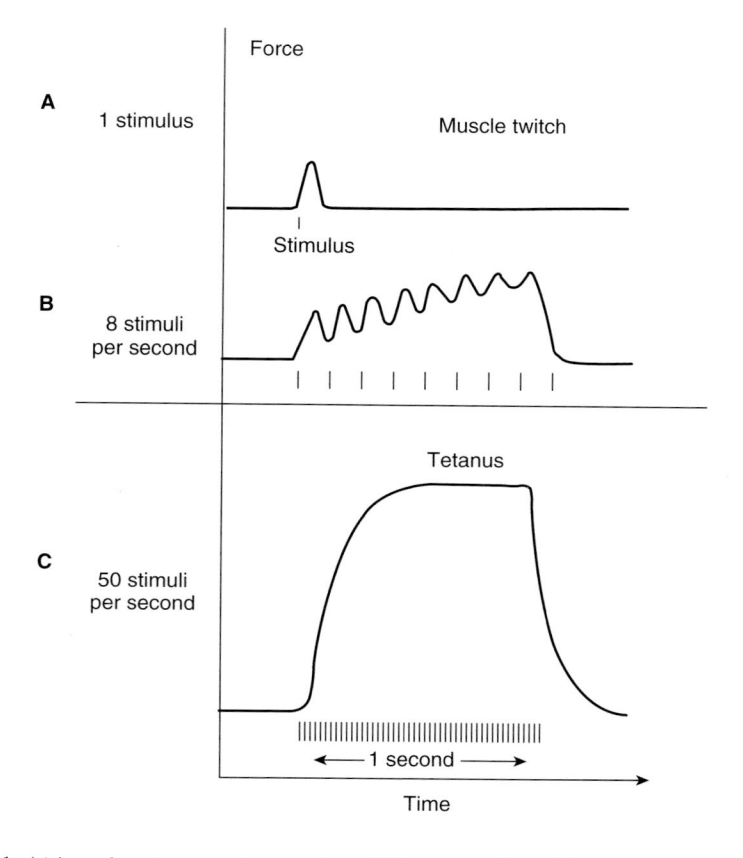

Frequent action potentials allow a muscle twitch (**A**) to fuse into an incomplete (**B**) or complete (**C**) tetanus.

Modified, with permission, from Berne RM, Levy MN: *Principles of Physiology*, 3rd ed. Mosby, 2000:158.

MUSCULAR DYSTROPHIES

Disorder	Etiology	Clinical Presentation
Duchenne	• X-linked recessive. • Dystrophin gene is absent.	• Occurs only in males. • Progressive muscle degeneration and weakness. • Often fatal by 20 years of age.
Becker	• X-linked recessive. • Dystrophin gene is altered or reduced.	• Presents in adolescence or adulthood. • Milder than Duchenne muscular dystrophy.
Limb-girdle	Defect in recessive gene on either autosomal or X chromosome.	• Slowly progressive weakening of pelvic and shoulder muscles. • Later stages of disease result in cardiac and pulmonary complications.
Myotonic Dystrophy (Steinert disease)	• Autosomal dominant. • Caused by abnormalities of Na^+ or Cl^- channels of sarcolemma, resulting in delayed relaxation and muscle spasm (myotonia).	• Slowly progressive weakening of both proximal (face and neck) and distal (hands and feet) muscles, myotonia. • Some patients are mentally disabled.
Periodic Paralysis	Attacks of muscle weakness triggered by exercise, drugs, cold temperatures.	• Periodic attacks of muscle weakening with normal muscle function in between attacks. • Number and severity of attacks decreases with increasing age.

IV. Body Fluids

BODY FLUID COMPARTMENTS

Main Compartment	Components of TBW	Components of ECF	Volume (70-kg Adult)	Volume (Body Weight; 70-kg Adult)	Important Points
TBW			42 L.	60%.	• TBW = ICF + ECF • Plasma osmolality is estimate of osmolality of ECF and ICF.
	ICF (⅔ of TBW).		28 L.	40%.	• *Major cation: K^+.* • Major anions: phosphates, protein, organic substances. • Composition is maintained by cell membrane, which mediates transport of substances between ICF and ECF by active transport, diffusion, osmosis, and vesicular transport.
	ECF (⅓ of TBW).		14 L.	20%.	• *Major cation: Na^+,* which also determines osmolality of ECF (double [Na+] estimates ECF osmolality). • Major anions: Cl^-, HCO_3^-. • ECF = interstitial fluid + plasma • Capillary wall separates interstitial fluid from blood plasma.
		Interstitial Fluid (¾ of ECF).	10.5 L.	15%.	Ionic composition similar to plasma, with less protein.
		Plasma (¼ of ECF).	3.5 L.	5%.	Ionic composition similar to interstitial fluid, with more protein. Total blood volume = plasma volume × (100/100 − hematocrit) Red cell volume = total blood volume − plasma volume

DIFFERENCES IN TERMS RELATED TO OSMOTIC PRESSURE AND OSMOLALITY OF SOLUTIONS

Prefix	Osmotic Pressure—-pressure necessary to prevent solvent migration.	Osmolality—-number of osmoles per kilogram of solvent.
Hyper-	**Hyperosmotic:** • Describes one solution that has greater osmotic pressure than another solution. • Water shifts out of cells in hyperosmotic solution. • Hyperosmotic plasma causes neurologic symptoms.	**Hypertonic:** • Describes extracellular solution that causes water to flow out of cell. • Hypertonic solution has greater osmolality than plasma.
Hypo-	**Hypo-osmotic:** • Describes one solution that has lower osmotic pressure than another solution. • Water shifts into cells, in hypo-osmotic solution. • Hypo-osmotic plasma causes neurologic symptoms.	**Hypotonic:** • Describes extracellular solution that causes water to flow into cell. • Hypotonic solution has lesser osmolality than plasma.
Iso-	**Iso-osmotic:** • Describes two solutions with the same osmotic pressure.	**Isotonic:** • Solution has same osmolality as plasma (~ 290 mOsm/L).

TRANSPORT ACROSS CELL MEMBRANES

Type of Transport	Mechanism	Clinical Example
Simple Diffusion	• Passive process by which atoms or molecules of two substances mix together because of their random thermal (brownian) motion. • Particles in solution flow down concentration (chemical) gradient, with tendency for mixture to attain uniform composition and to expand to fill all available volume.	Small intestine absorbs fat-soluble vitamins (A, D, E, K) via simple diffusion.
Facilitated Diffusion or Transport	• Carrier proteins enable particles too large for simple diffusion to move down their chemical or electrical gradients and pass through membranes. • Passive process.	Insulin increases sugar transport proteins, which in turn facilitate entry of glucose into muscle and fat cells.
Nonionic Diffusion	Diffusion of molecules of a substance from one side of membrane to another, where molecules dissociate.	NH_3 diffuses into renal collecting duct by nonionic diffusion, where it is protonated to NH_4^+ (ammonia), which is then excreted.
Osmosis	• Passage of substance (usually H_2O) from less concentrated to more concentrated solution through semipermeable membrane. • Continues until dynamic equilibrium is reached.	• Decreased osmotic pressure of ECF causes H_2O to enter cells. • Cells continue to swell until osmotic pressures of ECF and ICF are equal.
Primary Active Transport	• Carrier proteins actively move substances against their chemical and electrical gradients. • Energy source is required.	• Na^+-K^+ ATPase hydrolyzes ATP and uses its energy to pump Na^+ out of cell and K^+ into cell. • Digitalis inhibits Na^+-K^+ pump, causing decrease in concentration gradient of ions.
Secondary Active Transport	Transport protein obtains energy from concentration gradient of another substance that is actively transported.	Glucose is transported into small intestinal cells only if Na^+ binds to carrier protein and is transported down Na^+ electrochemical gradient at same time.

Endocytosis	• Process by which material enters cell without passing through its membrane. • Membrane invaginates and engulfs extracellular material, creating membrane-bound vesicle that buds off, bringing material into cell.	Uptake of neurotransmitters by muscle at neuromuscular junction.
	• Phagocytosis ("cell eating," or uptake of particulate material). • Pinocytosis ("cell drinking," or uptake of soluble molecules). • Receptor-mediated endocytosis by clathrin-coated pits.	• Receptor–low-density lipoprotein complexes aggregate to clathrin-coated pits on target cell membranes and are taken into cells by receptor-mediated endocytosis. • This is one process by which cholesterol is transported to cells.
Exocytosis	• Opposite of endocytosis. • Membrane of vesicle fuses with plasma membrane of cell, and contents of vesicle are ejected from cell.	• Release of neurotransmitters by neurons at neuromuscular junction. • Release of enzymes from pancreatic acinar cells.
Filtration	Process by which fluid is forced through membrane or other barrier because of difference in pressure on either side of barrier.	• Filtration between interstitial fluid and ICF across capillary wall. • Filtration of plasma across renal glomerulus.

EQUATIONS RELATING TO THE TRANSPORT OF IONS AND FLUIDS

Expression	Description	Equation and Meaning of Terms
Fick First Law of Diffusion	Diffusion rate across membrane is proportional to area of membrane and concentration gradient of diffusing substance.	$J = -DA \dfrac{\Delta c}{\Delta x}$ • J = net rate of diffusion (moles or grams per unit time). • D = diffusion coefficient of diffusing solute. • A = area of membrane. • Δc = concentration difference across the membrane. • Δx = membrane thickness.
Osmolality (mOsm/L)	• Number of osmoles per kilogram of solvent. • Not affected by volume of solutes or temperature.	Osmolality = $2[Na^+] + 0.055[glucose] + 0.36[BUN]$ • $[Na^+]$ measured in mEq/L. • [Glucose] measured in mg/dL. • [BUN] measured in mg/dL.
Van't Hoff Law of Osmotic Pressure	• Osmotic pressure of solution depends on number of particles in solution. • Ionization of solute must be taken into account. • Increased osmotic pressure means increased prevention of solvent (H_2O) migration, making solution more concentrated.	$\pi = RT(\phi ic)$ • π = osmotic pressure. • R = ideal gas constant. • T = absolute temperature. • ϕ = osmotic coefficient (*1 in ideal solution*; approaches 1 for all solutes as solution becomes more dilute). • i = number of ions formed by dissociation of solute molecule. • c = molar concentration of solute (moles of solute per liter of solution).

Osmotic Flow	• Membranes are more impermeable to larger solute molecules. • Therefore, larger solute molecules cause greater osmotic flow. • Reflection coefficient (σ) is relative obstruction to passage of substance through capillary membrane. • Value of σ for filterable solutes is 0 to 1, that of H_2O is 0, and that of albumin (to which endothelium is almost impermeable) is 1.	$\dot{V}w = \sigma L \Delta \pi$ • $\dot{V}w$ = osmotic flow of water across membrane. • σ = reflection coefficient. • L = hydraulic conductivity. • $\Delta \pi$ = osmotic pressure difference.
Electrochemical Potential Difference	Difference in potential energy of ion across membrane depends on differences in concentration and electrical potential across membrane.	$\Delta \mu(x) = RT \ln \dfrac{[X]_A}{[X]_B} + zF(E_A - E_B)$ • $\Delta \mu$ = electrochemical potential difference of ion between sides A and B of membrane. • R = ideal gas constant. • T = absolute temperature. • $\ln [X]_A/[X]_B$ = natural logarithm of concentration ratio of X^+ on each side of membrane. • z = charge number for ion. • F = Faraday constant. • $E_A - E_B$ = electrical potential difference across membrane.
Nernst Equation	• Calculates equilibrium potential for ion (membrane potential at which influx and efflux of ion are equal, such as when $\Delta \mu = 0$). • At this potential, ion is prevented from flowing down its concentration gradient. • When membrane potential of ion equals equilibrium potential, net flux of ion across membrane is 0. • Equilibrium potential of ion equals energy contained in concentration gradient (volts). • Nernst equation can be used to predict direction that ions tend to flow.	$E_x = (RT/FZ_x) \ln \dfrac{[x_o]}{[x_i]}$ • E_x = equilibrium potential of ion x. • R = gas constant. • T = absolute temperature. • F = Faraday constant. • Z_x = valence of ion x. • $[x_o]$ = concentration of ion x outside cell. • $[x_i]$ = concentration of ion x inside cell.

Continued

EQUATIONS RELATING TO THE TRANSPORT OF IONS AND FLUIDS (Continued)

Expression	Description	Equation and Meaning of Terms
Gibbs-Donnan Equation	• Demonstrates equilibrium that is established when membrane separating two solutions is permeable to some, but not all, ions. • In presence of nondiffusible ions, diffusable ions distribute themselves so that their concentration ratios at equilibrium are equal. • A cell in this case is not in osmotic equilibrium. • Intracellular proteins (nondiffusible anions) create osmotic gradient that causes H_2O to flow into cell. • Normally, Gibbs-Donnan equilibrium is prevented by Na^+-K^+ pump that keeps intracellular $[Na^+]$ and extracellular $[K^+]$ from reaching equilibrium. • In this case, membrane potential is called "steady state" or "resting membrane potential."	$[K^+]_x[Cl^-]_x = [K^+]_y[Cl^-]_y$ • K^+ and Cl^- are diffusible ions. • x and y are aqueous compartments on either side of semipermeable membrane.
Goldman Constant-field Equation	• Also known as chord conductance equation. • Calculates resting membrane potential, which depends on distribution of Na^+, K^+, and Cl^-, as well as on permeability of membrane to these ions. • Increased permeability to particular ion means increased strength of that ion in forcing membrane potential toward its own equilibrium potential (calculated from Nernst equation). • Goldman equation shows that resting membrane potential is determined mainly by concentration of extracellular K^+, to which resting membrane is more permeable. • Increased extracellular K^+ depolarizes membrane (makes it more positive). • Decreased extracellular K^+ hyperpolarizes membrane (makes it more negative).	$$V = \frac{RT}{F} \ln \frac{P_K^+[K_o^+] + P_{Na}^+[Na_o^+] + P_{Cl}^-[Cl_i^-]}{P_K^+[K_i^+] + P_{Na}^+[Na_i^+] + P_{Cl}^-[Cl_o^-]}$$ • V = membrane potential. • R = gas constant. • T = absolute temperature. • F = Faraday constant. • P_K^+, P_{Cl}^-, P_{Na}^+ = permeabilities of membrane to K^+, Cl^-, and Na^+. • i = inside of cell. • o = outside of cell.

CHAPTER 2
NERVOUS SYSTEM

V. MOTOR SYSTEM

Organization of the Motor System

Muscle Stretch Receptors

Components of Muscle Spindles

Components of Golgi Tendon Organs

Pathways Involved in Muscle Stretch

Spinal Cord Stretch Reflexes

Vestibular Apparatus

Membranous Labyrinth

Neural Circuit for the Vestibulo-ocular Reflex

Caloric Stimulation

Movement Disorders Caused by Lesions in the Basal Ganglia

Cerebellum

VI. AUTONOMIC NERVOUS SYSTEM

Divisions of the Autonomic Nervous System

Pathways of the Sympathetic Nervous System

Pathways of the Parasympathetic Nervous System

Neural Pathways in the Sympathetic and Parasympathetic Nervous Systems

Sympathetic and Parasympathetic Fibers

VII. HIGHER FUNCTIONS OF THE NERVOUS SYSTEM

Sleep Stages

Sleep Stages and EEG Patterns

Sleep Disorders

Classification of Epilepsy

Disorders of Consciousness

Types of Learning

Categories of Memory

Aphasia

ABBREVIATIONS

ACh = acetylcholine

cAMP = cyclic adenosine monophosphate

CN = cranial nerve

CNS = central nervous system

CSF = cerebrospinal fluid

EEG = electroencephalogram

ENS = enteric nervous system

GI = gastrointestinal

GTO = Golgi tendon organ

IOP = intraocular pressure

LGN = lateral geniculate nucleus

PNS = parasympathetic nervous system

REM = rapid eye movement

SNS = sympathetic nervous system

VPL = ventroposterolateral

VPM = ventroposteromedial

TERMS TO LEARN

Afferent Nerves	Sensory neurons that transmit information from receptors to the CNS; these neurons travel from organs to the CNS via a dorsal root or CN ganglia.
Agnosia	Brain disorder of parietal lobe in which the patient cannot interpret sensations correctly, although sensory modalities remain intact (eg, tactile agnosia [astereognosis] is the inability to identify objects by touch).
Alzheimer Disease	Progressive loss of short-term memory followed by general loss of cognitive function and death in middle age; associated with atrophy of hippocampus and cerebral cortex. *Hallmarks are intracellular neurofibrillary tangles and extracellular senile plaques.* Similar deterioration in elderly individuals is "senile dementia of the Alzheimer type."
Babinski Sign (reflex)	*Pathologic reflex associated with interruption of the lateral corticospinal tract;* reflex is normal in infancy. Extensor plantar reflex occurs (great toe goes up, other toes fan out) when the outer sole of foot is stroked.
Blood-Brain Barrier	Tight junctions between capillary endothelial cells in the brain and between epithelial cells in the choroid plexuses; keeps large molecules and highly charged ions in the circulating blood separate from brain tissue.
CSF (Cerebrospinal Fluid)	Clear, thin fluid contained within the subarachnoid space that surrounds the brain and spinal cord. CSF is isotonic to blood but has higher concentrations of Na$^+$ and Cl$^-$ and lower concentrations of K$^+$, glucose, and protein; in addition, it contains a *few white blood cells but no red blood cells.*
Decerebrate Rigidity	Pattern of spasticity resulting from transection of brainstem above superior border of pons; exaggerated extensor posture (extension and hyperpronation of arms, extension and internal rotation of legs, opisthotonos [arching of neck and back]).
Decorticate Rigidity	Pattern of spasticity resulting from lesion of cerebral cortex with most of brainstem intact; flexion of arms and extension and internal rotation of legs.
Efferent Nerves	Motor neurons that transmit information from the CNS via ventral roots or cranial nerves to muscles, glands, and other effectors.
Extrapyramidal System	Traditional name for descending motor pathways that do not pass through the pyramids and are concerned with postural control; *deficits due to corticospinal tract lesions are not as severe because of the descending extrapyramidal system.* The term is also applied to motor disorders caused by lesions of basal ganglia, without reference to the motor pathway involved.
Ganglion	Structure containing a collection of nerve cell bodies (may also contain synapses). Sympathetic ganglia are located on each side of the spinal cord, and parasympathetic ganglia are located near the organs they innervate.
Nystagmus	Rapid, involuntary movements of the eyes from side to side, up and down, or in circles.

Proprioception	Self-regulation of equilibrium, position, posture, and movement via stimuli sensed in receptors of joints, muscles, tendons, and the vestibular apparatus.
Pyramidal System	Traditional name for descending motor pathways that form the medullary pyramids and mediate voluntary movements of the distal parts of the extremities, facial muscles, and tongue; includes corticospinal and corticobulbar tracts. *All descending pathways communicate with the spinal cord through the brainstem except the pyramidal tracts.*
Receptive Field	Area of a sensory neuron that, when stimulated, causes the neuron to discharge; the smaller the receptive field, the more precise the of stimulus localization (eg, receptive fields in the fingertips are smaller than those on the arm).
Referred Pain	Pain produced by irritation of a viscus that is felt not in the viscus but in a somatic structure some distance away (eg, cardiac pain referred to the left arm).
Reticular Activating System	Polysynaptic pathway originating in midbrain and medulla that projects to the thalamus and diffusely (directly) to the neocortex; integrates information from all senses and regulates levels of consciousness and maintains awake state.
Sensory Transduction	Process in which stimulus energy is transformed into an electrical response, enabling a sensory receptor to respond usefully to a stimulus.
Somatotopic Organization	Characteristic of the brain and nervous system pathways in which each part of the body is controlled by a specific area of the cortex; that area is proportional to the amount of control (motor or sensory) exerted over that part. Medial/ventral motor pathways control muscles of trunk and proximal limbs and are concerned with postural adjustments and gross movements, and lateral/dorsal motor pathways control distal limbs and are concerned with fine, skilled movements.
Tinnitus	Ringing sensation in the ears caused by irritative stimulation of either the inner ear or the vestibule.

I. General Concepts

ORGANIZATION OF THE NERVOUS SYSTEM

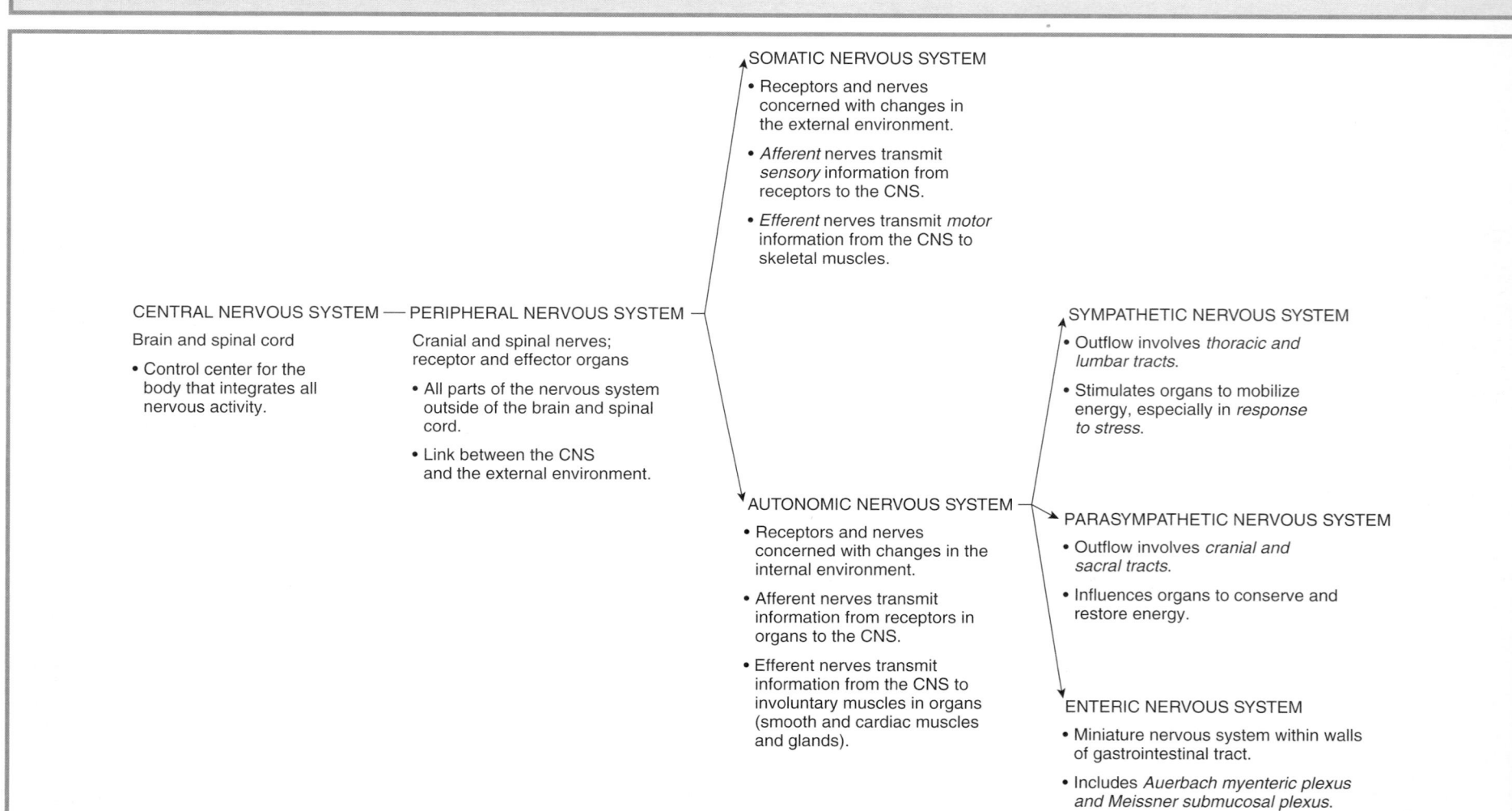

SOMATIC NERVOUS SYSTEM

- Receptors and nerves concerned with changes in the external environment.
- *Afferent* nerves transmit *sensory* information from receptors to the CNS.
- *Efferent* nerves transmit *motor* information from the CNS to skeletal muscles.

CENTRAL NERVOUS SYSTEM

Brain and spinal cord

- Control center for the body that integrates all nervous activity.

PERIPHERAL NERVOUS SYSTEM

Cranial and spinal nerves; receptor and effector organs

- All parts of the nervous system outside of the brain and spinal cord.
- Link between the CNS and the external environment.

AUTONOMIC NERVOUS SYSTEM

- Receptors and nerves concerned with changes in the internal environment.
- Afferent nerves transmit information from receptors in organs to the CNS.
- Efferent nerves transmit information from the CNS to involuntary muscles in organs (smooth and cardiac muscles and glands).

SYMPATHETIC NERVOUS SYSTEM

- Outflow involves *thoracic and lumbar tracts*.
- Stimulates organs to mobilize energy, especially in *response to stress*.

PARASYMPATHETIC NERVOUS SYSTEM

- Outflow involves *cranial and sacral tracts*.
- Influences organs to conserve and restore energy.

ENTERIC NERVOUS SYSTEM

- Miniature nervous system within walls of gastrointestinal tract.
- Includes *Auerbach myenteric plexus and Meissner submucosal plexus*.

DIVISIONS OF THE CNS

Part of Brain	Subdivisions	Function	Effects of Lesions
Cortex	Frontal, parietal, temporal, occipital lobes.	Responsible for "higher functioning": consciousness, movement, memory, emotions, comprehension, speech, the five senses.	Aphasia, tremor, paralysis, memory loss, visual field defects, altered sexual behavior.
Cerebellum	• Lateral cerebellar hemispheres. • Medial vermis. • Superior, middle, inferior peduncles.	Coordination of voluntary movement, balance and equilibrium, memory for reflexive motor acts.	Ataxia, tremor, vertigo, slurred speech, loss of coordination of fine movements.
Brainstem	Midbrain, pons, medulla oblongata.	• Control of sleep and alertness, blood pressure, heart rate, and respiratory drive. • Medulla oblongata is responsible for following reflexes: coughing, gagging, sneezing, swallowing, and emesis (contains *chemoreceptor trigger zone*).	Dysphagia, vertigo, alterations in consciousness, emesis.

FUNCTIONAL DIVISIONS OF THE CEREBRAL CORTEX

Lobe	Cortical Area	Function
Frontal	Prefrontal cortex.	Emotions, complex thought, problem solving.
	Motor association cortex (premotor and supplementary cortex): • Located in front of primary motor cortex, on lateral cortex (Brodmann area 6).	Coordination of complex movement.
	Primary motor cortex: • Located within precentral gyrus (Brodmann area 4). • Body parts represented in order along gyrus: legs on top, head at bottom. • Amount of body cortex representing body part is proportional in size to amount of skill needed for its movement (eg, cortical areas for hand movement are much larger than those for trunk).	Initiation of voluntary movement; receives sensory input from spinal cord and other cortical areas which it uses to modify motor commands.
	Broca area—at inferior frontal gyrus, anterior to inferior end of motor cortex (Brodmann areas 44 and 45).	Production and articulation of speech.
Parietal	Primary somatosensory cortex: • Located within postcentral gyrus (Brodmann areas 1, 2, 3). • Body parts represented in order along gyrus: legs on top, head at bottom. • Size of cortical receiving area for impulses from a body part is proportional to the number of receptors in that part (eg, cortical areas for hands are much larger than those for trunk).	Receives tactile information from the body.
	Sensory association cortex.	Processing of multisensory information.
Temporal	Auditory cortex: • Located in superior temporal lobe in sylvian fissure (Brodmann area 41).	Detection of sound quality.

Lobe	Cortical Area	Function
	Auditory association cortex.	Complex processing of auditory information.
	Wernicke area: • Supramarginal and angular gyri and posterior part of superior temporal gyrus (Brodmann area 22).	Comprehension of language.
	Limbic system: • Includes cingulate, parahippocampal, and subcallosal gyri; hippocampus; amygdala; dentate gyrus; subiculum; hypothalamus; basal ganglia. • Papez circuit: closed circuit of the limbic system: hippocampus → fornix → mamillary bodies → anterior nuclei of thalamus (mamillothalamic tract) → cingulate cortex → hippocampus.	Behavior (aggression, feeding, sexuality). Emotions, olfaction, memory. Autonomic responses (blood pressure, respiration).
Occipital	Visual cortex: occipital eye fields (Brodmann area 17).	Detection of visual stimuli.
	Visual association area overlaps posterior parietal and temporal areas.	Complex processing of visual information.

MAJOR SENSORY AND MOTOR AREAS OF THE CEREBRAL CORTEX

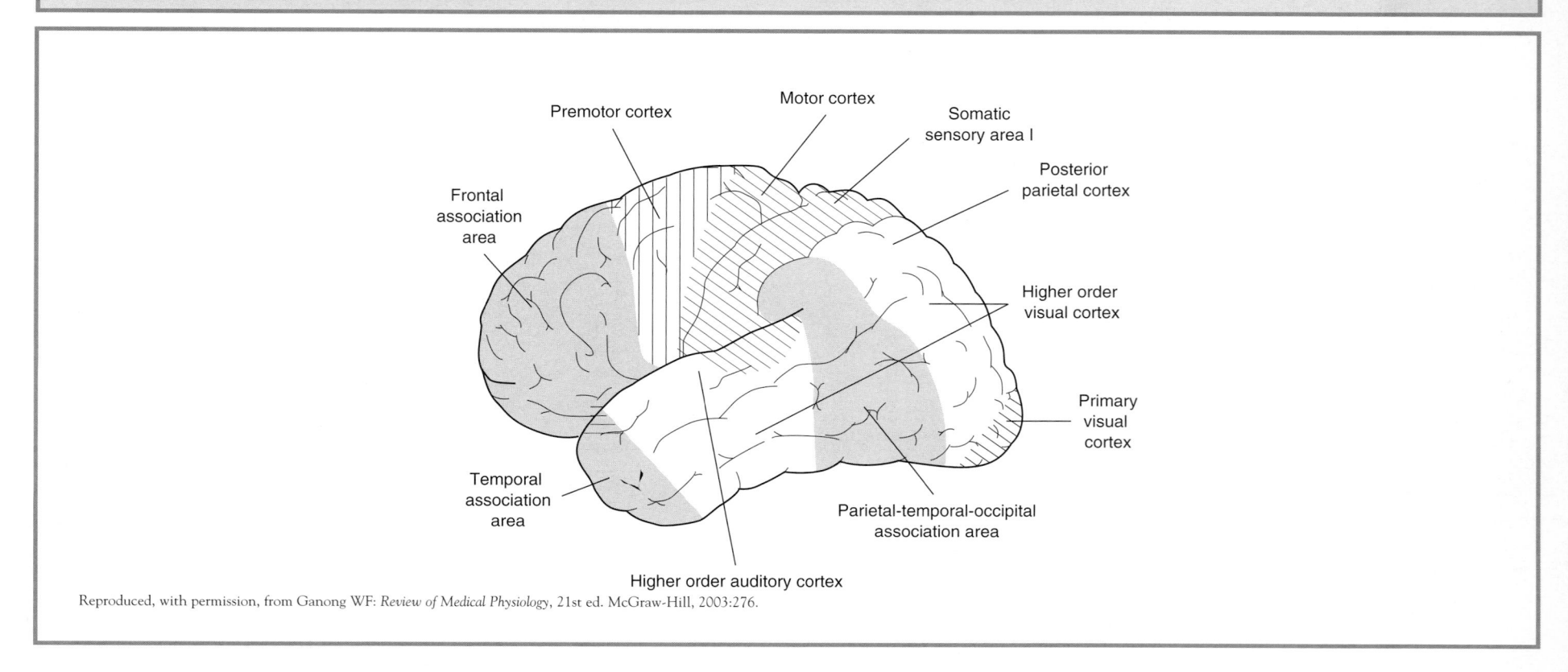

Reproduced, with permission, from Ganong WF: *Review of Medical Physiology*, 21st ed. McGraw-Hill, 2003:276.

CRANIAL NERVES

CN No.	Name	Predominant Nerve Type	Function
I	Olfactory.	Sensory.	Smell.
II	Optic.	Sensory.	Vision.
III	Oculomotor.	Motor.	Pupillary constriction, lens accommodation.
			Eye movement (innervation of extraocular muscles): • Superior rectus—elevation of abducted eye. • Inferior rectus—depression of abducted eye. • Medial rectus—adduction. • Inferior oblique—elevation of adducted eye.
IV	Trochlear.	Motor.	Eye movement: superior oblique—depression of adducted eye.
V	Trigeminal.	Motor.	Muscles of mastication: • Mandibular division (V3)
		Sensory.	Mouth and face: • Ophthalmic (V1), maxillary (V2), and mandibular (V3) divisions.
VI	Abducens.	Motor.	Eye movement: lateral rectus—abduction.
VII	Facial.	Motor.	Facial movements.
		Sensory.	Taste (anterior two thirds of tongue)
VIII	Vestibulocochlear	Sensory.	• Hearing (cochlear nucleus). • Balance (vestibular nucleus).
IX	Glossopharyngeal.	Motor.	Pharynx, stylopharyngeus muscle (for swallowing).
		Sensory.	Taste (posterior one third of tongue).
X	Vagus.	Motor.	Larynx, pharynx, soft palate, heart, GI tract.
		Sensory.	Taste.
XI	Accessory.	Motor.	Neck and shoulder movement (trapezius and sternocleidomastoid muscles).
XII	Hypoglossal.	Motor.	Movement of tongue.

ORGANIZATION OF THE SPINAL CORD

Composition	Description	Major Subdivisions	Components
Gray Matter (Central)	• Contains descending tracts from brain. • Primary afferent fibers make synaptic connections here.	Dorsal horns (posterior columns).	• Lamina I–VI. • *Ascending tracts (afferent input).* • Each fiber is central process of dorsal root ganglion cell.
		Intermediate gray commissure (cross bar of **H**).	Lamina X.
		Ventral horns (anterior columns).	• Lamina VII–IX. • *Descending tracts (efferent output).* • Somatic motor axons. (Note: those axons innervating distal muscles are lateral, and those innervating proximal muscles are medial.) • Some preganglionic and primary afferent fibers.
White Matter (Peripheral)	• Contains long ascending and descending pathways between the spinal cord and brain. • Axons of primary afferent fibers and spinal cord interneurons also present.	Dorsal (posterior) funiculi.	Ascending tracts.
		Posterior lateral sulcus.	Site of entry of dorsal root.
		Lateral and ventral (anterior) funiculi.	Ascending and descending tracts.
		Anterior lateral sulcus.	Site of exit of ventral root.

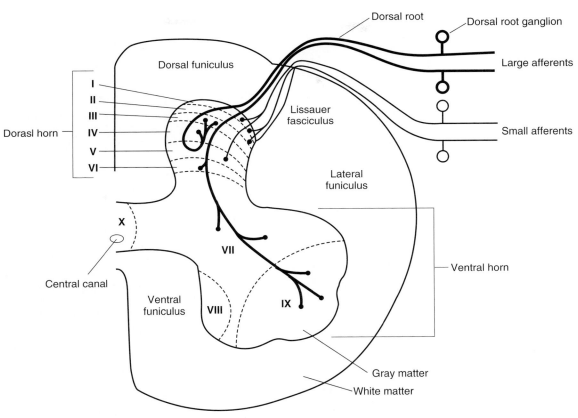

Primary afferent fibers are shown entering the posterior lateral sulcus.

Modified, with permission, from Berne RM, Levy MN: *Principles of Physiology*, 3rd ed. Mosby, 2000:86.

CLINICAL PRESENTATION OF UPPER AND LOWER MOTOR NEURON LESIONS

Type of Neuron	Description	Deep Tendon Reflexes	Signs of Denervation	Muscle Response to Active Stretching
Upper Motor Neurons	• First-order neurons in cerebral (motor) cortex of CNS. • Includes neurons in pyramidal and extrapyramidal tracts.	• Increased (reflex arc is intact). • Spastic paralysis. • *Babinski reflex present.*	• None. • Muscles are hypotonic and weak.	Greater stretch, greater muscle response: • Clonus—regular, rhythmic contractions of muscle subjected to suddenly applied and maintained stretch (eg, ankle clonus). • Clasp knife reaction—resistance followed by give when limb is moved passively.
Lower Motor Neurons	Second-order neurons, including cranial motor neurons in brainstem and motor neurons in spinal cord.	• Decreased or absent (reflex arc is damaged). • Flaccid paralysis.	• Initial fasciculations, followed by muscle atrophy. • Muscles are contracted. • Antagonistic muscles are shortened because of lack of opposition from paralyzed muscles.	None.

ASCENDING SENSORY PATHWAYS

Pathway	Function	Input	First-Order Neuron	Second-Order Neuron	Third- and Fourth-Order Neurons	Termination
Dorsal column–medial lemniscus	Discriminative touch and conscious proprioception (flutter-vibration, touch-pressure, joint movement, position sense, visceral distention).	Sensory receptors in upper trunk and upper extremities (cranial–T6).	Fasciculus cuneatus (lateral).	Nucleus cuneatus (synapses then crosses) [dorsal column nuclei].	Via medial lemniscus to VPL nucleus of thalamus.	Somatosensory cortex.
		Sensory receptors in lower trunk and lower extremities (caudal–T7).	Fasciculus gracilis (medial).	Nucleus gracilis (synapses then crosses).		
Ventrolateral Spinothalamic	• Ventral (touch, pressure). • Lateral (superficial pain and temperature sensation).	Nociceptors, mechanoreceptors, chemoreceptors, thermoreceptors.	Laminas I and V of dorsal horn (synapses then crosses).	Spinothalamic tract in ventrolateral funiculus.	Several nuclei, including VPL nucleus.	Somatosensory cortex.
Spinoreticular	Deep (somatovisceral) pain sensation.	Ill-defined, multisynaptic, bilateral pathway.				
Spinocerebellar (dorsal and ventral)	*Ipsilateral* proprioception.	Muscle spindles, GTOs, joint receptors.	Lumbar and sacral dorsal columns.	Clarke nucleus in upper lumbar spinal cord.		Via spinocerebellar tract and inferior cerebellar peduncle to cerebellum.
			Cervical dorsal columns.	External cuneate nucleus in medulla.		

ASCENDING VISUAL PATHWAYS

Function	Input	First-Order Neuron	Second-Order Neuron	Termination
Normal Vision	Photoreceptors in retina.	• Optic nerve (CN II). *Fibers from nasal retina cross at optic chiasm, and those from temporal retina do not.*	• Via optic tract to lateral geniculate nucleus in thalamus. • Magnocellular pathway: layers 1 and 2 of LGN carry signals for detection of movement, location, and spatial organization to superficial layer 4C of occipital cortex. • Parvocellular pathway: layers 3–6 of LGN carry signals for color, shape, texture, and fine detail to deep layer 4C of occipital cortex.	Via optic radiations to primary visual cortex in occipital lobe.
Eye Positioning, Reflex Movements of Head and Neck	Photoreceptors in retina.	• Optic nerve (CN II). • Cerebral cortex.	• Superior colliculus.	Via tectopontine tract to cerebellum and tectospinal tract to cervical spine.

ASCENDING PATHWAYS FOR SPECIFIC SENSES

Pathway	Function	Input	First-Order Neuron	Second-Order Neuron	Third- and Fourth-Order Neurons	Termination
Auditory	Audition.	Outer hair cell receptors in cochlea.	Spiral ganglion joins auditory/cochlear nerve (branch of vestibulocochlear nerve, CN VIII).	Cochlear nucleus in brainstem.	• Ventral cochlear nucleus → superior olivary nucleus in medulla (for localization of sound). • Dorsal cochlear nucleus (for quality of sound).	Both tracts via lateral lemniscus → inferior colliculus → medial geniculate nucleus of thalamus → primary auditory cortex.
Vestibular	Equilibrium.	Inner hair cell receptors in semicircular canals, utricle, and saccule.	Via vestibular nerve (branch of CN VIII) to vestibular nuclei.			Several routes: • Reticular formation and cerebellum. • Oculomotor nuclei. • Spinal cord. • Cortex.
Trigeminal	Discriminatory touch for face.	Mechanoreceptors via trigeminal ganglion.	Principal nucleus in brainstem (synapse then cross).	Via medial lemniscus to VPM nucleus of thalamus.		Somatosensory cortex.
	Pain and temperature sensation for face.	Trigeminal ganglion.	Via midpons and spinal tract of V to spinal nucleus of V in medulla.	Spinothalamic tract in ventrolateral funiculus.	Via medial lemniscus to VPM of thalamus.	Somatosensory cortex.
	Proprioception for muscles of mastication.	Mesencephalic nucleus in brainstem.	Motor nucleus of V in pons.			Efferent fibers exit via mandibular division of CN V.

Continued

ASCENDING PATHWAYS FOR SPECIFIC SENSES (Continued)

Pathway	Function	Input	First-Order Neuron	Second-Order Neuron	Third- and Fourth-Order Neurons	Termination
Olfactory	Smell.	Odorant molecules.	Olfactory receptor cells.	Via olfactory nerve to olfactory bulb (primary afferent, mitral and tufted cells form olfactory glomeruli).	• Via olfactory tract to base of brain. • Lateral inhibition by periglomerular and granule cells help discriminate between odors.	Orbitofrontal gyri ("olfactory cortex"), limbic system.
Gustatory	Taste.	CN V, VII, IX, X to taste buds.	Via ipsilateral solitary tract to nucleus of solitary tract in medulla (synapse, then cross).	Via medial lemniscus to VPM of thalamus.		Somatosensory cortex.

DESCENDING MOTOR PATHWAYS

Pathway	Origin	Site of Crossing	Termination	Muscles Controlled
Lateral Corticospinal (80% of fibers)	Motor, pre-motor, and somatosensory cortices.	Medullary pyramids.	On motor neurons in *lateral* part of lamina IX of ventral horn.	Contralateral *distal limb muscles for fine movements*.
Medial Corticospinal (20% of fibers)		At level of motor neurons.	Mostly on interneurons that then synapse on motor neurons in *medial* part of lamina IX of ventral horn.	Contralateral axial and *proximal limb muscles for gross movements, posture,* balance, and locomotion.
Lateral Corticobulbar		Midbrain, pons, or medulla.	Cranial motor nuclei in brainstem.	*Bilateral* muscles of *upper face, contralateral* muscles of *lower face* and tongue.
Medial Corticobulbar		Midbrain, pons, or medulla.	Cranial motor nuclei in brainstem.	Contralateral postural support of voluntary movements of face.
Pontine (medial) Reticulospinal (*excitatory*)	• Input from motor cortex. • Pontine reticular formation (input from motor cortex).	Does not cross.	Motor neurons in *medial* part of lamina IX of ventral horn.	Maintains postural muscle tone and direct voluntary movement by *enhancing antigravity reflexes* of spinal cord (facilitates upper limb flexors and lower limb extensors).
Medullary (Lateral) Reticulospinal (Inhibitory)	• Input from other motor pathways. • Medullary reticular formation.	Some cross in medulla.	Motor neurons in *lateral* part of lamina IX of ventral horn.	Maintains postural muscle tone and direct voluntary movement by *reducing antigravity reflexes* of spinal cord.

Continued

DESCENDING MOTOR PATHWAYS (Continued)

Pathway	Origin	Site of Crossing	Termination	Muscles Controlled
Corticovestibulospinal (Medial and Lateral)	• Input from motor cortex. • Vestibular nuclei in medulla.	Does not cross.	Motor neurons in *medial* part of lamina IX of ventral horn.	• Maintains head position and keeps body upright by innervating antigravity muscles of neck and back. • Keeps eyes on target when head turns.
Rubrospinal	• Input from motor cortex. • Red nucleus in midbrain.	Pons.	Ventrolateral spinal cord.	Voluntary control of skeletal muscle.
Tectospinal	• Input from somatosensory systems. • Superior colliculus in midbrain.	Pons.	Cervical spinal cord.	Postural control of head and neck.
Olivospinal	• Input from cerebellum. • Olivary nucleus in medulla.	Pons.	Thoracic spinal cord.	Muscle coordination, posture, equilibrium.

Continued

II. Sensory System: Visual Sensation

STRUCTURES IN THE EPITHELIAL LAYERS OF THE EYE

Structure	Description/Function
Outer Layer (Fibrous Coat)	
Conjunctiva	Mucous membrane. • Avascular, transparent area covers front of eye. • Vascular area lines inside of eyelids.
Cornea	• Avascular, *transparent*. • Provides converging power for eye. • Main refractive surface of eye, which, unlike lens, is not subject to physiologic alteration.
Sclera	White, fibrous layer that becomes cornea at front of eye.
Middle Layer (Vascular Coat)	
Iris	• Colored portion. • Regulates amount of light that reaches retina: smooth muscle forms pupillary sphincter and dilator. • *Sympathetic nervous system activates dilator.* • *Parasympathetic nervous system activates sphincter.*
Choroid	Blood supply to outer retina.

Continued

STRUCTURES IN THE EPITHELIAL LAYERS OF THE EYE (Continued)

Structure	Description/Function
Inner Layer (Neural Coat/Layers of Retina)	
Pigment Epithelium	Absorbs light, reduces light scatter, stores vitamin A (retinol), and clears debris from photoreceptors by phagocytosis (each layer of eye contains pigment that reduces light scatter).
Rods and Cones (Outer and Inner Segments)	• Photoreceptors. • Outer segment contains photopigment *rhodopsin* in membranous disks. • Inner segment contains organelles.
Outer Nuclear Layer	Contains nuclei of rods and cones.
Outer Plexiform Layer	Horizontal cells connect receptor cells.
Inner Nuclear Layer	Contains nuclei of retinal neurons (bipolar, horizontal, and amacrine cells).
Inner Plexiform Layer	Amacrine cells connect ganglion cells to one another.
Ganglion Cell Layer	Axons of ganglion cells form *optic nerve*.

IMPORTANT STRUCTURES OF THE EYE

Structure	Description	Significance
Macula Lutea	• "Yellow spot" in center of retina. • Surrounds fovea. • Contains high concentration of cones.	• Area of high visual acuity. • Macular degeneration is common cause of blindness.
Fovea	• Depressed area in center of macula lutea that contains highest concentration of cones. • Serves as fixation point of retina on which light rays are focused.	*Area of highest visual acuity.*
Optic Disk (Blind Spot)	Area on medial retina where fibers from photoreceptors merge to form optic nerve.	• Absence of rods or cones. • Light does not register in this area.
Lens	Avascular, transparent, crystalline structure behind pupil that refracts light and helps focus images on retina.	• Refractive power is under physiologic control. • Process by which curvature of lens is increased is *accommodation*. • Opacities called *cataracts* may develop and interfere with vision as person ages.
Suspensory Ligaments (zonule fibers)	Attach to wall of eye by ciliary processes and hold lens in place behind iris.	• Sympathetic stimulation (no accommodation): ciliary muscles relaxed, suspensory ligaments tense, lens flat.
Ciliary Body (ie, ciliary ring, processes, muscle)	• Ciliary ring connects the choroid with the iris • Ciliary processes secrete aqueous humor • Ciliary muscle contraction alters the curvature of the lens in accommodation	• Parasympathetic stimulation (accommodation): ciliary muscles contracted, suspensory ligaments relaxed, lens spherical.

Continued

IMPORTANT STRUCTURES OF THE EYE (Continued)

Structure	Description	Significance
Aqueous Humor	• Watery fluid surrounding iris that provides O_2 and nutrients to cornea and helps maintain shape of eye. • Circulation: posterior chamber → pupil → anterior chamber → canal of Schlemm → venous system.	• Increased IOP is caused by imbalance in secretion and absorption of aqueous humor. • *Increased IOP is not equivalent to glaucoma*, which is a degenerative disease or loss of ganglion cells that is worsened by increased IOP.
Vitreous Humor	Gelatinous material behind lens in posterior chamber.	Helps maintain shape of eye.

COMPARISON OF RODS AND CONES

Photoreceptor	Location	Opsins	Stimuli	Response	Function
Rods	Peripheral retina.	Rhodopsin: protein *opsin* plus 11-*cis* retinal (analog of vitamin A); visual purple, encoded on chromosome 3.	• More sensitive to light. • Can respond to single photon of light. • Respond to scattered light.	• Absorb more light and produce greater response for each photon of light absorbed. • Remain polarized longer.	Vision in dim light (*scotopic vision*).
Cones	Fovea.	• Red and green opsin: encoded on X chromosome. • *Red-green color blindness is X-linked.* • Blue opsin: encoded on chromosome 7.	• Less sensitive to light. • Do not respond to scattered light. • Respond over large range of light intensities.	Brisk response to light.	• Vision in daylight (*photopic vision*). • Visual acuity. • Color perception.

PRINCIPLES OF IMAGE FORMATION

Principle	Description	Mechanism
Refractive Power (also known as converging power, optical power)	• Degree to which lens bends light rays passing through it. • *Greater curvature of lens means greater refractive power.*	• Cornea contributes two thirds of refractive power of eye. • Lens contributes one third of refractive power and can undergo accommodation.
Accommodation	• Adjustment of shape of lens to focus images of nearby objects on retina. • Refractive power increases. • Focal length decreases.	Bulging of lens: contraction of ciliary muscle releases tension on zonular fibers, and elastic capsule surrounding lens contracts, increasing convexity (and thus power) of lens.
Near Response	• Reflex that occurs when one looks at near object. • Includes accommodation, convergence of the visual axes, and pupillary constriction.	• Pupillary constriction (parasympathetic) reduces spherical aberration and increases depth of focus (squinting also increases depth of focus). • Convergence of the eyes: the gaze of the eyes shifts toward center to keep both eyes focused on object. • *Argyll Robertson pupil:* pupil contracts normally for near vision, but *pupillary light reflex is absent*; this is seen in some CNS lesions (eg, CNS syphilis).
Direct Pupillary Light Reflex	When light is directed into one eye, its pupil constricts.	Light → retina → optic nerve (CN II) → pretectal nuclei in midbrain → nucleus of Edinger-Westphal (CN III) → ciliary ganglion → pupillary sphincter.
Consensual Pupillary Light Reflex	When light is directed into one eye and it constricts, the pupil of the other eye also constricts.	Light shined into one eye produces pupillary constriction in both eyes because of bilateral projections from pretectal nuclei to Edinger-Westphal nuclei.

EYE MOVEMENTS

Movement	Description/Significance
Conjugate	Movement of both eyes in same direction and through same angle.
Convergent	• Inward turning of both eyes, bringing visual axes toward each other to focus on near point so that single image is formed on both retinas. • A *convex lens* causes light rays to converge.
Divergent	• Outward turning of both eyes, separating the visual axes. • A *concave lens* causes light rays to diverge.
Saccades and Microsaccades	• Rapid, jerky, conjugate movements of eyes that cause visual target to be imaged on fovea. • Occurs as gaze shifts from one object to another. • Reduces adaptation (and visual loss of target) that would occur if gaze were fixed on single object for long periods. • *Can occur in dark.*
Smooth Pursuit	• Tracking of moving visual targets. • Once eyes have located target, fixation is maintained. • Cannot occur in dark (target is required).
Nystagmus	• Rapid, involuntary eye movements (side to side, up and down, or rotatory). • Alternate from slow to fast. • *Optokinetic nystagmus* occurs normally when one tries to look at a succession of objects moving quickly across line of sight. • *Nystagmoid jerks* occur when a person is tired. • Nystagmus may also occur related to neural disease.
Vestibular	• Adjustments that occur in response to stimuli initiated in semicircular canals. • Help maintain visual fixation as head moves.

IMAGE FOCUSING

Condition	Description	Corrective Measures
Normal Sight		
Emmetropia	• Near point: nearest point at which object can be seen clearly. • Far point: distance from the eye that object must be placed so that it can be seen clearly without accommodation (6 feet for normal person).	Not applicable.
Disorders		
Presbyopia	• Loss of accommodative power that occurs with age. • Near point is farther than normal.	Converging lenses.
Myopia/ Nearsightedness	• *Focal point is in front of retina.* • *Eye is disproportionately long.* • Distant objects are not focused on the retina. • Far point is closer than normal. • Near point is closer than normal.	• Diverging lenses. • Radial keratotomy.
Hyperopia/ Farsightedness	• *Focal point is behind retina.* • *Eye is disproportionately short.* • Close objects are not focused on retina. • Near point is farther than normal.	Converging lenses.
Astigmatism	• Asymmetrical focusing due to uneven cornea. • Cornea lacks radial symmetry (is egg-shaped rather than spherical), causing lens power to be different in different axes.	Cylindrical lenses (increase converging power in only one axis).

GLAUCOMA AND OTHER VISION DISORDERS

Condition	Description	Corrective Measures
Glaucoma	• Degenerative disease leading to loss of ganglion cells. • Primary: associated with increasing age. • Secondary: impaired circulation of aqueous humor by another ocular disease. • Increases in IOP worsen glaucoma. • Normal IOP occurs in minority of cases.	• β-Blockers or carbonic anhydrase inhibitors that decrease production of aqueous humor. • Cholinergic agonists (eg, pilocarpine) that constrict pupil, decreasing resistance to drainage of aqueous humor • Surgery to create channel through which aqueous humor can drain.
Open-Angle Glaucoma	Permeability through trabeculae is decreased.	
Angle-Closure Glaucoma	Iris is moved forward, obliterating angle between iris and cornea.	
Nyctalopia	• *Night blindness caused by avitaminosis* A. • Initial degeneration of rods and cones. • Eventual destruction of neural layers of retina.	Vitamin A, which is important in synthesis of rhodopsin, helps restore retinal function if given before photoreceptors are destroyed.
Strabismus	• *Cross-eye caused by weakness of muscles of one eye* leading to misalignment of two visual axes, causing *diplopia* (double vision). • Over time, misaligned eye may lose visual acuity (*amblyopia*), which is not correctable.	• Lenses with prisms that bend light rays enough to compensate for abnormal position of affected eye. • Training exercises or surgical shortening of eye muscles.

VISUAL PATHWAYS

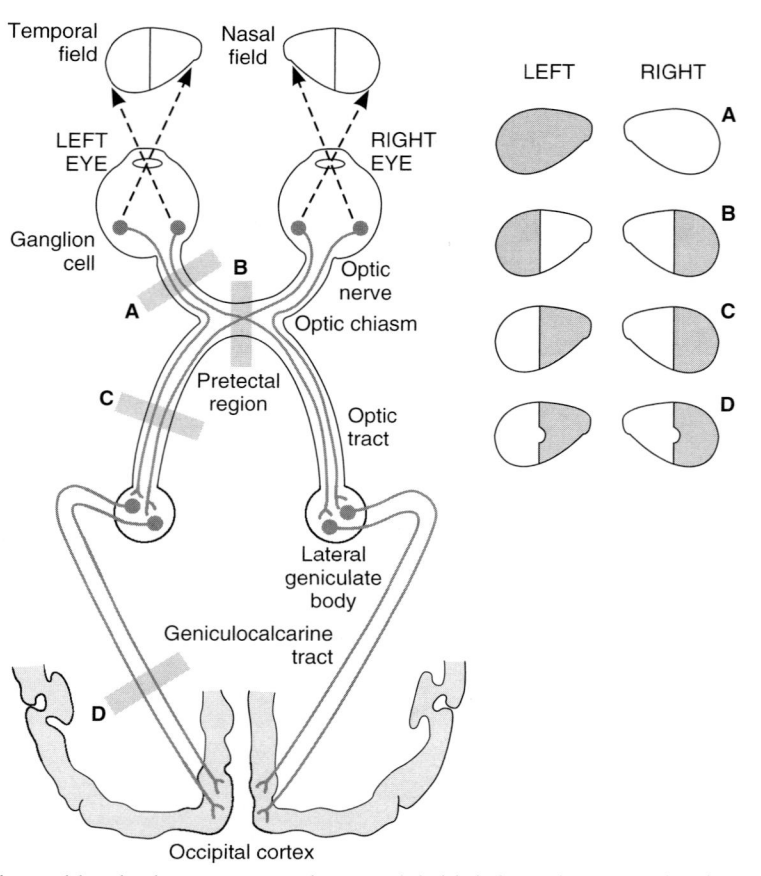

Transection of the pathways at the locations indicated by the letters causes the visual field defects shown in the diagrams on the right.

Reproduced, with permission, from Ganong WF: *Review of Medical Physiology*, 21st ed. McGraw-Hill, 2003:153.

VISUAL FIELD DEFECTS

Type of Defect	Level of Lesion	Visual Field Abnormality	Example
Scotoma	Retina.	Partial blindness in one visual field.	Macular degeneration.
Unilateral Blindness	Unilateral optic nerve.	Complete loss of vision in ipsilateral eye.	Left optic neuritis causing complete blindness in left eye.
Bitemporal Heteronymous Hemianopsia	Optic chiasm (prevention of passage of impulses from nasal halves of each retina to optic chiasm).	Loss of vision in temporal (lateral) fields of both eyes.	Pituitary tumor.
Binasal Heteronymous Hemianopsia (extremely rare)	Bilateral lesion affecting uncrossed optic fibers.	Loss of vision in nasal (medial) fields of both eyes.	Atheroma of internal carotid siphon.
Homonymous Hemianopsia	Unilateral optic tract, lateral geniculate nucleus, optic radiations, or primary visual cortex.	Loss of vision in contralateral half of visual field of each eye.	Right-sided lesion in primary visual cortex causing loss of vision in nasal field of right eye and in temporal field of left eye.

III. Sensory System: Auditory Sensation

ANATOMY OF THE EAR

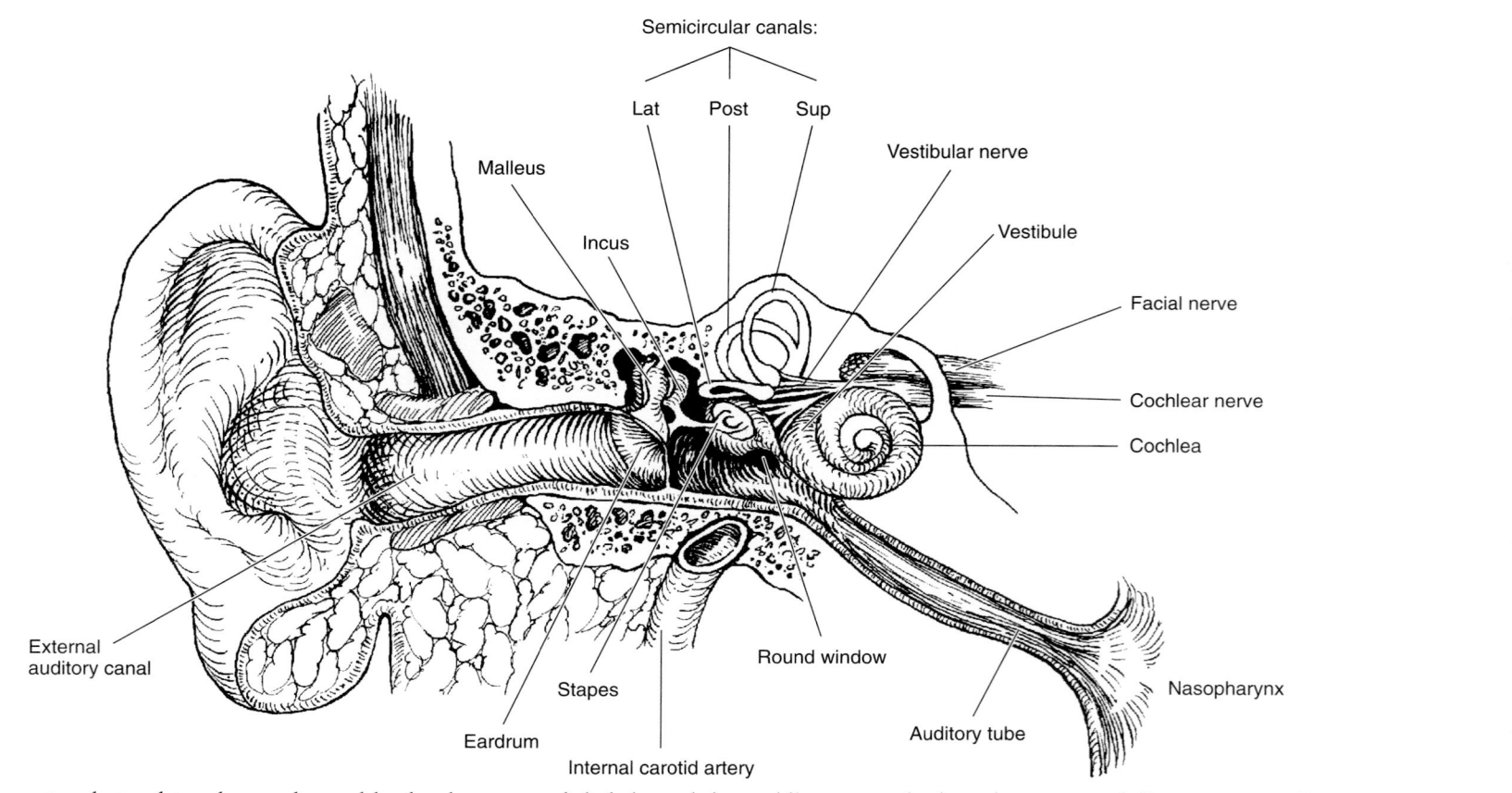

To make the anatomic relationships clearer, the cochlea has been turned slightly, and the middle ear muscles have been omitted. Sup = superior; Post = posterior; Lat = lateral.

Reproduced, with permission, from Ganong WF: *Review of Medical Physiology*, 21st ed. McGraw-Hill, 2003:173.

STRUCTURES OF THE OUTER EAR

Structure	Description	Function(s)
Pinna (Auricle)	Skin and cartilage that projects from head at external opening of external auditory meatus.	• Helps identify source of sound. • Funnels sound waves to external auditory meatus.
External Auditory Meatus	Opening to auditory canal.	Allows sound waves to enter auditory canal.
Auditory Canal	Passage between external auditory meatus and tympanic membrane.	Conduit for sound waves.

STRUCTURES OF THE MIDDLE EAR

Structure	Description	Function(s)
Tympanic Membrane (Eardrum)	Membrane at inner end of auditory canal that separates outer and middle ears.	Transmits sound wave vibration to ossicles.
Auditory Ossicles	• Malleus ("mallet"). • Incus ("anvil"). • Stapes ("stirrup").	• Sound wave vibration travels through ossicular chain to cochlea. • Footplate of stapes contacts cochlea at oval window. • Leverage of auditory ossicles and force produced by sound on tympanic membrane is concentrated and, therefore, *amplified at oval window*.
Middle Ear Muscles	Two skeletal muscles.	Contract reflexively in response to intense sounds (*tympanic reflex*).
	• Tensor tympani inserts on malleus. • Innervated by CN V.	Contraction reduces sound pressure and transmission by dampening movement of ossicular chain.
	• Stapedius inserts on stapes. • Innervated by CN VII.	Contraction pulls footplate of stapes out of oval window.
Eustachian Tube	Opening from middle ear to nasopharynx.	• Equalizes pressure differences between environment and middle ear. • Normally closed, but opens during chewing, swallowing, and yawning.

STRUCTURES OF THE INNER EAR

Structure	Description	Function(s)
Cochlea (auditory receptor apparatus)	• Spiral organ that contains auditory hair cell receptors. • Bony and membranous labyrinths are separated into two compartments (scala vestibuli and scala tympani) by cochlear duct (scala media).	Scalae vestibuli and tympani communicate via opening called helicotrema at apex of cochlea.
Reissner Membrane	Roof over cochlear duct.	Separates scala vestibuli and scala media.
Perilymph	Fluid similar to extracellular fluid (high Na$^+$, low K$^+$) contained in scalae vestibuli and tympani.	Transmits sound vibrations.
Endolymph	Fluid similar to intracellular fluid (high K$^+$, low Na$^+$) contained in scala media (no communication with other two compartments).	Transmits sound vibrations.
Oval Window	Opening between scala vestibuli and middle ear.	Sound vibration of oval window causes round window to bulge outward, causing basilar membrane to vibrate and stimulating organ of Corti.
Round Window	Opening between scala tympani and middle ear.	
Organ of Corti	• Sense organ for hearing. • Located in cochlear duct on basilar membrane.	• Converts sound signals into impulses that are transmitted to brain via cochlear nerve. • *When organ of Corti moves up, hair cells depolarize.* • *When organ of Corti moves down, hair cells hyperpolarize.*
Hair Cells	• Receptor cells for sound located in organ of Corti on basilar membrane. • Stereocilia protrude from apices and into overlying tectorial membrane. • Single row of inner hair cells innervated by over 90% of auditory nerve fibers. • Three rows of outer hair cells innervated by only 10% of auditory nerve fibers.	• Oscillation of basilar membrane causes shear forces on stereocilia at junction with tectorial membrane. • *Bending of stereocilia toward longest cilia causes depolarization.*

Continued

STRUCTURES OF THE INNER EAR (Continued)

Structure	Description	Function(s)
Basilar Membrane	Base of cochlear duct, separating scala vestibuli and scala tympani.	Detects sound based on frequency.
	Most *stiff and narrow at base* of cochlea (near oval and round windows)	Detection of *high-frequency sounds*.
	Most *compliant and wide at apex* of cochlea.	Detection of *low-frequency sounds*.
Modiolus	Bony core around which cochlea is wound.	Contains spiral ganglion (cell bodies of afferent neurons).
Vestibular Apparatus	Part of membranous labyrinth of inner ear involved in proprioception.	See Vestibular Apparatus chart on p. 101.

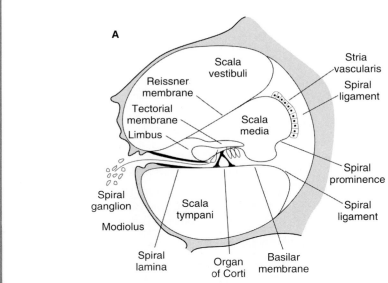

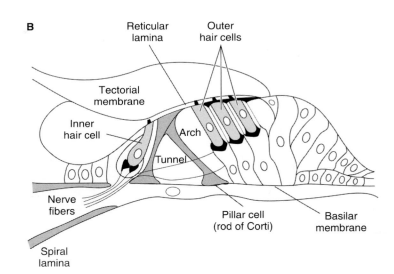

A. Cross-section of the cochlea. **B.** Structure of the organ of Corti.

Reproduced, with permission, from Pickels JO: *An Introduction to the Physiology of Hearing,* 2nd ed. Academic Press, 1988.

TESTING FOR AUDITORY IMPAIRMENT

Condition	Weber Test: (place vibrating tuning fork on top of skull)	Rinne Test: (place vibrating tuning fork on mastoid process)
Normal Hearing	Sound is heard equally in both ears.	• When patient can no longer hear sound through bone, he or she can hear it in air if fork is placed near ear. • Shows that *air conduction is greater than bone conduction*.
Conduction Deafness • Defect in sound conduction system (ie, external or middle ear) interferes with transmission of sound to inner ear.	Sound localized to deaf ear (masking effect of environmental noise is absent on diseased side).	• Sound is not restored when tuning fork moved near ear. • Shows that *bone conduction is greater than air conduction*.
Sensory/Nerve Deafness • Defect in initial stages of auditory pathway (ie, inner ear, cochlear nerve, or cochlear nucleus).	Sound localized to normal ear.	When patient can no longer hear sound through bone, he or she can hear it in air if fork is placed near ear (as long as nerve deafness is partial).

IV. Sensory System: Gustatory and Cutaneous Sensation

DISTRIBUTION OF TASTE BUDS

Area of Tongue	Primary Taste Sensation	Effect of Stimulus	Papillae Types Most Sensitive to Particular Taste	Innervation of Taste Buds
Tip	Sweet.	Opens amiloride-sensitive Na^+ channels and activates adenylate cyclase and cAMP, leading to closing of K^+ channels.	Fungiform: anterior two thirds of tongue.	Anterior two thirds of tongue innervated by facial nerve (CN VII).
Side: Front Half	Salty.	Opens amiloride-sensitive Na^+ channels.		
Side: Back Half	Sour.	Raises intracellular $[H^+]$, which blocks K^+ channels.	Foliate: lateral border of tongue, anterior to circumvallate.	Posterior one third of tongue innervated by glossopharyngeal nerve (CN IX).
Back	Bitter.	Stimulates inositol triphosphate, leading to increased intracellular $[Ca^{2+}]$, which leads to release of neurotransmitter.	Circumvallate: V-shaped row on posterior tongue.	Pharyngeal area innervated by vagus nerve (CN X).
			Filiform: mechanical papilla (not gustatory).	Tactile and temperature receptors innervated by trigeminal nerve (CN V).

TASTE SENSATION BY THE TONGUE

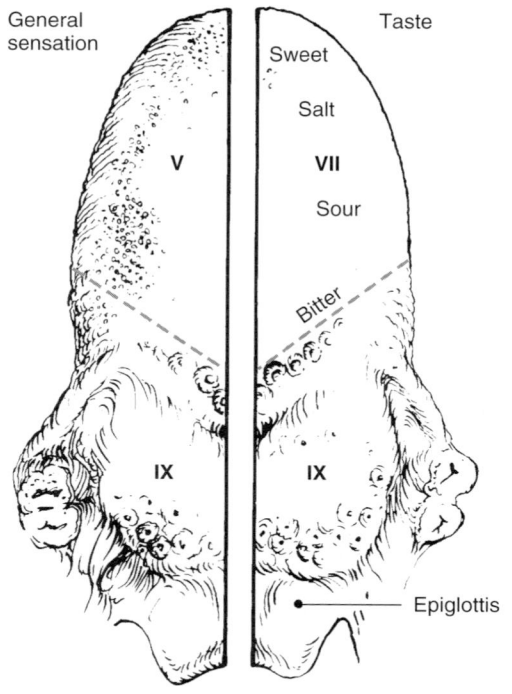

The taste qualities associated with different parts of the tongue, innervation of anterior two thirds and posterior one third of the tongue, and arrangement of the taste buds on the three different types of papillae are shown.

Reproduced, with permission, from Ganong WF: *Review of Medical Physiology*, 20th ed. McGraw-Hill, 2001:184.

Sensation/Receptor	Location	Types	Characteristics
Touch/ Mechanoreceptors	At ends of large, *myelinated* group II afferent fibers located in hairless regions of skin.	Pacinian corpuscle: onion-like lamellar capsule surrounding end of group II afferent fiber.	• *Large* receptive field. • *Very rapid* adaptation. • Encodes *vibration*.
		Meissner corpuscle: small capsule surrounding end of group II afferent fiber.	• *Small* receptive field. • *Rapid* adaptation. • Encodes *speed of stimulus application*.
		Merkel disk: disk on epithelial sensory cells that synapse with branches of a single group II afferent fiber.	• *Small* receptive field. • *Slow* adaptation. • Encodes *location of stimulus*.
		Ruffini corpuscle: • Located on end of group II fiber covered by liquid-filled collagen capsule. • Collagen strands contact nerve fiber and overlying skin.	• *Large* receptive field. • *Slow* adaptation. • Encodes *magnitude and duration of stimulus*.
Temperature/ Thermoreceptors	On free nerve endings of small, *unmyelinated* (C) fibers.	Warm fibers: active when skin is 30 °C–43 °C.	*Firing rate and skin temperature are directly related* (ie, firing rate transiently increases and decreases with skin temperature).
	On free nerve endings of small, *myelinated* (Aδ) fibers.	Cold fibers: active when skin is 15 °C–38 °C.	• *Firing rate and skin temperature are inversely related* (ie, firing rate transiently increases as skin temperature decreases). • Temperatures 45°C–49 °C simultaneously stimulate cold and pain fibers.

Continued

CUTANEOUS SENSATION (Continued)

Sensation/Receptor	Location	Types	Characteristics
Pain/Nociceptors	On free nerve endings of small, *myelinated* (Aδ) fibers.	Aδ mechanical nociceptors.	Respond to strong, noxious mechanical stimuli.
	On free nerve endings of *unmyelinated* (C) fibers.	Polymodal nociceptors.	Respond to noxious mechanical, chemical, and thermal stimuli.
		Central pathways: pain sensation is conveyed to CNS through *anterolateral quadrant* of spinal cord.	Many of specific mechanisms are not well understood.
		Peripheral pathways: *somatic fast pain* travels to brain via *spinothalamic tract* and is topographically represented on cortex.	• *Fast (initial) pain*: well-localized, pinprick sensation that results from activating nociceptors on Aδ fibers. • Evokes withdrawal reflex and sympathetic response.
		• *Somatic slow pain* travels to brain via *spinoreticulothalamic tract*. • Fiber tracts for emotional perceptions of pain are activated.	• *Slow (delayed) pain*: poorly localized, dull, burning sensation that results from activating nociceptors on C fibers. • Evokes hypotension, nausea, sweating, and decreased skeletal muscle tone.
		• *Visceral pain is referred pain*. • Pain originating in visceral organs is referred to sites on skin	• *Skin is topographically mapped and viscera are not mapped*. • Example: pain due to a kidney stone is referred to flank and abdomen.
		Projected pain occurs as result of directly stimulating fibers within pain pathway.	• *Labeled line mechanism* is used to encode location of pain. • Stimulation anywhere along path results in same perception (eg, *phantom limb sensation*).

V. Motor System

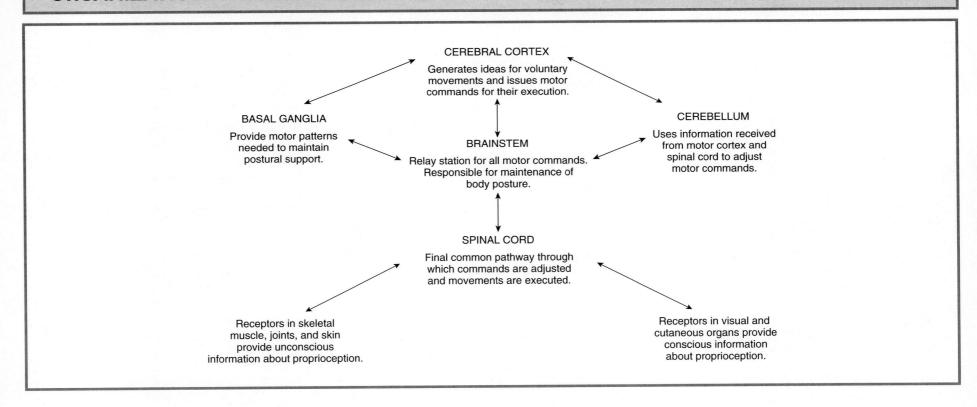

CEREBRAL CORTEX

Generates ideas for voluntary movements and issues motor commands for their execution.

BASAL GANGLIA

Provide motor patterns needed to maintain postural support.

CEREBELLUM

Uses information received from motor cortex and spinal cord to adjust motor commands.

BRAINSTEM

Relay station for all motor commands. Responsible for maintenance of body posture.

SPINAL CORD

Final common pathway through which commands are adjusted and movements are executed.

Receptors in skeletal muscle, joints, and skin provide unconscious information about proprioception.

Receptors in visual and cutaneous organs provide conscious information about proprioception.

MUSCLE STRETCH RECEPTORS

Feature	Muscle Spindle	GTO
Description	• Intrafusal muscle fibers. • Organized *in parallel* with extrafusal muscle fibers. • Attached to tendons at either end of muscle or to sides of extrafusal fibers.	• Net-like collection of knobby nerve endings. • Organized *in series* with muscle fibers. • Found in tendons of skeletal muscles and around joint capsules.
	• Passive stretch of muscle causes stretch of spindle, which leads to muscle contraction. • *Electrical stimulation of muscle does not stretch spindle, and muscle relaxes.*	• Stimulated by *both* passive stretch and active contraction of muscle. • *GTOs stretch when muscle contracts.*
Function	*Stretch reflex: muscle stretch causes muscle contraction.*	• *Inverse stretch reflex* (autogenic inhibition): *relaxation in response to stretch.* • Autogenic inhibition allows GTOs to regulate muscle tension during normal activity.
Innervation	Afferent (sensory) nerves: • Single, large, myelinated, *group Ia fiber with a primary ending* (spiral terminals on both nuclear bag and nuclear chain fibers). • *Dynamic/phasic response* signals velocity of muscle stretch. • *Static response* signals change in muscle length. • Multiple, smaller group II fibers with one or more *secondary endings* (flower-spray terminals on nuclear chain fibers) carry out only static response.	Afferent (sensory) nerves: • Increase in muscle force activates myelinated, group Ib fibers that enter dorsal root and excite spinal cord inhibitory interneurons, which inhibit α-motor neurons that supply same extensor muscle from which force arises. • Ib fibers also make excitatory connections with motor neurons that supply antagonists to acting muscle. • Flexor muscles are relatively unaffected by this pathway.
	Efferent (motor) nerves: • *Dynamic γ motor neurons* innervate primarily nuclear bag fibers and increase phasic activity of Ia afferent fibers. • *Static γ motor neurons* innervate nuclear chain fibers and increase tonic activity of Ia afferents. • During normal movement, motor control system activates both α and γ neurons, which allows constant level of Ia input to CNS without unloading.	Efferent (motor) nerves: • *There is no efferent innervation.*

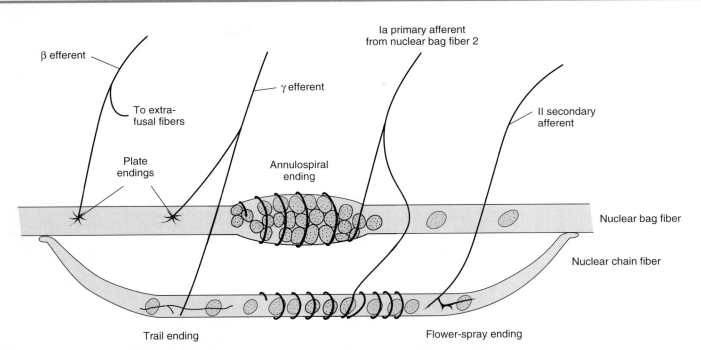

There are two types of intrafusal fibers in mammalian muscle spindles: nuclear bag fibers and nuclear chain fibers.

Reproduced, with permission, from Ganong WF: *Review of Medical Physiology*, 21st ed. McGraw-Hill, 2003:131.

COMPONENTS OF GOLGI TENDON ORGANS

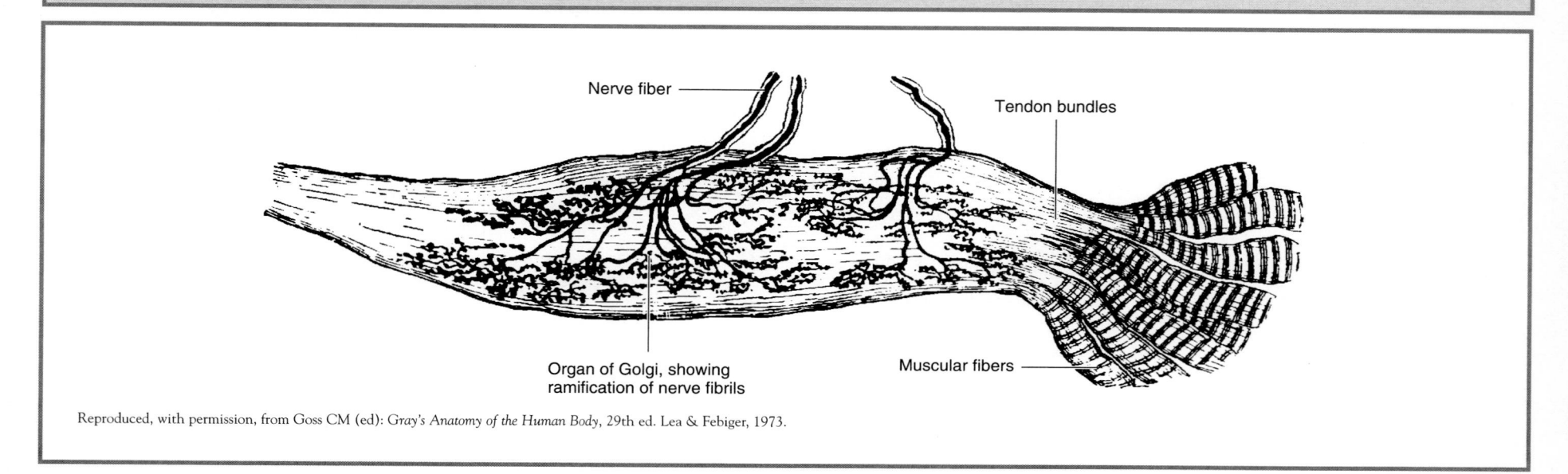

Nerve fiber

Tendon bundles

Organ of Golgi, showing
ramification of nerve fibrils

Muscular fibers

Reproduced, with permission, from Goss CM (ed): *Gray's Anatomy of the Human Body*, 29th ed. Lea & Febiger, 1973.

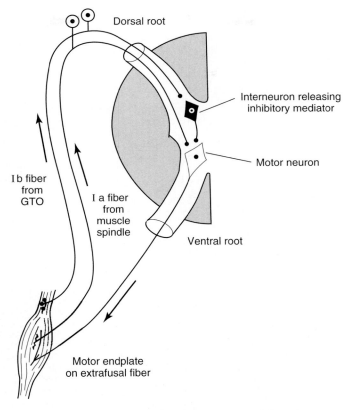

Dorsal root

Interneuron releasing
inhibitory mediator

Motor neuron

I b fiber
from
GTO

I a fiber
from
muscle
spindle

Ventral root

Motor endplate
on extrafusal fiber

- Stretch reflex: Stretch stimulates the spindle, and excitatory impulses pass via the Ia fiber to stimulate the α motor neuron. γ Efferents then initiate muscle contraction.
- Inverse stretch reflex: Stretch also stimulates the GTO. Excitatory impulses passing via the Ib fiber stimulate the interneuron to release the inhibitory mediator glycine.

Reproduced, with permission, from Ganong WF: *Review of Medical Physiology*, 21st ed. McGraw-Hill, 2003:134.

SPINAL CORD STRETCH REFLEXES

Type of Reflex	Receptor	Description/Example	Reflex Characteristics
Stretch	Muscle spindle.	• Stretch of muscle causes reflex contraction of that muscle and reflex relaxation of antagonist muscles. • Phasic stretch reflex: results from stretching muscle quickly (eg, in knee jerk reflex: reflex hammer strike on patellar tendon stretches quadriceps muscle). • Tonic stretch reflex: results from slow stretch of muscle (eg, posture maintenance or passive movement).	• Monosynaptic pathway. • No aftercharge or irradiation. • Reciprocal innervation. • Short latency. • Integration at α-motor neuron.
Inverse Stretch	GTO.	• Stretch or contraction of muscle causes reflex relaxation of that muscle. • Example: when standing, there is force in patella tendon, and the inverse stretch reflex prevents contraction of quadriceps so that posture is maintained.	• Autogenic inhibition: force generated when muscle contracts is stimulus for its own relaxation. • Disynaptic pathway. • Can override stretch reflex.
Withdrawal (flexor or pain)	Cutaneous nociceptors.	• Removal of body part from noxious stimulus. • Stimulation of flexor muscles and inhibition of extensor muscles. • Crossed extensor reflex occurs simultaneously. • Example: withdrawal of hand from hot surface (flexor muscles contract, extensor muscles relax).	• Polysynaptic pathway involving many interneurons with integration at α-motor neuron. • Irradiation (stronger stimulus activates larger number of muscles [eg, entire arm withdraws instead of just the hand]). • Local sign (dependence of exact response on location of stimulus).
Crossed Extensor	Cutaneous nociceptors.	• Stimulation of extensor muscles and inhibition of flexor muscles of opposite limb during withdrawal (flexor) reflex. • Example: stepping on tack with right foot. Right foot undergoes withdrawal reflex (flexor muscles contract, extensor muscles relax). Left foot undergoes crossed extensor reflex to maintain balance (flexor muscles relax, extensor muscles contract).	• Long latency: afferent pathway uses small, slowly conducting fibers and involves many synapses. • Reciprocal innervation (eg, reflex pathway allows contraction of joint flexors as antagonist extensors relax). • Reverberating circuits produce aftercharge (response outlasts the stimulus).

VESTIBULAR APPARATUS

Structure	Description	Function
Otolith Organs: Saccule and Utricle	• Each has *macula*, which contains sustentacular and *hair cells*, and is covered by gelatinous membrane in which *otoliths* (crystals of calcium carbonate) are embedded. • Saccular macula is oriented vertically. • Utricular macula is oriented horizontally.	When hair cells move from their vertical, or resting position, otoliths bend stereocilia.
Semicircular Canals (three)	• Membranous labyrinth containing endolymph and suspended in perilymph within bony labyrinth of petrous portion of temporal bone. • Three canals are perpendicular to each other.	• Angular acceleration in plane of given semicircular canal bends hair cells and stimulates its crista ampullaris. • This displaces endolymph in direction opposite direction of rotation, which deforms cupula and bends stereocilia.
	Contain *crista ampullaris*: hair cell receptor structure, which is located in ampulla of each semicircular canal.	Movements to right (clockwise) stimulate hair cells in the right horizontal canal and inhibit those in left horizontal canal (and vice versa).
	Contain *cupula*: gelatinous structure that fills ampullar space of semicircular canals in which hair cell cilia are embedded.	Constant speed causes hair cells to return to their vertical, or resting position.
Hair (Receptor) Cells	• *Polarized cells* with bases near afferent fibers of vestibular division of vestibulocochlear nerve (CN VIII). • Processes embedded in otolith membrane in saccule and utricle, and in cupula in semicircular canals. • Have many stereocilia and one large kinocilium on one end (called *outer* hair cells in cochlea and *inner* hair cells in vestibular apparatus). • Kinocilium of each hair cell is oriented in different plane so that some hair cells are stimulated and some inhibited no matter in what direction head is moved.	• *When stereocilia bend toward kinocilium, cell depolarizes.* • *When stereocilia bend away from kinocilium, cell hyperpolarizes.* • Hair cells in otolith organs detect *linear acceleration* and the *static position* of the head. • Otolith reflex helps muscles of lower extremities contract before making impact to prevent injury. • Hair cells in semicircular canals detect *angular accelerations* of head. These cells are *insensitive* to movements at *constant* angular velocity.

MEMBRANOUS LABYRINTH

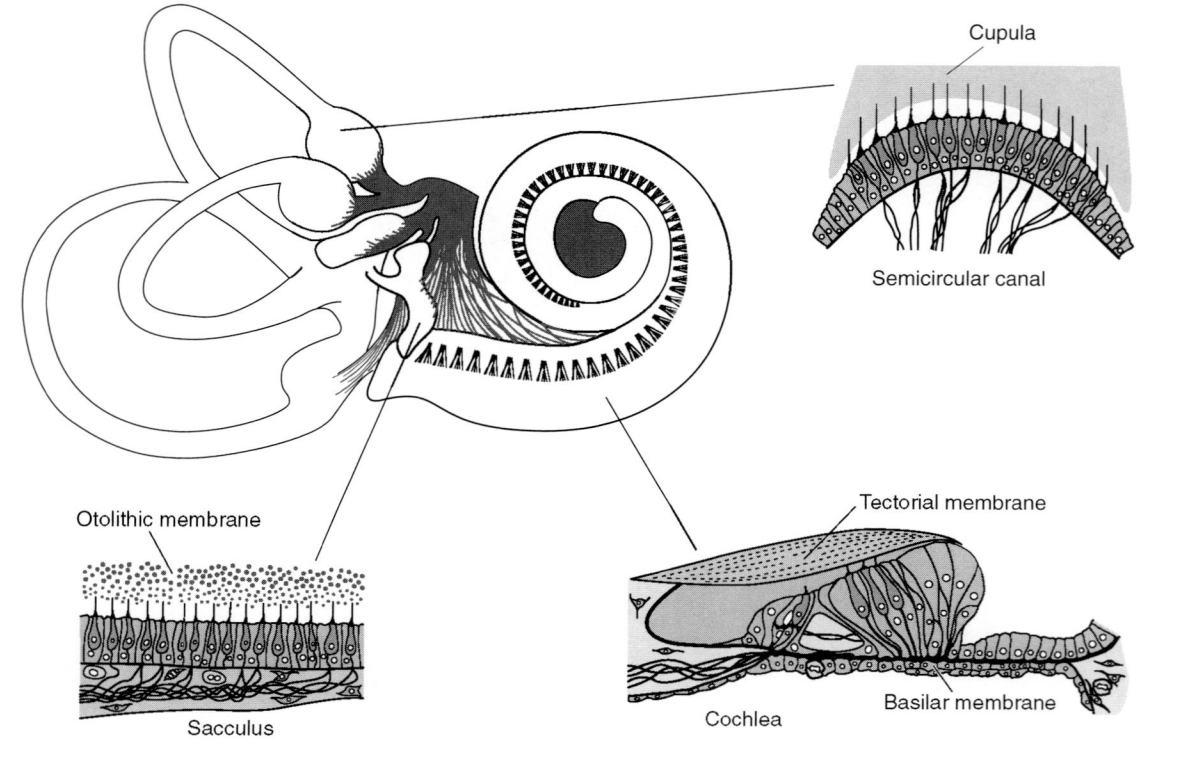

The structures in which hair cells are embedded have been enlarged.

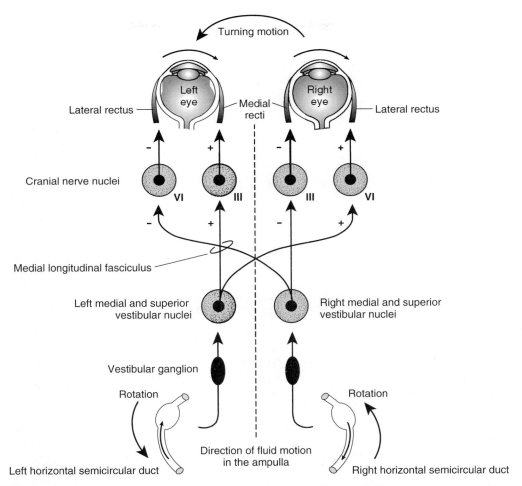

The vestibulo-ocular reflex maintains visual fixation during head movement. If the head rotates to the left, the eyes move slowly toward the right to keep the image on the fovea. When the eyes have rotated as far as possible, they quickly return to the center (nystagmus).

Modified, with permission, from Berne RM, Levy MN: *Principles of Physiology,* 3rd ed. Mosby, 2000:126.

CALORIC STIMULATION

Patient's Level of Consciousness	Test/Purpose	Water Temperature	Ear Injected	Primary Movement	Secondary Movement
Awake	• Warm and cold calorics.	Cold.	Right.	Left: fast.	Right: slow.
	• Used to assess acoustic nerve status.	Warm.	Right.	Right: fast.	Left: slow.
	☞ Remember COWS:	Cold.	Left.	Right: fast.	Left: slow.
	• Cold = Opposite				
	• Warm = Same	Warm.	Left.	Left: fast.	Right: slow.
Comatose	• Cold calorics.	Cold.	Right.	Right: sustained deviation.	None.
	• Used to assess oculovestibular reflex ("doll's eyes").	Cold.	Left.	Right: sustained deviation.	None.

MOVEMENT DISORDERS CAUSED BY LESIONS IN THE BASAL GANGLIA

Location of Lesion	Associated Disorders of Posture and Movement
Striatum (caudate nucleus and putamen)	• Athetosis: continuous, slow, writhing movements of limbs, hands, and fingers. • Chorea: rapid, "dancing" movements of distal muscles; often bilateral. • Dystonia: slow, twisting movements of head and trunk. • *Huntington chorea*.
Globus Pallidus (putamen + globus pallidus = lenticular nucleus)	• Inability of trunk muscles to maintain postural support. • Head is bent forward, and body bends at waist. • Patient can stand upright on request.
Subthalamic Nucleus	Hemiballismus: wild, flailing movement of limbs *on opposite side of lesion*, caused by loss of GABA-ergic inhibition from subthalamic nucleus → thalamus → cortex.
Substantia Nigra (Pars Compacta and Pars Reticulata)	• Akinesia: difficulty initiating movement, decreased spontaneous movement. • Bradykinesia: slowness of movement. • Cogwheel rigidity: when moved, limb periodically gives way, then reestablishes its resistance to movement. • Lead pipe rigidity: when moved, the rigid limb stays where it is placed. • Tremor: "pill rolling" movement that disappears during voluntary activity. • *Parkinson disease*.

CEREBELLUM

Lobe	Description	Microscopic Layers	Effects of Lesion
Neocerebellum	• Receives input from opposite motor cortex. • Helps plan and program motor movements. • Third lobe to evolve. • Also known as flocculonodular lobe or cerebrocerebellum.	• *Granule cell layer* is inner layer with granule and Golgi cell interneurons. • Axons of granule cells form parallel fibers.	• Adiadochokinesia: inability to make rapidly alternating movements. • Decomposition of movement; muscles act individually. • Dysmetria: inability to stop movement at proper time or to direct it appropriately. • Intention tremor: as one approaches object and tries to touch it, movements become more uncontrolled.
Paleocerebellum	• Receives input from spinal cord and smooths and coordinates ongoing movements. • Second lobe to evolve. • Also known as anterior lobe or spinocerebellum.	*Purkinje cell layer* is middle layer, with dendrites extending into outer cortex and axons extending into granule cell layer.	No obvious effects because functions are assumed by cerebrocerebellum.
Archicerebellum	• Receives input from vestibular apparatus. • Helps control axial muscles, maintains equilibrium, and coordinates head and eye movements. • First lobe to evolve. • Also called posterior cerebellum or vestibulocerebellum.	*Molecular layer* is outer layer, with basket and stellate cell interneurons.	Ataxia, loss of equilibrium.

VI. Autonomic Nervous System

DIVISIONS OF THE AUTONOMIC NERVOUS SYSTEM

Division	Description/Function	Neurotransmitters	Effects of Stimulation	Important Points
SNS	Rapidly adapts to "fight-or-flight" situation.	• ACh for preganglionic motor neurons. • Norepinephrine for postganglionic motor neurons.	• Increased heart rate. • Elevated blood pressure. • Dilated pupils. • Dilated bronchi. • Conversion of glycogen to glucose.	• Preganglionic neurons in intermediolateral cell column, ventral horn, and T1–L2. • Pathway includes white communicating rami.
PNS	Assists with body's return to normal "rest-and-digest" status.	ACh for most pre- and post-ganglionic motor neurons.	• Decreased heart rate. • Decreased blood pressure. • Decreased size of bronchi. • Decreased conversion of glycogen to glucose.	• Main parasympathetic nerve: vagus (CN X). • Preganglionic neurons located in CN nuclei (III, VII, IX, X) in brainstem.
ENS	• Ganglia within walls of GI tract. • Organizes movements of GI tract smooth muscle (peristalsis) and GI secretions. • Considered to be independent component of ANS.	• ACh. • ATP. • Endorphins. • Enkephalins. • Nitric oxide. • Serotonin. • Somatostatin. • Substance P. • Vasoactive intestinal polypeptide.	• SNS stimulation decreases activity of ENS. • PNS stimulation increases activity of ENS.	Includes Auerbach myenteric plexus: • Located between outer longitudinal and middle circular layers. • Innervates longitudinal and circular smooth muscle. • Motor control. Includes Meissner submucosal plexus: • Located between middle circular layer and mucosa. • Innervates glandular epithelium, intestinal endocrine cells, and submucosal blood vessels. • Controls intestinal secretion.

PATHWAYS OF THE SYMPATHETIC NERVOUS SYSTEM

Preganglionic Neuron	Route	Postganglionic Neurons/Route	Visceral Effectors
Cell Bodies (intermediolateral cell column, ventral horn, T1–L2)	White communicating rami.	• Cell body in cranial extension of sympathetic chain to superior, middle, and inferior cervical sympathetic ganglia. • Travels via plexus around great vessels.	Head: smooth muscles and glands of face, eyes, and other structures, including carotid.
		• Cell body in paravertebral sympathetic chain ganglia. • Travels via gray communicating rami and splanchnic nerves.	• Body wall. • Body viscera.
	Splanchnic nerve.	• Cell body in prevertebral ganglia: celiac, superior mesenteric, inferior mesenteric. • Travels via sympathetic plexuses near target organs.	Body viscera.
	Direct innervation.		Chromaffin cells of adrenal medulla.

PATHWAYS OF THE PARASYMPATHETIC NERVOUS SYSTEM

Preganglionic Nucleus	Route	Postganglionic Ganglion	Visceral Effectors
Cell Bodies in Sacral Parasympathetic Nucleus, S2–S4	Appropriate nerves.	• Ganglia in abdominal and pelvic cavities. • *Splenic flexure is boundary between GI organs supplied by vagus nerve and those supplied by sacral parasympathetics.*	Body viscera.
CN Nuclei in Brainstem	Appropriate CN.	Appropriate cranial parasympathetic ganglia.	Structures in head.
• Edinger-Westphal	• CN III.	• Ciliary.	• Ciliary body and pupillary sphincter.
• Superior Salivatory	• CN VII.	• Sphenopalatine.	• Lacrimal glands, mucosal glands of paranasal sinuses, oral cavity salivary glands.
	• CN VII.	• Submandibular.	• Submandibular and sublingual glands.
• Inferior Salivatory	• CN IX.	• Otic.	• Parotid gland.
• Nucleus Ambiguus and Dorsal Motor	• CN X.	• Ganglia in or near walls of target viscera.	• Pharynx, soft palate, heart, GI tract.

NEURAL PATHWAYS IN THE SYMPATHETIC AND PARASYMPATHETIC NERVOUS SYSTEMS

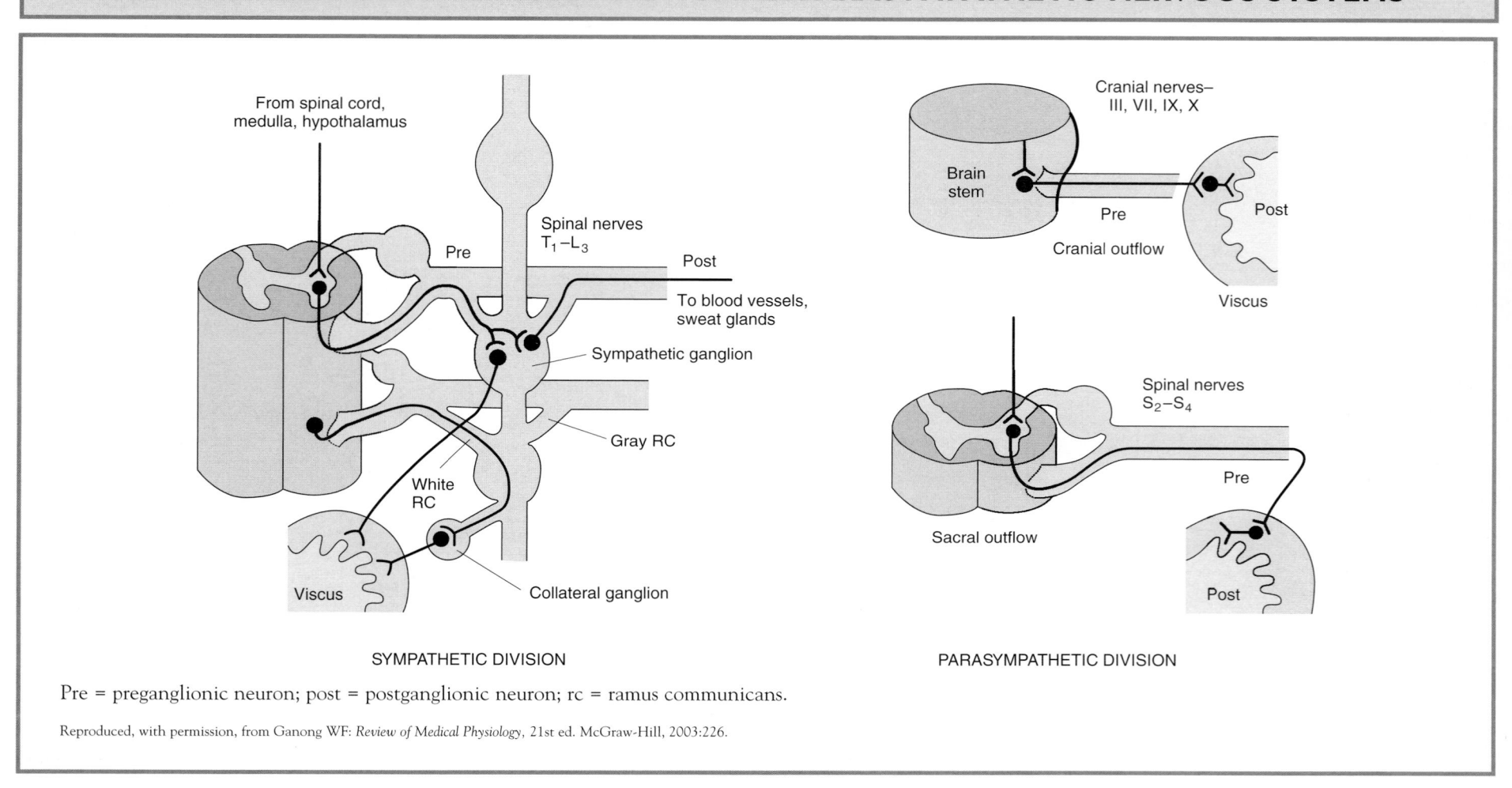

SYMPATHETIC DIVISION

PARASYMPATHETIC DIVISION

Pre = preganglionic neuron; post = postganglionic neuron; rc = ramus communicans.

Reproduced, with permission, from Ganong WF: *Review of Medical Physiology*, 21st ed. McGraw-Hill, 2003:226.

SYMPATHETIC AND PARASYMPATHETIC FIBERS

Neurotransmitter	Receptor Activated by:	Receptor Blocked by:	Effector Cell Receptor	Effector Cell Response
Preganglionic Sympathetic And Parasympathetic Fibers From CNS				
ACh	Low doses of nicotine.	Curare.	Cholinergic/nicotinic postganglionic receptor.	Stimulation.
	Muscarine.	Atropine.	Cholinergic/ muscarinic postganglionic receptor.	
Postganglionic Sympathetic Fibers				
Norepinephrine	Epinephrine > norepinephrine >> isoproterenol.	Phenoxybenzamine.	α-Adrenergic.	• Contraction of vascular smooth muscle. • Contraction of GI tract sphincters. • Relaxation of other GI tract smooth muscle.
	Isoproterenol > epinephrine > norepinephrine.	Propranolol.	β-Adrenergic.	• Relaxation of bronchial and vascular smooth muscle. • Contraction of ventricular muscle.
ACh	Muscarine.	Atropine.	Cholinergic/muscarinic.	• Sweat gland secretion. • Relaxation of blood vessels in skin and skeletal muscle.
Postganglionic Parasympathetic Fibers				
ACh	Muscarine.	Atropine.	Cholinergic/muscarinic.	• Relaxation of GI tract sphincters and contraction of other GI tract smooth muscle. • Slowed conduction through sinoatrial and atrioventricular nodes. • Secretion from secretory cells.

VII. Higher Functions of the Nervous System

SLEEP STAGES

Stage	Description	EEG Waves
Non-REM Sleep		
Stage 1	• Drowsy. • Initial 90 minutes of sleep.	Alpha waves: highly synchronized waves of increased amplitude and voltage and decreased frequency (8–12 Hz).
Stage 2	• Light sleep. • Progressive reduction in consciousness and increasing resistance to being awakened.	Alpha waves with bursts of *sleep spindles*, which are high-amplitude waves that periodically interrupt alpha rhythm (12–15 Hz).
Stage 3	• Moderate sleep. • Muscle tone decreases, heart and respiratory rates decrease, blood pressure falls, heart rate and metabolism slow, and pupils constrict.	Theta waves: slower and larger waves (4–7 Hz).
Stage 4	• Deepest sleep. • Progressive relaxation. • Individual is extremely difficult to arouse. • Amount of time spent in this stage decreases with age and may disappear by 60 years of age.	Delta waves: very slow, very large waves (1–3 Hz).

Stage	Description	EEG Waves
REM Sleep		
Paradoxical Sleep, Dream Sleep	• *Vivid dreams occur*, muscles twitch, muscle tone disappears, reflexes are inhibited, eyes move rapidly, respiration is irregular, and blood pressure fluctuates. • Penile erection occurs in males. • Five cycles of non-REM–REM sleep per night. • After second cycle, intervals between REM shorten, and duration spent in REM lengthens. • As morning approaches, less time is spent in deep, slow-wave sleep, and individual periodically awakens. • Amount of time spent in REM is greatest in newborns and declines with age.	• Desynchronized, rapid, low voltage wave pattern similar to beta waves that occur in alert individual. • Beta waves (similar to those seen during arousal) are asynchronous waves of low amplitude and voltage and high frequency (18–30 Hz).

 Behold All The Details (brain waves from most conscious to deepest sleep)—**B**eta, **A**lpha, **T**heta, **D**elta

SLEEP STAGES AND EEG PATTERNS

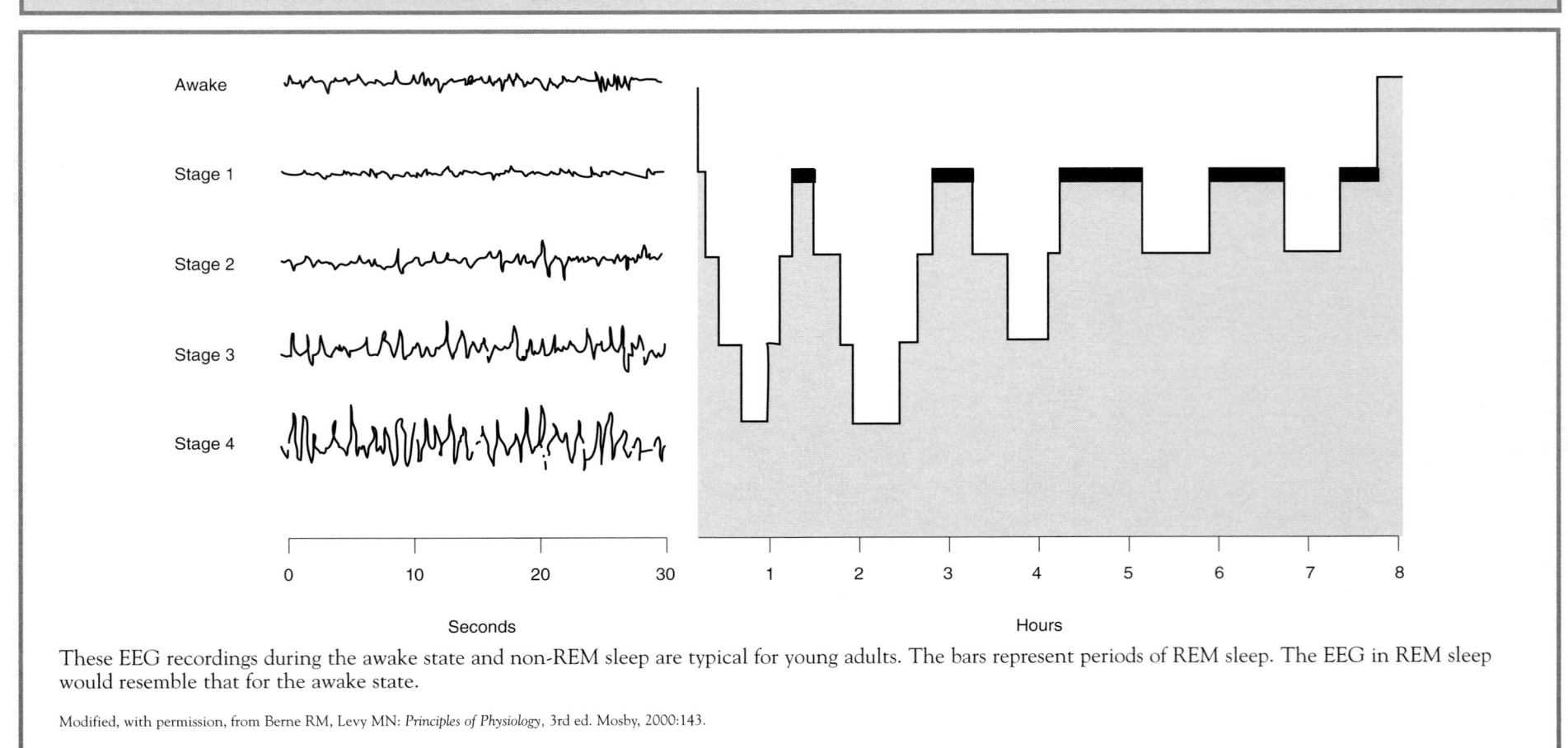

These EEG recordings during the awake state and non-REM sleep are typical for young adults. The bars represent periods of REM sleep. The EEG in REM sleep would resemble that for the awake state.

Modified, with permission, from Berne RM, Levy MN: *Principles of Physiology*, 3rd ed. Mosby, 2000:143.

SLEEP DISORDERS

Type of Disorder	Characteristic Features	Time During Sleep Cycle
Insomnia	• Subjective problem of insufficient or nonrestorative sleep. • Example: fatal familial insomnia, a progressive prion disease (encephalopathic disease such as Creutzfeldt-Jakob) of worsening insomnia, impaired autonomic and motor functions, dementia, and death.	
Somnambulism	Sleepwalking.	Arousal from slow-wave sleep.
Nocturnal Enuresis	Bed-wetting.	Arousal from slow-wave sleep.
Pavor Nocturnes	Nightmares.	Slow-wave sleep.
Narcolepsy	Episodic sudden loss of muscle tone and eventually irresistible urge to sleep during daytime activities.	• Sudden onset of REM sleep. • REM entered directly from waking state.
Cataplexy	• Occurs in individuals with narcolepsy. • Profoundly reduced muscle tone that is characteristic of REM occurs *without* loss of consciousness. • Individual becomes paralyzed, falls to ground, and cannot move.	Sudden onset of REM.
Sleep Apnea	• Caused by obstruction of the airway during inspiration. • Repeated occurrence causes loss of sleep, tiredness, and poor performance during daytime.	Most common during REM, when pharyngeal muscles are most relaxed.
REM Behavior Disorder	• Hypotonia fails to occur during REM. • Patients act out their dreams.	REM.

CLASSIFICATION OF EPILEPSY

Type	Description	Characteristic Seizures	EEG Changes
Partial or Local	• Repetitive attacks of uncontrollable, focal neurologic dysfunction. • May be primarily motor (*Jacksonian march*), sensory, or psychological. • *Symptoms are experienced contralaterally to lesion.* • May be preceded by sensory *aura* (first symptom is often olfactory or visual and usually reflects seizure focus).	• Simple: single symptom expressed without loss of consciousness. • Complex: changing symptoms expressed with a loss of consciousness. • Partial complex: behavioral seizure with loss of consciousness, usually originates in limbic lobe. • Lesion in temporal uncus area results in aura of foul odor called "uncinate" fit.	• Focal EEG spike train.
Generalized	• Involves large regions of brain, both hemispheres. • Symptoms expressed bilaterally. • Consciousness is lost at onset.	• Nonconvulsive: petit mal or absence, atonic, myoclonic (brief, uncontrollable jerk). • Convulsive: grand mal or tonic-clonic, with prodromal warnings (not auras) such as change in mood or loss of appetite may precede attack by hours.	• Repeated bursts and runs of symmetric 3.5 Hz activity. • Rapidly repeating spikes during tonic phase, followed by sharp-slow waves during clonic phase. • Slow waves persist for hours postictally

DISORDERS OF CONSCIOUSNESS

Disorder	Description
Syncope (fainting)	Transient pathologic loss of consciousness caused by temporarily insufficient blood flow to the brain from which person can be aroused.
Stupor	More persistent loss of consciousness from which arousal cannot be obtained.
Coma	• Lesion blocking connection between ascending reticular activating system and thalamus. • Stimulation of sensory pathways causes momentary desynchronization of EEG, but there are no behavioral signs of arousal. • O_2 consumption is reduced.
Brain Death	• Loss of consciousness is accompanied by flat EEG (no brain waves) and loss of all brainstem regulatory systems. • By definition, must be present for 6–12 hours and be due to traumatic or ischemic anoxia and not hypothermia or metabolic poisons, from which later recovery is possible.

TYPES OF LEARNING

Type	Description	Subtype	Description	Example
Nonassociative	Learning about single stimulus.	Habituation.	• Response to particular stimulus diminishes with repetition of that stimulus. • Learning that *stimulus is not important*.	Sleeping through sound of morning alarm clock.
		Sensitization.	• Repeated stimulus produces greater response if it is coupled with pleasant stimulus (positive reinforcement) or unpleasant stimulus (negative reinforcement). • Learning that *stimulus is important*.	Mother who sleeps through many noises but wakes at first sound of her baby crying.
Associative	Learning about relationship between two stimuli.	Classical conditioning.	• Conditioned stimulus is paired with unconditioned stimulus until conditioned stimulus alone produces response originally evoked only by unconditioned stimulus. • Extinction: if conditioned stimulus is presented repeatedly without unconditioned stimulus, conditioned reflex eventually disappears. • If conditioned stimulus is reinforced from time to time, it persists indefinitely.	Pavlov's dog: • Food (unconditioned stimulus) that normally caused salivation in dog (reflex) was paired with bell (conditioned stimulus) until dog salivated with only bell (now conditioned reflex). • If bell is presented repeatedly without food, dog will eventually stop salivating with only the bell.
		Operant conditioning.	• Subject is taught to perform task in order to obtain reward or punishment. • Subject develops conditioned reflex. • Reinforcement of response changes probability of response.	• Animal steps on wire grid and receives shock. • Thereafter, animal avoids grid, thus showing conditioned avoidance reflex.

CATEGORIES OF MEMORY

Category	Description	Type	Characteristics of Memory Types
Explicit (Declarative or Recognition Memory)	Associated with consciousness.	Episodic memory.	Memory for events and experiences in serial form.
	• Dependent on hippocampus and medial temporal lobes for retention. • Explicit memories required for activity to become implicit once task is thoroughly learned. • Example: riding a bike.	Semantic memory.	Memory for facts (words, rules, language).
Implicit (Nondeclarative or Reflexive Memory)	• Consciousness is not involved. • Retention not solely dependent on hippocampus. • Examples: skills, habits, conditioned reflexes.	Short-term memory.	• Small capacity memory that lasts seconds to hours and is stored in hippocampus. • Depends on ongoing neural activity. • Easily disrupted by trauma or drugs. • Example: retrograde amnesia is loss of memory for events immediately preceding brain injury, in which days of memory may be lost but remote memories remain intact.
		Long-term memory.	• Memory of limitless capacity that lasts a lifetime and is stored in various parts of neocortex • Resistant to disruption. • Depends on permanent changes in structure or function of widely distributed sets of neurons.

Continued

CATEGORIES OF MEMORY (Continued)

Category	Description	Type	Characteristics of Memory Types
		Working memory.	Information available for very short periods while individual plans actions based on it.
		Recent memory.	• Process by which information in short-term memory is transformed into long-term memory. • Dependent on hippocampus.
		Priming.	Facilitation of recognition of words or objects by prior exposure.

APHASIA

Type	Location of Lesion in Dominant Hemisphere	Description
Fluent	Wernicke area (in superior temporal gyrus, where auditory and visual information is comprehended).	• Normal to excessive amount of speech filled with jargon and neologisms. • Decreased ability to comprehend meaning of spoken or written words and visual and auditory information.
Nonfluent	Broca area (in frontal lobe, anterior to motor cortex, where information from Wernicke area is processed for vocalization, then projected to speech articulation area and motor cortex).	• Slow speech, limited vocabulary (often reduced to expletives). • Decreased ability to write. • Normal ability to understand spoken and written words.
Conduction	In and around auditory cortex.	• Normal ability to speak, with good auditory comprehension. • Decreased ability to put words together or conjure up words.
Anomic	Angular gyrus, without damage to Wernicke or Broca area.	• Difficulty understanding written language or pictures (information is not processed and transmitted to Wernicke area). • No difficulty with speech or with understanding auditory information.
Global	Lesion involving more than one area of left brain.	Difficulty with both receptive and expressive functions of speech, which is nonfluent.

CHAPTER 3
CARDIOVASCULAR SYSTEM

ABBREVIATIONS

ACE = angiotensin-converting enzyme

ADP = adenosine diphosphate

AV = atrioventricular

bpm = beats per minute

CAD = coronary artery disease

cAMP = cyclic adenosine monophosphate

cGMP = cyclic guanosine monophosphate

CO = cardiac output

CHF = congestive heart failure

CNS = central nervous system

COPD = chronic obstructive pulmonary disease

CVP = central venous pressure

DDAVP = 1-deamino-8-D-arginine vasopressin

ECG = electrocardiogram

EF = ejection fraction

G6PD = glucose-6-phosphate dehydrogenase

GI = gastrointestinal

HR = heart rate

HTLV-I = human T-cell leukemia/lymphoma virus type I

LBBB = left bundle branch block

LVF = left ventricular failure

LVH = left ventricular hypertrophy

MAP = mean arterial pressure

MHC = major histocompatibility complex

MI = myocardial infarction

NADPH = reduced nicotinamide adenine dinucleotide phosphate

PEEP = positive end-expiratory pressure

PT = prothrombin time

PTT = partial thromboplastin time

RBBB = right bundle branch block

RBC = red blood cell

RV = residual volume

RVF = right ventricular failure

RVH = right ventricular hypertrophy

SA = sinoatrial

SV = stroke volume

SVR = systemic vascular resistance

t-PA = tissue-type plasminogen activator

u-PA = urokinase-type plasminogen activator

VEDV = ventricular end-diastolic volume

VESV = ventricular end-systolic volume

vWF = von Willebrand factor

WBC = white blood cell

Autoregulation	Capacity of tissues to compensate for changes in perfusion pressure by changing vascular resistance in order to maintain relatively constant blood flow.
Baroreceptors	Stretch receptors in pulmonary circulation, atrial walls, carotid sinus, and aortic arch innervated by glossopharyngeal and vagus nerves; discharge of baroreceptors increases when the pressure in the structures in which they are located rises, causing bradycardia, decreased blood pressure, decreased CO, and vasodilation.
Automaticity	Ability of the heart to initiate its own beat; continues for some time without any neural or hormonal regulation.
Capacitance (vascular compliance)	Quantity of blood that can be stored in a given part of the circulation for each mm Hg rise in pressure, calculated by distensibility multiplied by volume for a vessel; the capacitance of a vein is about 24× that of its corresponding artery (the vein is about 8 times as distensible and its volume is 3 times as great) .
Class I Antigens	Proteins found on all nucleated cells; genes that encode them are on short arm of chromosome 6 (A, B, C).
Class II Antigens	Proteins found on antigen-presenting cells, including B cells and activated T cells; genes that encode them are on short arm of chromosome 6 (DP, DQ, DR).
Complement System	Plasma enzymes C1–C9 that work in sequence to mediate the cell-killing effects of innate and acquired immunity; the *classic pathway* is activated by an antigen-antibody reaction, the *alternative pathway* is not (and, therefore, is one of the first lines of defense against invading organisms).
Cytokines	Hormone-like molecules secreted by endothelial cells, fibroblasts, lymphocytes, macrophages, and monocytes that regulate immune responses; examples include colony-stimulating factors, interleukins, and tumor necrosis factors.
Diastolic Pressure	Lowest pressure in the arterial system during any cardiac cycle; occurs just before the onset of ventricular ejection; normal systemic arterial diastolic pressure = 80 mm Hg.
Erythroblastosis Fetalis (hemolytic disease of newborn)	Complication due to Rh-incompatibility that occurs when an Rh-negative mother develops anti-Rh antibodies against an Rh-positive fetus; there is no effect on first pregnancy, but subsequent babies may suffer from anemia, jaundice, edema, and kernicterus unless mother is given Rh immunoglobulin with first pregnancy.
Erythropoietin	Hormone secreted by the kidney in response to tissue hypoxia that increases the rate of RBC production.
Fick Law	Amount of O_2 used by the heart depends on the amount of work performed; used to measure CO, where $CO = VO_2/(CaO_2 - CvO_2)$; $VO_2 = O_2$ consumption, $CaO_2 =$ coronary arterial O_2 content, and $CvO_2 =$ mixed venous content.

Continued

Hypercapnia	Abnormally high arterial P_{CO_2} that *causes central vasoconstriction and peripheral vasodilation*; moderate hyperventilation lowers the CO_2 tension of blood.
Hypertrophy	Increase in size of organ or tissue due to increase in size of its cells; any increase in work of the heart (eg, pulmonary or systemic hypertension) causes ventricular muscle to enlarge–*first dilate, then hypertrophy*. Ischemia occurs if blood supply does not increase proportionately.
Laminar Flow	Normal blood flow; streamlined and silent. *Fluid moves in one direction* as a series of infinitesimally thin layers, parallel to the axis of the tube; each layer moves at a different velocity, with that of the fluid next to the tube's wall being zero and that at the center of the stream being maximum.
Poiseuille Law	$Q = \pi(P_i - P_o)r^4/8\eta L$; laminar flow of newtonian fluids is directly proportional to the difference between inflow (P_i) and outflow (P_o) pressures to the fourth power of the radius of a tube (r). It varies inversely with the viscosity of fluid (η) and the length of the tube (L).
Reactive Hyperemia	Condition after a period of ischemia in which vessels are dilated and blood flow is higher than normal, with a magnitude and duration that depends on the duration of the prior occlusion; after blood flow is reestablished, skin becomes fiery red.
Reentry/Circus Movement	Reexcitation phenomenon; a cardiac impulse reexcites an area of myocardium through which the impulse had previously passed (eg, Wolff-Parkinson-White syndrome); HR is excessively fast and CO declines.
Systolic Pressure	Highest pressure in the arterial system, occurs during ventricular ejection, normal = 120 mm Hg.
Turbulent Flow	Irregular movement of fluid in a tube characterized by radial and circumferential mixing and development of vortices.

I. Circulation

STRUCTURE AND FUNCTION OF BLOOD COMPONENTS

Type of Blood Cell	Description	Function	Clinical Significance
Erythrocytes (RBCs)	• Biconcave disks. • No nucleus. • Contain hemoglobin. • Life span: 120 days.	Hemoglobin carries O_2 to body tissues.	• Anemia and chronic hypoxia can produce polycythemia. • Hemolytic anemia caused by dapsone, sulfonamides, nitrofurantoin, primaquine, probenecid, and vitamin K may occur in patients with G6PD deficiency.
Leukocytes (WBCs)	• Larger than erythrocytes. • Nucleus present. • Life span: 6 hours. • Three subtypes: granulocytes (65%), lymphocytes (30%), monocytes (5%).	• Participate in immune defense system inflammatory response. • Stimulated by colony-stimulating factors and interleukins.	• Before birth: all subtypes originate in bone marrow. • After birth: lymphocytes originate from lymph nodes, spleen, and thymus.
Granulocytes	• Horseshoe-shaped nuclei that become multilobed as cells become older. • Present on endothelial cell surfaces. • Named for different types of granules they contain. • Three subtypes: neutrophils (95%), eosinophils (4%), basophils (1%).	Granulocytes defend against infection by phagocytizing bacteria and other foreign bodies and destroying them via release of proteolytic enzymes, cytokines, and toxic O_2 metabolites.	• Eosinophils are especially important in responding to allergens. • Eosinophils are abundant in mucosa of respiratory, GI, and urinary tracts. • Basophils also release histamine and heparin and are essential in immediate-type hypersensitivity reactions.
Lymphocytes	• Large, round nuclei with scanty cytoplasm. • Subtypes: B cells, T cells.	• *B cells confer humoral immunity.* • *T cells confer cellular immunity.*	• B cells differentiate into plasma cells that produce antibodies. • T cells are responsible for delayed allergic reactions and rejection of transplanted organs.

Continued

STRUCTURE AND FUNCTION OF BLOOD COMPONENTS (Continued)

Type of Blood Cell	Description	Function	Clinical Significance
Monocytes	Kidney-shaped nuclei with abundant, agranular cytoplasm.	Tissue macrophages (reticuloendothelial system).	Examples: alveolar macrophages, Kupffer cells in liver, microglia.
Mast Cells	<ul><li>Heavily granulated.</li><li>Present in connective tissue.</li><li>Contain histamine, heparin, proteases, leukotrienes, and prostaglandins.</li><li>Have IgE receptors on their membranes.</li></ul>	<ul><li>Role in acquired immunity: inflammatory responses initiated by IgE and IgG.</li><li>Role in natural immunity: release tumor necrosis factor α by antibody-independent mechanism.</li></ul>	Marked mast cell degranulation produces clinical manifestations of allergy that may be equivalent to anaphylaxis.
Platelets	<ul><li>Small, anuclear cell fragments of megakaryocytes.</li><li>Have membrane receptors for collagen, fibrinogen, and vWF.</li><li>Contain clotting factors, actin, myosin, lysosomes, and serotonin.</li><li>Half-life: 4 days.</li></ul>	Hemostasis.	Drugs such as carbamazepine, digoxin, heparin, quinidine, and rifampin are associated with thrombocytopenia (platelet count < 150,000/μL).

PLASMA, SERUM, AND LYMPH

Fluid	Description	Contents	Clinical Significance
Plasma	• Straw-colored, fluid portion of blood in which blood cells are suspended. • Makes up 5% of normal body weight.	• Ions, organic and inorganic molecules. • Clotting factors such as fibrinogen. • Other proteins (eg, albumin, globulins, hemoglobin).	Hypoproteinemia: • Low plasma protein causes decreased oncotic pressure and subsequent edema. • Seen in prolonged starvation and malabsorption syndromes, liver disease (protein synthesis depressed), and nephrosis (large amounts of albumin are lost in urine).
Serum	Fluid remaining if whole blood or blood plasma is allowed to clot and clot is removed.	Same as plasma, except no fibrinogen or other clotting factors (II, V, or VII).	
Lymph	Tissue fluid that enters lymphatic vessels and drains into venous circulation via thoracic and right lymphatic ducts.	• Clotting factors. • Other proteins. • Water-insoluble fats (mostly from GI tract). • Lymphocytes.	Lymphedema: • Accumulation of lymph in tissues, producing swelling. • Caused by congenitally abnormal lymph vessels or obstruction of vessels due to tumor, parasites, inflammation, or injury.

TYPES OF HEMOGLOBIN

Type	Description	Important Points
Hemoglobin A	Normal adult hemoglobin, with two α and two β subunits, each containing heme moiety.	Hemoglobin A_{1C} increases in individuals with poorly controlled diabetes mellitus.
Hemoglobin F	Fetal hemoglobin, with two α and two γ subunits.	Compared to hemoglobin A, does not bind 2,3-diphosphoglycerate as much and has greater affinity for O_2.
Hemoglobin S	Abnormal hemoglobin (valine in position 6 of β chain instead of glutamate).	• Present in sickle cell anemia. • Polymerizes at low O_2 tensions, which causes RBCs to become sickle-shaped, hemolyze, and form aggregates that block blood vessels.
Carboxyhemoglobin	Carbon monoxide reacted with hemoglobin.	• Affinity of hemoglobin for O_2 is lower than its affinity for carbon monoxide. • This displaces O_2 on hemoglobin, reducing its O_2-carrying capacity.
Methemoglobin	Present when normal ferrous iron of hemoglobin is converted to ferric iron.	• Occurs when blood is exposed to various drugs and other oxidizing agents. • Darkens color of blood.
Oxyhemoglobin	• Hemoglobin bound to oxygen via iron in heme. • Affected by pH, temperature, and 2,3-diphosphoglycerate	• 2,3-Diphosphoglycerate and H^+ compete with O_2 for binding to deoxygenated hemoglobin, decreasing affinity of hemoglobin for O_2. • Note difference with myoglobin, a pigment found in red (slow) muscles and respiratory chain enzymes that contains heme and acts as an oxygen reservoir.

ABO BLOOD GROUPS

Blood Type	Antigens (Agglutinogens) on RBCs	Antibodies (Agglutinins) in Plasma	Possible Genotypes	Frequency in United States
O	Neither A nor B.	Anti-A, anti-B (universal donor).	OO.	45%.
A	A.	Anti-B.	• AA, AO. • A antigen: Mendelian dominant inheritance.	41%.
B	B.	Anti-A.	• BB, BO. • B antigen: Mendelian dominant inheritance.	10%.
AB	A, B.	None (universal recipient).	AB.	4%.

NATURAL VERSUS ACQUIRED IMMUNITY

Feature	Natural (Innate) Immunity	Acquired Immunity
Function	• Provides first line of defense against foreign bodies (infections, cancer cells, transplanted organs). • Participating cells react to substances unique to cell walls of foreign bodies by activating complement and proteolytic cascades, producing antibacterial peptides, releasing interferons, and phagocytosis. • Foreign cells are killed by osmotic lysis or apoptosis. • Cytokine release from participating cells activates *slower but more specific acquired immune response*.	• B and T cells are activated by specific antigens to form clones of cells that attack foreign proteins. • B and T cells act and communicate by secreting cytokines and activating complement system. • B and T cells persist in small numbers as memory cells after invasion is prevented so that second exposure to same antigen triggers a *prompt, magnified immune response*.
Types of Cells Involved	• Neutrophils. • Macrophages. • Natural killer cells (cytotoxic cells that are not T cells).	• B cells. • T cells.

☞ It's good for what **AIL**s you (acquired immunity involves the B and T lymphocytes):
Acquired
Immunity
Lymphocytes

B CELLS VERSUS T CELLS

Feature	B Cells	T Cells
Characteristics	• Made in liver and bone marrow, both from bone marrow precursors. • Differentiate into plasma cells and memory B cells.	• Made in thymus from bone marrow precursors. • Differentiate into cytotoxic T cells (CD8), helper T cells (CD4), suppressor T cells, and memory T cells.
Function	• *Humoral immunity* is major defense against bacterial infections. • Plasma cells secrete antibodies, also known as immunoglobulins (IgA, IgD, IgE, IgG, IgM). • Antibodies function as antigen-binding receptors on B-cell membrane.	• *Cellular immunity* is defense against viruses, fungi, a few bacteria (tubercle bacillus), and cancer cells. • Cellular immunity is also responsible for delayed allergic reactions and rejection of transplants. • *Cytoxic T cells recognize class I MHC proteins.* • *Helper T cells recognize class II MHC proteins.* • T_H1 cells are primarily involved in cellular immunity. • T_H2 cells are primarily involved in humoral immunity (help activate B cells). • Suppressor T cells inhibit B cells.

INTRINSIC AND EXTRINSIC PATHWAYS OF THE COAGULATION SYSTEM

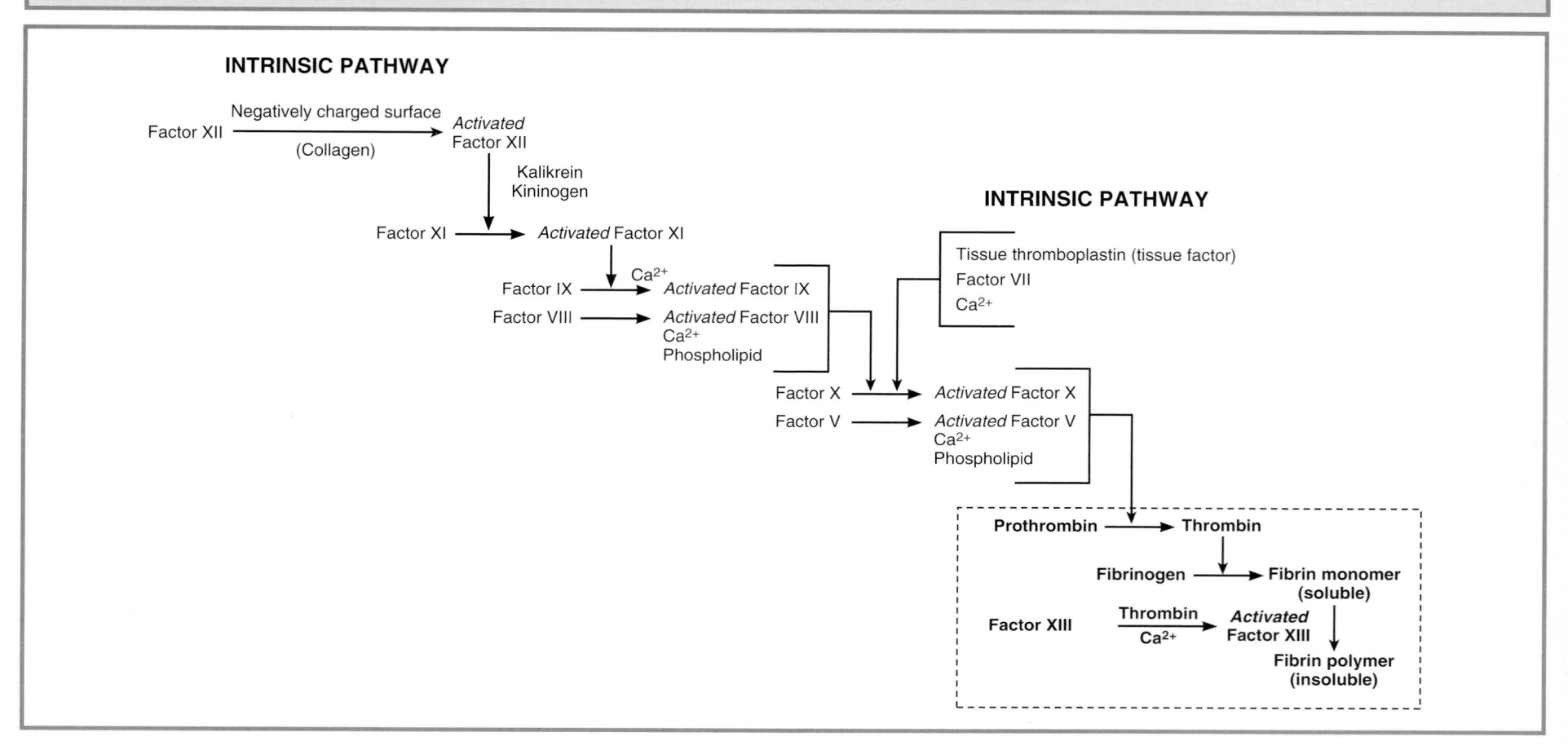

INTRINSIC PATHWAY

Factor XII →(Negatively charged surface / (Collagen))→ Activated Factor XII

Kalikrein
Kininogen

Factor XI → Activated Factor XI

Factor IX → Ca^{2+} → Activated Factor IX

Factor VIII → Activated Factor VIII
Ca^{2+}
Phospholipid

INTRINSIC PATHWAY

Tissue thromboplastin (tissue factor)
Factor VII
Ca^{2+}

Factor X → Activated Factor X

Factor V → Activated Factor V
Ca^{2+}
Phospholipid

Prothrombin → Thrombin

Fibrinogen → Fibrin monomer (soluble)

Factor XIII →(Thrombin / Ca^{2+})→ Activated Factor XIII

Fibrin polymer (insoluble)

EVENTS IN HEMOSTASIS

Step No.	Event	Mechanism
1	Physical injury to blood vessel.	
2	Vasoconstriction.	Mechanical stimulation of penetrating object provokes a contractile response in vascular smooth muscle.
3	Platelet aggregation.	• Damaged endothelium encourages platelet adherence at injury site; binding to collagen initiates platelet activation; aggregation is fostered by platelet-activating factor (cytokine from neutrophils, monocytes, and platelets). • Platelets bind collagen and form temporary hemostatic plug. • Adherent platelets release ADP and thromboxane A_2, which cause adherence of additional platelets; serotonin, which enhances vasoconstriction; and thromboplastin, which hastens blood coagulation. • Extension of platelet aggregate along vessel is prevented by prostacyclin, which is released from endothelial cells in adjacent, uninjured part of vessel.
4	Blood coagulation.	• *Conversion of soluble fibrinogen to insoluble fibrin by thrombin is key step.* • Intrinsic pathway is initiated by exposure of blood to negatively charged surface such as collagen from damaged endothelium or glass from outside body. • Extrinsic pathway initiated by tissue damage and release of tissue thromboplastin. • Intrinsic and extrinsic pathways converge on activation of factor X, which catalyzes cleavage of prothrombin to thrombin. • Presence of Ca^{2+} and other cofactors are required.
5	Clot retraction.	After clot is formed, actin and myosin from platelets cause contraction that pulls fibrin strands toward platelets, extruding serum and shrinking clot.
6	Clot lysis.	• Thrombin, t-PA, and u-PA convert soluble plasminogen to its active, soluble form, proteolytic enzyme plasmin (fibrinolysin). • Plasmin lyses fibrin and fibrinogen. • Fibrinogen degradation products inhibit thrombin.

DISORDERS OF HEMOSTASIS

Disorder	Epidemiology and Etiology	Symptoms	Laboratory Findings	Therapy
Factor VII Deficiency	• Autosomal recessive. • 1/500,000 births.	• Mild: easy bruising, increased tendency to bleed following trauma, GI hemorrhage. • Severe: recurrent bleeding episodes, such as epistaxis; hemarthroses; intramuscular hematomas; hematuria; menorrhagia; gingival, mucosal, GI, and intracranial bleeding.	Prolonged PT.	Fresh frozen plasma.
Hemophilia A (Factor VIII Deficiency)	• X-linked hemorrhagic disorder. • No family history in 30% of cases. • 1/5000 births. • Gene on long arm of X chromosome.		Prolonged PTT that corrects with normal plasma.	• Mild: DDAVP stimulates vascular endothelium to release factor VIII. • Severe: replacement with factor VIII.
Von Willebrand Disease	• Both autosomal dominant and recessive inheritance. • vWF factor binds and stabilizes factor VIII. • Also binds exposed subendothelial collagen, so plays role in platelet adhesion.		• ± Prolonged PTT, depending on associated factor VIII deficiency. • Prolonged bleeding time.	Depends on severity: • Mild: DDAVP may help. • Severe: replacement with vWF.
Hemophilia B (Factor IX Deficiency)	• X-linked hemorrhagic disorder. • 1/30,000 births. • Gene on long arm of X chromosome.		• Prolonged PTT that corrects with normal plasma. • Decreased factor IX.	Factor IX replacement.
Factor X Deficiency	• Autosomal recessive. • Fewer than 1/500,000 births.		Prolonged PT and PTT.	Fresh frozen plasma.

Vitamin K Deficiency	• Affects production of factors II, VII, IX, and X, and proteins C and S. • Caused by vitamin K deficiency of newborn, malabsorption syndromes, prolonged parenteral feeding, ingestion of oral anticoagulants.		• Early: prolongation of PT due to short half-life (2–6 hours) of factor VII. • Late: prolonged PTT.	Vitamin K replacement.
Antithrombin III Deficiency	• Autosomal dominant disorder. • 1/2000–5000 births. • Risk of venous thrombosis that increases with age. • Acquired with liver disease, nephrotic syndrome, medications such as heparin and L-asparaginase, and thrombohemorrhagic states.	Venous thrombosis.	Functional and antigenic assays.	Anticoagulation.
Protein C Deficiency	• Autosomal dominant (suggested autosomal recessive). • Type I: decreased protein C levels. • Type II (rare): decreased protein C function with normal levels.	• Homozygous: patients may die of thrombosis in early infancy. • Heterozygous: clotting is common (eg, deep venous thrombosis, retinal vein thrombosis). • Neonatal purpura fulminans can occur (usually fatal).	Decreased level protein C in patients who are not taking warfarin or who are not vitamin K–deficient.	Long-term anticoagulant therapy for patients who have had venous thromboembolic events.
Protein S Deficiency	• Autosomal dominant. • Heterozygotes have increased risk of thromboembolic events.	• Deep venous thrombosis. • Superficial thrombophlebitis. • Pulmonary embolism. • Thrombosis of cerebral, axillary, or mesenteric veins.	Decreased level protein S in patients who are not taking warfarin or who are not vitamin K–deficient.	Long-term anticoagulant therapy for patients who have had venous thromboembolic events.

Continued

DISORDERS OF HEMOSTASIS (Continued)

Disorder	Epidemiology and Etiology	Symptoms	Laboratory Findings	Therapy
Disseminated Intravascular Coagulation	• Secondary response to primary disorder such as infection, malignancy, trauma, or transfusion reaction. • Fibrin is deposited in vascular system, and small-and medium-sized vessels are thrombosed. • Increased consumption of platelets and coagulation factors causes simultaneous bleeding.	Hemorrhage.	Acute: • Elevated PT and PTT. • Decreased factors II, V, and VII. • Decreased platelets.	• Treatment of underlying disease. • Replacement of clotting factors and platelets may help decrease risk of hemorrhage.

ANTICOAGULANTS

Drug	Mechanism of Action/Use
Antithrombin III	Serine protease inhibitor that blocks thrombin and clotting factors IX, X, XI, and XII.
Chelating Agents (eg, deferoxamine)	Bind calcium and iron.
Citrate, Oxalate	Used in vitro, they form insoluble salts with Ca^{2+}, removing it from solution and preventing coagulation.
Coumarin Derivatives: Dicumarol and Warfarin	• Inhibit action of vitamin K, a cofactor for activation of clotting factors II, VII, IX, X, protein C and S. • Used for long-term anticoagulation (eg, status post–deep venous thrombosis or after placement of artificial cardiac valves).
Heparin	• Naturally occurring substance. • Used clinically for rapid anticoagulation. • Facilitates antithrombin III.
Low-Molecular-Weight Heparin	• Works similarly to unfractionated heparin but has longer half-life. • Produces a more predictable anticoagulant response.
Recombinant t-PA (eg, alteplase)	• Activates plasminogen, leading to formation of plasmin. • Used in treatment of early MI.
Streptokinase	• Bacterial enzyme that activates plasminogen, leading to formation of plasmin. • Used in treatment of early MI.
Thrombomodulin	• Made by endothelial cells. • Complex of thrombomodulin-thrombin activates protein C. • Protein C and protein S inactivate an inhibitor of t-PA, increasing formation of plasmin.

REGULATION OF THE FIBRINOLYTIC SYSTEM BY PROTEIN C

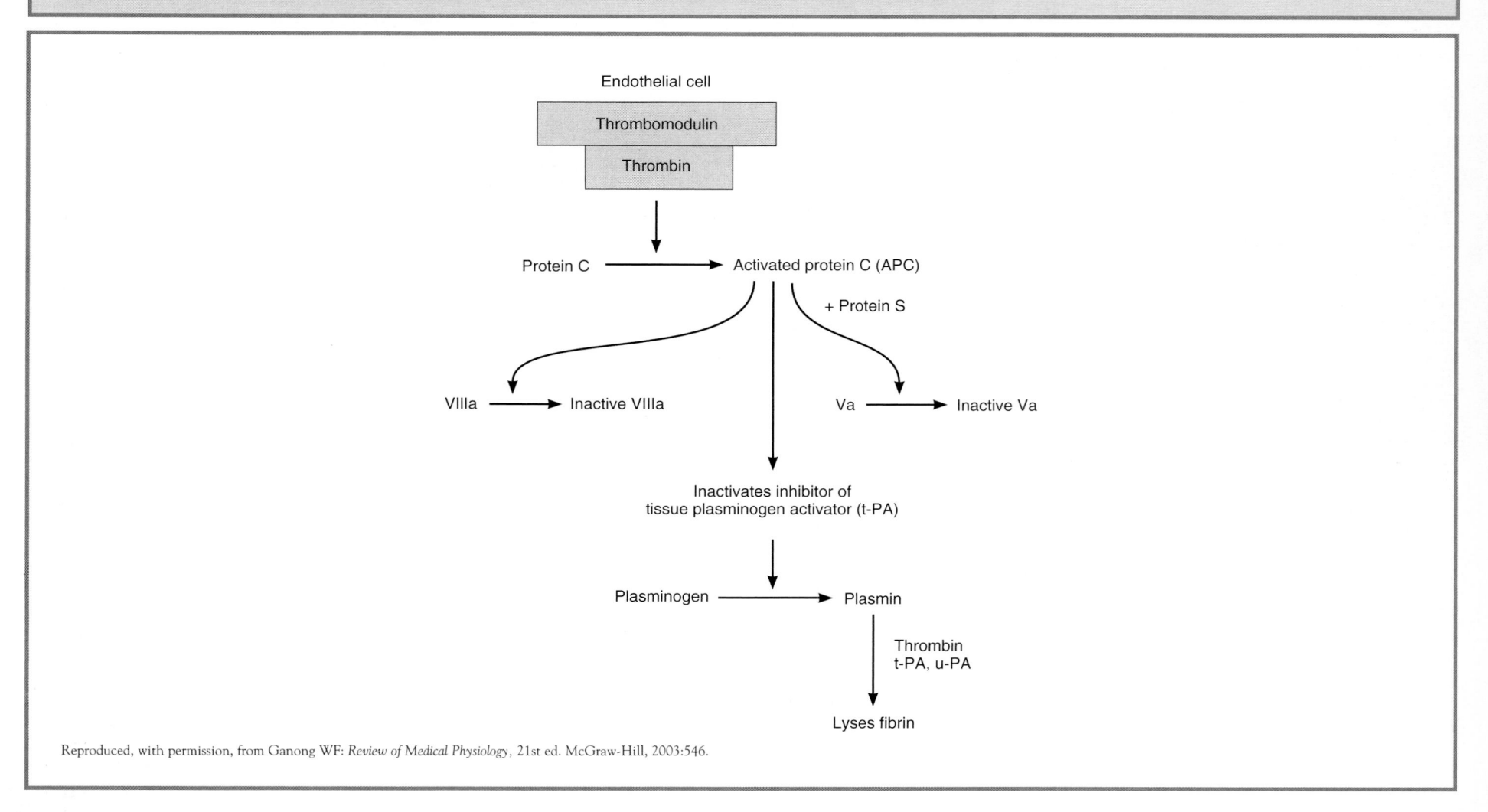

SELECTED BLOOD CELL DISORDERS

Cell Type	Disorder	Description
Stem Cells	Polycythemia vera.	• Chronic myeloproliferative disease of older patients of unknown cause. • Elevated RBCs, WBCs, and platelets. • Hyperviscous blood with impaired flow to organs. • Symptoms may include cyanosis, thrombosis, pruritus, headaches, and splenomegaly.
	Essential thrombocythemia.	• Abnormal proliferation of megakaryocytes that leads to increased platelets in blood. • Increased platelets cause tendency to clot. • Platelet dysfunction causes tendency to bleed (especially from GI tract). • Symptoms may include transient ischemic attacks, amaurosis fugax, MI, gangrene of extremities, and splenomegaly.
Erythrocytes	G6PD deficiency.	• G6PD catalyzes first step in oxidation of glucose via hexose monophosphate shunt (NADPH generated is needed for maintenance of normal red cell fragility). • Predisposes RBCs to hemolysis associated with drugs and infections. • More severe in persons of Mediterranean descent.
	Hereditary spherocytosis.	• Common cause of hereditary hemolytic anemia. • Caused by abnormality of protein network that maintains shape and flexibility of RBC membrane. • Cells are spherocytic in normal plasma and hemolyze more readily than normal cells in hypotonic NaCl solutions.
	Polycythemia.	• Increased number of RBCs in blood. • Relative polycythemia: decreased plasma volume. • Absolute polycythemia: increased production of RBCs. • May also occur secondarily as result of respiratory or other disorder (eg, chronic hypoxia stimulates RBC production; renal carcinoma accelerates erythropoietin production, which causes increased RBC production).

Continued

SELECTED BLOOD CELL DISORDERS (Continued)

Cell Type	Disorder	Description
	Sickle cell anemia.	• Hereditary disease that affects persons of African and Mediterranean descent. • Abnormal hemoglobin (hemoglobin S) becomes insoluble when blood is deprived of O_2 and it precipitates, forming elongated crystals that distort RBCs into characteristic sickle shape, causing anemia. • Heterozygous patients have sickle cell *trait*, which is usually asymptomatic; these patients are resistant to infection with *Plasmodium falciparum* (malaria). • Supportive treatment includes oxygen supplementation and blood transfusion.
	Thalassemias.	• Globin gene defects (eg, α, β, γ) cause low amounts or absence of polypeptide chains. • Result is abnormal RBC function, anemia, and splenomegaly. • Autosomal dominant inheritance. • Homozygous state is thalassemia major, and heterozygous state is thalassemia minor.
Lymphocytes	Chronic lymphocytic leukemia.	• *Most common form of leukemia.* • Usually occurs in individuals > 50 years of age, in men more than women, and in whites more than blacks. • B-cell disease more common than T-cell disease, which has worse prognosis.
Plasma Cells	Multiple myeloma.	• Monoclonal production of immunoglobulins (IgG, A, D, or E) or light chains (κ or λ) that are found in serum and urine (Bence Jones proteins). • Serum electrophoresis shows monoclonal spike. • Focal plasma cell tumors cause bone destruction. • Patients are usually older than 50 years of age and have bone pain and anemia.
	Waldenström macroglobulinemia.	• Monoclonal production of IgM. • Chronic disease that occurs in older persons. • Symptoms may include anemia, increased plasma viscosity associated with epistaxis, retinal hemorrhages, CHF, mental confusion, and cyanosis.

Platelets	Idiopathic thrombocy-topenic purpura.	• Immune-mediated destruction of platelets that occurs after viral infection and in absence of exposure to drugs or other toxins.
		• Symptoms may occur at any age and include ecchymoses and petechiae (especially in lower extremities); epistaxis; and cranial, GI, or mucosal bleeding.
		• Spleen is usually normal, as are coagulation studies.
		• Treatment is prednisone of splenectomy if no response to steroids.
	Thrombotic thrombocy-topenic purpura.	• Diffuse microvascular occlusion of arterioles and capillaries causes ischemic dysfunction of multiple organs.
		• Symptoms may include fever; CNS involvement with mental status changes, seizures, and focal deficits; and renal failure.
		• Medical emergency that must be treated immediately with plasma exchange; mortality in untreated cases is greater than 90%.

II. Dynamics of Blood Flow

STRUCTURE AND FUNCTION OF THE VASCULAR SYSTEM

Structure	Description	Function
Arteries	• *High-resistance system.* • *Distensibility and compliance* allow accommodation of stroke volume with only moderate increase in pressure. • *Elastic recoil* (Windkessel effect) creates pressure that maintains blood flow during diastole.	• Serve as conduits for blood flow between heart and arterioles. • Normally carry 10–15% of blood volume.
Arterioles	• Terminal components of arterial system. • Structure similar to arteries, except with more narrow lumen. • Narrow lumen provides greatest resistance to blood flow in vascular system.	• *Resistance vessels: site of major pressure drop in cardiovascular system.* • *"Stopcocks of the circulation."* • Convert pulsatile blood flow in arteries to steady flow in capillaries. • Rigid walls of *arteriosclerosis* cause pulsatile capillary flow, leading to increased capillary flow during systole and little or no flow during diastole.
Microcirculation	Includes metarterioles, capillaries, postcapillary venules, and arteriovenous anastomoses (arteriovenous anastomoses).	Exchange of diffusible substances (gases, solutes, water) between blood and tissue.
	• Capillaries have narrow lumens, thin walls, and no smooth muscle, maximizing cross-sectional area. • Diameter is controlled by alterations in capillary resistance. • Capillary venous ends are more permeable than arterial ends. • Capillary endothelium has fenestrations (except in blood-brain barrier).	• Capillaries can withstand high internal pressures without bursting (see Law of Laplace, p. 149). • Capillary endothelium controls blood flow by releasing vasodilators (nitric oxide, prostacyclin) and vasoconstrictors (endothelin).

	Arteriovenous anastomoses (in fingertips, toes, palms, soles, ears, nose, and lips) have no basal tone or tonic activity, are very sensitive to vasoconstrictors, and are not under metabolic control (no reactive hyperemia or autoregulation).	Arteriovenous anastomoses shunt blood from arterioles to venous plexuses, bypassing capillary bed.
Veins	• *Low-resistance, low pressure, highly distensible system.* • Because veins are not normally fully distended, small changes in pressure can cause large changes in volume.	• Serve as reservoirs, capacitance vessels, and conduits. • As much as 75% of circulating blood volume is in veins at any one time. • Venoconstriction, respiration and pumping of skeletal muscles all help increase venous return. • Standing, PEEP, and Valsalva maneuver all impede venous return.
	Veins in dependent parts of body have valves.	• Valves prevent backflow of venous blood, and their support helps minimize increases in capillary hydrostatic pressure. • Varicose veins are caused by incompetent valves.
Lymph Vessels	• Highly permeable (endothelial cells lack tight junctions). • Fine filaments anchor them to surrounding connective tissue. • Normal lymph flow is 2 L/d, and the rate varies with organ (highest in GI tract and liver). • Lymph flow increased by any mechanism that enhances rate of blood capillary filtration. • *Thoracic duct is largest lymph vessel.* • Bone, cartilage, CNS tissues, and epithelium lack lymphatic vessels.	• Return fluid and solutes from capillaries to circulatory system. • Filter lymph at lymph nodes and remove foreign matter such as bacteria. • *Only mechanism for returning protein (mainly albumin) to circulatory system (prevents edema).*

MICROCIRCULATION

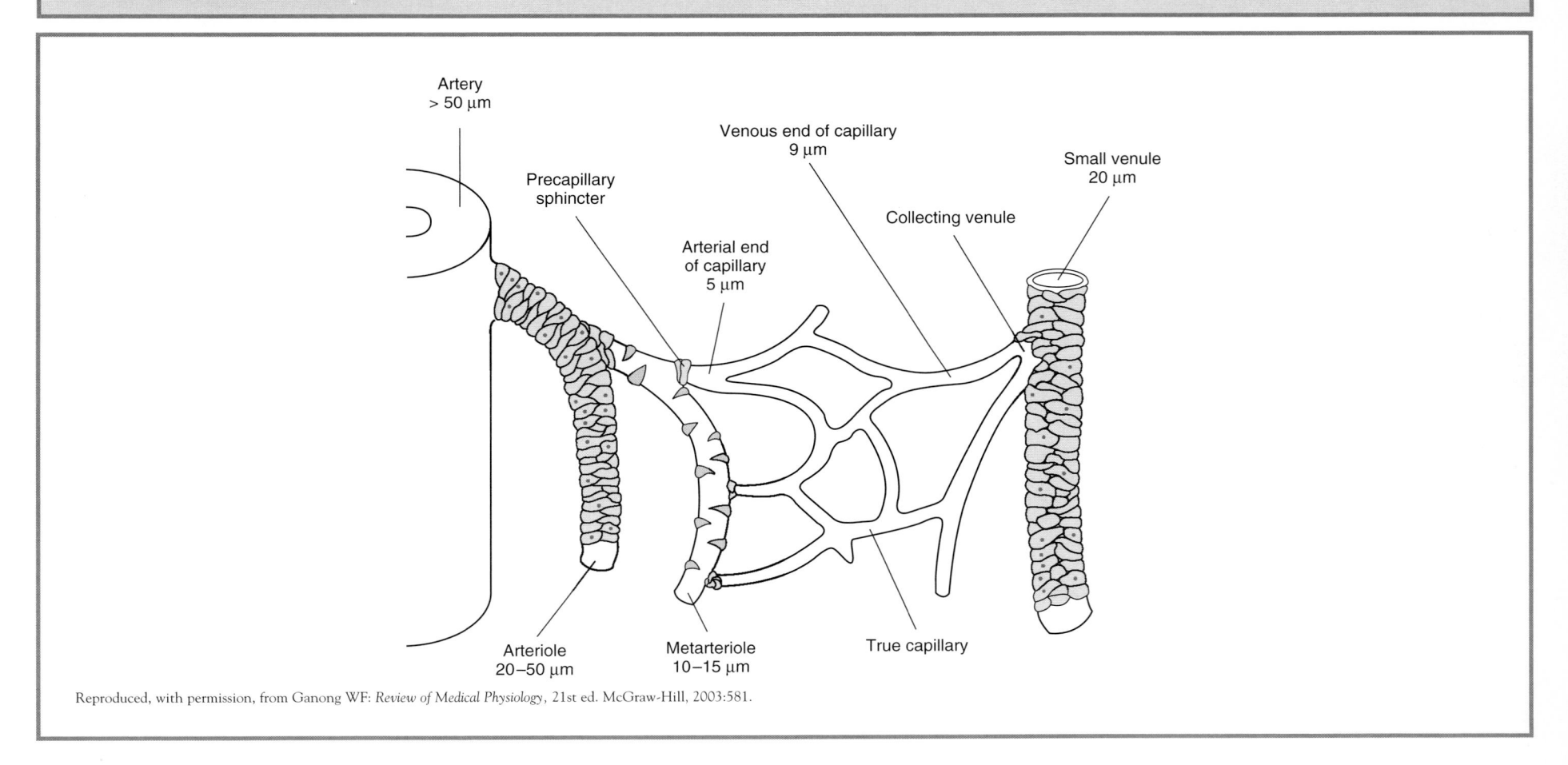

Artery
> 50 µm

Precapillary
sphincter

Venous end of capillary
9 µm

Small venule
20 µm

Collecting venule

Arterial end
of capillary
5 µm

Arteriole
20–50 µm

Metarteriole
10–15 µm

True capillary

Reproduced, with permission, from Ganong WF: *Review of Medical Physiology*, 21st ed. McGraw-Hill, 2003:581.

HEMODYNAMICS

Factors That Influence Blood Flow	Principles	Formula	Clinical Significance
Velocity	• Given rigid tube and incompressible fluid, fluid velocity is inversely proportional to cross-sectional area of tube. • *Larger cross-sectional area means slower flow of fluid.*	$Q = \dot{V} \times A$ • Q = blood flow. • V = fluid velocity. • A = tube cross-sectional area. When cross-sectional area along tube varies: $\dot{V}_1 / \dot{V}_2 = A_2 / A_1$.	• Blood flow is slowest through capillaries, which have greatest cross-sectional area. • This allows time for exchange of materials between tissues and bloodstream.
Pressure	Ohm law: current (or flow) is voltage (or pressure gradient) divided by resistance.	$Q = (P_i - P_o)/R$ • Q = blood flow. • $P_i - P_o$ = difference in pressure between two points in vascular system. • R = resistance to flow.	• Increased arterial pressure causes increase in pressure gradient which increases blood flow. • Increased resistance decreases blood flow. • CO = MAP/SVR.
Hydraulic Resistance	Applying Poiseuille law (see Terms to Learn), resistance to flow depends on length and radius of tube and viscosity of fluid.	$R = 8\eta L/\pi r^4$ • R = resistance to flow. • η = viscosity of fluid. • L = tube length. • r = tube radius.	• *Principal determinant of resistance to blood flow through any individual vessel is its caliber.* • *Major resistance to blood flow in vascular beds is in arterioles.*
Vessel Radius	Law of Laplace: tension in wall of cylinder equals product of its transmural pressure and its radius divided by its wall thickness.	$T = Pr/w$ • T = wall tension of vessel. • P = transmural pressure. • r = vessel radius. • w = thickness of vessel wall.	• Capillaries can withstand high pressure without bursting because of their narrow lumens and thin walls. • Increased wall tension of dilated aortic aneurysm increases its risk of rupturing.

Continued

HEMODYNAMICS (Continued)

Factors That Influence Blood Flow	Principles	Formula	Clinical Significance
Vessel Arrangement	In series: • Total system resistance equals sum of individual resistances. • *Total resistance increases as number of tubes increases.*	$R_{total} = R_1 + R_2 + R_3$ • R = resistance to flow.	Renal and splanchnic vasculature are in series.
	In parallel: • Total resistance of system is less than any of individual resistances. • *Total resistance decreases as number of tubes increases.*	$1/R_{total} = 1/R_1 + 1/R_2 + 1/R_3$ • R = resistance to flow.	Pulmonary and systemic capillaries are in parallel.
Turbulence	More pressure is required to force given fluid through tube when flow is turbulent than when it is laminar.	$N_R = \rho D \dot{V}/\eta$ • N_R = Reynold's number. • ρ = fluid density.	Examples of turbulent flow: Korotkoff sounds heard during auscultation of blood pressure, murmur caused by stenotic cardiac valve, bruit associated with carotid artery stenosis.
Viscosity	• Physical property of fluids that determines internal resistance to shear forces. • *Large diameter tubes, high velocities, and low viscosities predispose to development of turbulence.*	• D = tube diameter. • V = fluid velocity. • η = fluid viscosity. $N_R < 2000$ = laminar flow. $N_R > 3000$ = turbulent flow.	• *Hematocrit is the major factor that changes viscosity of blood.* • Higher hematocrit = greater viscosity = greater resistance to flow.
Shear Stress	Flowing blood creates force on endothelium that is parallel to long axis of vessel and varies directly with viscosity and shear rate.	$\gamma = \eta(dy/dr)$ • γ = shear stress. • η = viscosity. • dy/dr = shear rate.	At slow rates of shear, suspended blood cells tend to aggregate, increasing viscosity and decreasing flow.
Gravity	Gravity gives fluid a weight that generates force, which is proportional to its vertical height.	$P_c = \delta \times h \times g$ • P_c = hydrostatic pressure. • δ = fluid density. • g = gravitational constant.	• Pressure in any vessel below heart level is increased. • Pressure in any vessel above heart level is decreased.

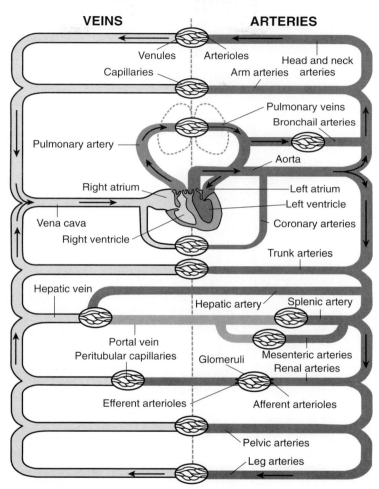

The capillary beds are represented by thin lines connecting the arteries and the veins.

Modified, with permission, from Green HD. In Glasser O, ed. *Medical Physics*, Vol 1, Mosby, 1944.

STARLING HYPOTHESIS

Description	Formula	Important Points
<ul><li>Fluid movement across capillary wall depends on balance between hydrostatic and osmotic forces across capillary endothelium.</li><li>Net filtration occurs when sum of all pressures (Q_f) is positive.</li><li>Net absorption occurs when sum of all pressures (Q_f) is negative.</li></ul>	$$Q_f = k\,[(P_c + \pi_i) - (P_i + \pi_p)]$$ <ul><li>Q_f = fluid movement across capillary wall.</li><li>k = filtration constant for capillary membrane.</li><li>P_c = capillary hydrostatic pressure (tends to pull fluid out of vessels).</li><li>π_i = interstitial fluid oncotic pressure (tends to pull fluid out of vessels).</li><li>P_i = interstitial fluid hydrostatic pressure (tends to pull fluid into vessels).</li><li>π_p = plasma oncotic pressure (tends to pull fluid into vessels).</li></ul>	Capillary hydrostatis pressure (P_c): <ul><li>Principal force in capillary filtration.</li><li>Increased capillary hydrostatic pressure favors movement of fluid out of vessels and into interstitial space.</li><li>($P_c - P_i$) is the driving force for filtration.</li></ul> Interstitial fluid pressure outside the capillaries (P_i): <ul><li>Opposes capillary filtration.</li><li>If no edema is present, $P_i = 0$.</li></ul> Colloid osmotic pressure or oncotic pressure (π_p): <ul><li>Increase in concentration of osmotically active molecules within vessels favors movement of fluid into vessels from interstitial space.</li><li>Albumin is the plasma protein that mainly determines π_p.</li></ul>

DISTURBANCES IN THE BALANCE OF HYDROSTATIC AND OSMOTIC FORCES

Disorder	Mechanism of Disturbance
Burn	• Capillary injury causes increased capillary permeability and capillary hydrostatic pressure. • Large amounts of fluid and protein leak from capillaries into interstitial space. • May lead to severe vascular hypovolemia.
CHF, Pregnancy	Elevated venous pressures enhance filtration beyond capacity of lower extremity lymphatics to remove filtrate, causing lower extremity edema.
Dehydration	• Plasma protein concentration is increased, causing increased plasma oncotic pressure. • This causes H_2O to move from tissues to vascular system.
Hemorrhage	• Low blood pressure decreases capillary hydrostatic pressure. • Decreased blood flow causes arteriolar dilation and relaxation of precapillary sphincters. • This causes absorption to predominate over filtration.
LVF, Mitral Valve Stenosis	Pulmonary capillary hydrostatic pressure greater than plasma oncotic pressure causes pulmonary edema.
Nephrosis	Decreased plasma protein concentration decreases plasma oncotic pressure, causing edema.

HYPERTENSION

Type	Description	Clinical Significance
Essential	• Sustained increase in systemic arterial blood pressure of unknown cause. • Comprises more than 90% of all cases of hypertension. • Heart adapts initially to generalized arteriolar vasoconstriction and increased afterload by increasing diastolic ventricular volume. • May progress to cardiac hypertrophy and LVF	• Possible results of untreated or uncontrolled essential hypertension include atherosclerosis, cerebral hemorrhage, cerebrovascular accident, LVF, MI, and renal damage.
Secondary	• Sustained increase in systemic arterial blood pressure that results from another (primary) disease.	• Examples of associated conditions: primary aldosteronism, Cushing syndrome, pheochromocytoma, coarctation of aorta, chronic renal disease, and chronic treatment with estrogens.
Malignant	• Accelerated phase of chronic hypertension in which necrotic arteriolar lesions develop.	• Rapid downhill course with papilledema, cerebral symptoms, and progressive renal failure. • Fatal in less than 2 years if not treated. • May be reversed with antihypertensive therapy.
Renal	• Hypertension that is result of constriction of renal arterial blood supply or compression of kidney.	• Unilateral: renin production is increased in stenosed kidney and decreased in normal kidney. • Bilateral: renin production is increased in both kidneys. • May lead to renal failure.
Pulmonary	• Sustained increase in blood pressure within (narrowed) pulmonary arteries. • Heart and lungs are otherwise normal.	• Primary: most commonly occurs in females 20–40 years of age. • Without correction, secondary heart failure may occur. • Secondary: occurs associated with atrial septal defect, ventral septal defect, and exposure to high altitudes.

III. The Heart as a Pump

STRUCTURE AND FUNCTION OF THE HEART

Structure	Description	Function
Left and Right Atrium	Thin-walled, low-pressure chambers.	Reservoir and conduit of blood for ipsilateral ventricle.
SA Node	• Located on posterior right atrium, near its junction with superior vena cava. • Specialized cells with *automaticity* initiate each cardiac contraction. • Electrical conduction rate: 0.05 m/s.	• *Cardiac pacemaker.* • Noradrenergic (sympathetic postganglionic) neurons increase pacemaker rate. • Cholinergic (parasympathetic) neurons decrease pacemaker rate via the vagus nerve.
Internodal Tracts	• Specialized muscle fibers between SA and AV nodes • Includes: Bachman (anterior), Wenckebach (middle), and Thorel (posterior).	• Rapidly conduct impulses from SA node to AV node. • If destroyed, conduction proceeds from right to left atrium along ordinary myocardial fibers.
AV Node	Located on subendocardium in posterior right atrium near interatrial septum and ostium of coronary sinus associated with tricuspid valve.	• Along with its continuation, bundle of His, it is *the only functional electrical connection between atria and ventricles*. • AV nodal delay: delay of impulse conduction from atrial to ventricular myocardial cells allows time for ventricles to fill adequately and protects them from excitation at excessive contraction frequencies.
Mitral and Tricuspid Valves	• Also known as AV valves. • Thin flaps of tough, flexible, fibrous tissue covered with endothelium that separate atria from ventricles. • Mitral valve has two cusps and lies between left atrium and left ventricle. • Tricuspid valve has three cusps and lies between right atrium and right ventricle.	• Responsible for unidirectional flow of blood through heart. • Open during ventricular diastole to allow blood to fill ventricles. • Close during ventricular systole to prevent regurgitation of blood from ventricles to atria.

Continued

STRUCTURE AND FUNCTION OF THE HEART (Continued)

Structure	Description	Function
Chordae Tendineae	Fine, strong filaments that arise from papillary muscles and attach to free edges of valves.	Prevent eversion of valves during systole.
Left and Right Ventricles	• Continuum of muscle fibers from base of heart that includes papillary muscles. • Left ventricle has thicker wall than right ventricle. • Electrical conduction rate: 1 m/s.	• Left ventricle pumps blood through systemic circulation. • Right ventricle pumps blood at low pressures through lungs for exchange of O_2 and CO_2.
Aortic Valve	• Also known as semilunar valves. • Three cusps. • Eddy currents that develop in sinus of Valsalva behind each valve keep cusps away from vessel walls. • Orifices of right and left coronary arteries are behind right and left cusps of aortic valve.	• Located between left ventricle and aorta. • Opens during systole, and left ventricle ejects blood into aorta. • Closes during diastole to prevent regurgitation of blood into left ventricle.
Pulmonary Valve		• Located between right ventricle and pulmonary artery. • Opens during systole, and left ventricle ejects blood into pulmonary artery. • Closes during diastole to prevent regurgitation of blood into left ventricle.
Bundle of His	• Continuation of AV node located on subendocardium in right ventricle near interventricular septum. • Electrical conduction rate: 1 m/s. • Splits into right and left bundle branches on either side of interventricular septum. • Left bundle branch divides into anterior and posterior fascicles. • Includes *Purkinje fibers* with electrical conduction rate of 4 m/s.	Conducts electrical impulses from AV node throughout ventricles.

Pericardium	• Epithelialized fibrous sac that invests heart.	• Prevents sudden overdistention of heart chambers.
	• Visceral layer is adherent to epicardium.	• Fluid layer provides lubrication for continuous movement of heart.
	• Parietal layer is separated from visceral layer by thin layer of fluid.	• Progressive, sustained enlargement of heart (hypertrophy) or slow, progressive increase in pericardial fluid (pericardial effusion) can gradually stretch intact pericardium.

ANATOMY OF THE HEART

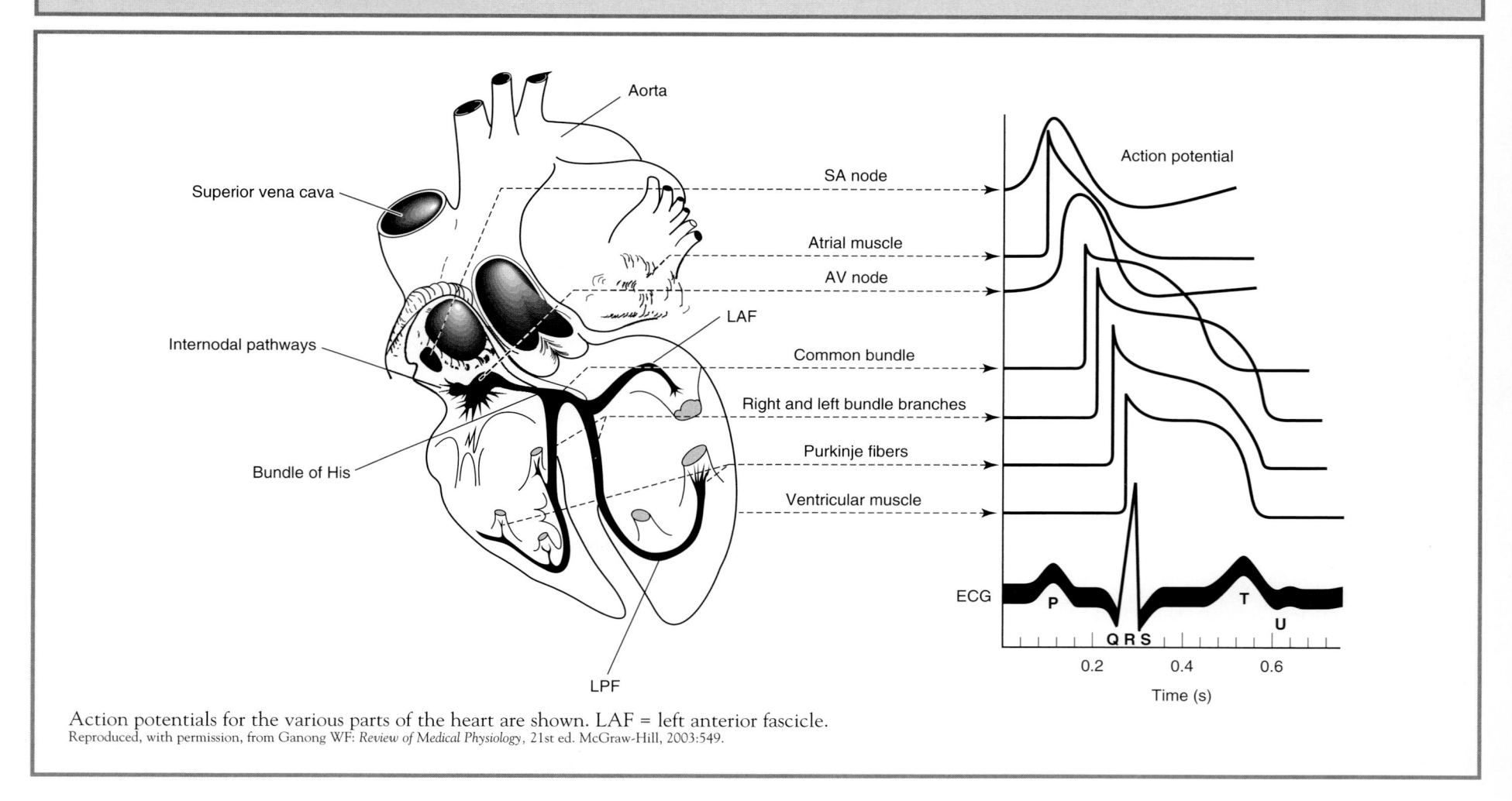

Action potentials for the various parts of the heart are shown. LAF = left anterior fascicle.
Reproduced, with permission, from Ganong WF: *Review of Medical Physiology*, 21st ed. McGraw-Hill, 2003:549.

HEART VOLUMES

Volume	Description	Normal Values
EF	• Ratio of volume of blood ejected from left ventricle per beat. • Declines with ventricular dysfunction. EF = SV/VEDV	60–70%.
RV	• Volume of blood approximately equal to that ejected during systole that remains in ventricles at end of ejection. • RV is constant in normal hearts. • RV is smaller when HR increases or when outflow resistance is reduced. • In heart failure, RV may > SV.	50 mL.
SV	Volume of blood ejected with each beat. SV = VEDV − VESV	75–80 mL.
VEDV	• Volume of blood in ventricles just before onset of ventricular contraction. • Greater VEDV means stronger contraction and larger SV at any one level of contractility. • Increases when filling pressure in atria or central veins increases (higher pressure stretches ventricular walls). • Increases if distensibility of ventricles increases or if HR slows, allowing more time for blood to enter ventricles during diastole.	120–140 mL.
VESV	Volume of blood remaining in ventricle at end of ejection.	40–70 mL (left VESV).

IMPORTANT CARDIAC MEASUREMENTS[1]

Measurement	Description	Normal Value
CI	CO per minute divided by BSA (m^2). CI = CO/BSA	2.5–4 L/min/m^2.
CO	Output of heart over time. CO = SV × HR	4–8 L/min.
CVP	• Pressure in right atrium and thoracic vena cava. • Right ventricular preload.	–2 cm H$_2$O inspiration. +4 cm H$_2$O expiration.
EF	• Ratio of volume of blood ejected from left ventricle per beat. • Declines with ventricular dysfunction. EF = SV/VEDV	60–70%.
MAP	Arterial pressure averaged over time. • MAP = CO × SVR + CVP (or CO × SVR, assuming CVP = 0) • MAP = (SBP + 2DBP)/3	Minimum: 60 mm Hg.
Mean Circulatory Pressure (Static Pressure)	• Equilibrium pressure/highest venous pressure that exists in absence of flow (ie, when CO or venous return = 0). • Reflects total volume of blood and overall compliance of system.	7 mm Hg.
Pulmonary Vascular Resistance	Resistance to blood flow due to pulmonary vasculature. PVR = [(PA – PCWP) × 80]/CI	100–240 dyne/s/cm^5.
Arterial Pulse Pressure	Difference between systolic and diastolic pressures for a given heartbeat. Pulse pressure = SBP – DBP	40 mm Hg (aortic pulse pressure).
SV	Volume of blood ejected with each beat. • SV = CO/HR • SV = VEDV – VESV	40 ± 7 mL/beat/m^2, or 75–80 mL.

SVR	• Also known as total peripheral resistance.	800–1200 dyne/s/cm^5
	• Resistance to blood flow due to systemic vasculature, excluding pulmonary vasculature.	
	SVR = 80[(MAP − CVP)/CO], or 80(MAP/CO) assuming CVP = 0	

[1]BSA = body surface area; CI = cardiac index; DBP = diastolic blood pressure; PA = pulmonary artery pressure; PCWP = pulmonary capillary wedge pressure; SBP = systolic blood pressure.

SUMMARY OF THE CARDIAC CYCLE

Step	Step No.	Mechanism	Important Points
Ventricular Contraction (Systole)			
AV Valve Closure	1	Ventricular contraction causes increased ventricular pressure.	• Normal aortic systolic pressure: 120 mm Hg.
	2	When ventricular pressure exceeds atrial pressure, AV valves close.	• Normal pulmonary artery systolic pressure: 15–18 mm Hg.
Isovolumetric Contraction	3	Closed AV valves isolate ventricles from atria	• Arterial diastolic pressure is the lowest arterial pressure.
	4	Ventricular volume stays constant while ventricular pressure rises.	• *It occurs just before onset of ventricular ejection.*
Ventricular Ejection	5	When ventricular pressure exceeds arterial pressure semilunar valves open.	• Arterial systolic pressure is the peak arterial pressure.
	6	Ejection starts, and arterial volume and pressure begin to increase.	• *It occurs at the end of rapid ejection.*
	7	Rapid ejection: two thirds of stroke volume ejected during first third of systole (ventricular pressure > aortic pressure).	• Right ventricular ejection occurs before left because pressure in pulmonary artery is low compared to that in aorta.
	8	Reduced ejection: one third of stroke volume ejected during last two thirds of systole (ventricular pressure < aortic pressure).	
	9	Ventricles relax.	
Semilunar Valve Closure	10	Closure of aortic and pulmonic valves prevents flow of blood back into ventricles.	*Incisura:* notch on descending limb of aortic pressure curve produced by closure of aortic valve, indicates end of ventricular systole.
Ventricular Relaxation (Diastole)			
Isovolumetric Relaxation	11	Ventricles relax and ventricular pressure rapidly falls without change in ventricular volume.	Systemic arterial pressure declines as blood continues to flow.

AV Valve Opening	12	Rapid filling: high atrial pressure (due to continued venous return during ventricular systole) causes initial rapid passive ventricular filling (80% of blood volume).
	13	Pressure in atria and ventricles decreases and ventricular relaxation continues during rapid filling.
	14	Slow filling or *diastasis*: as blood continues to return to heart, atrial and ventricular pressures slowly rise.
	15	Ventricular filling of blood stops when ventricles reach their volume limit.
	16	Atrial contraction forces blood into ventricles to complete ventricular filling.

- Normal diastolic pressure in aorta: 80 mm Hg.

- Normal diastolic pressure pulmonary artery: 8–10 mm Hg.

- Tachycardia (>180 bpm) results in decreased CO; ventricular filling time is markedly reduced, which lowers VEDV and SV.

- Atrial contraction is not essential for ventricular filling, as evidenced by adequate ventricular filling in patients without atrial contraction (eg, atrial fibrillation or heart block).

- Contribution of atrial contraction to ventricular volume is more important when HR is rapid and duration of diastasis is short (eg, mitral stenosis).

PHASES OF THE CARDIAC CYCLE

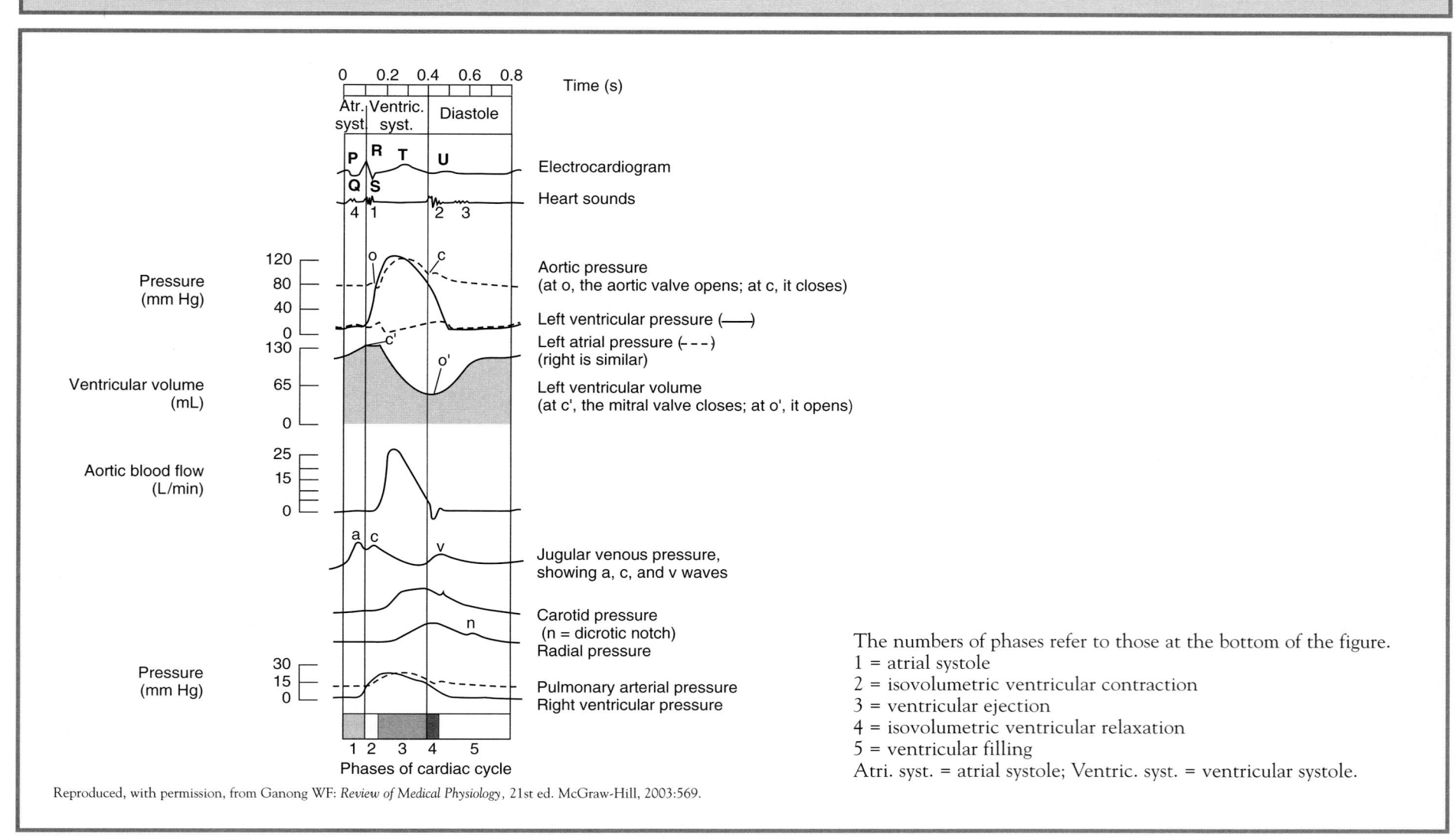

The numbers of phases refer to those at the bottom of the figure.
1 = atrial systole
2 = isovolumetric ventricular contraction
3 = ventricular ejection
4 = isovolumetric ventricular relaxation
5 = ventricular filling
Atri. syst. = atrial systole; Ventric. syst. = ventricular systole.

Reproduced, with permission, from Ganong WF: *Review of Medical Physiology*, 21st ed. McGraw-Hill, 2003:569.

HEART SOUNDS

Sound	Cause of Sound	When Sound is Heard
S_1	Closure of AV valves.	• Just after onset of ventricular contraction. • Signals onset of ventricular systole.
S_2	Closure of semilunar valves.	Signals end of systole and onset of ventricular diastole. • Normal splitting: during inspiration, increased venous return causes prolongation of right ventricular EF and an increased separation between aortic valve closure (A_2) and pulmonic valve closure (P_2). • *Aortic valve closes first* because ejection rate from left ventricle is higher than that from right ventricle. • Paradoxical splitting occurs if splitting of S_2 decreases during inspiration, indicating P_2 precedes A_2. • Delayed aortic valve closure indicates a disease process affecting left ventricle (LBBB, aortic stenosis).
S_3	Rapid, passive ventricular filling.	• At start of ventricular diastole. • Heard best at apex. • Usually not heard in adults but may be heard in children or patients with LVF.
S_4	Forcing of additional blood into distended ventricle.	• Atrial contraction. • Occasionally heard in healthy individuals. • Individuals with CHF have triple sound called gallop rhythm.

ATRIAL PRESSURE CHANGES VIA JUGULAR VENOUS TRACING

Wave	Timing of Wave	Cause of Wave
a	Atrial contraction at end of ventricular diastole.	• Small amount of blood regurgitates into great veins. • Venous inflow stops, causing rise in venous pressure.
c	Isovolumetric contraction.	Rise in atrial pressure produced by bulging of AV valves into atria.
v	Ventricular diastole.	Rise in atrial pressure before AV valves open during diastole.

EFFECTS OF SYSTOLIC AND DIASTOLIC DYSFUNCTION ON PRESSURE-VOLUME RELATIONSHIPS IN THE LEFT VENTRICLE

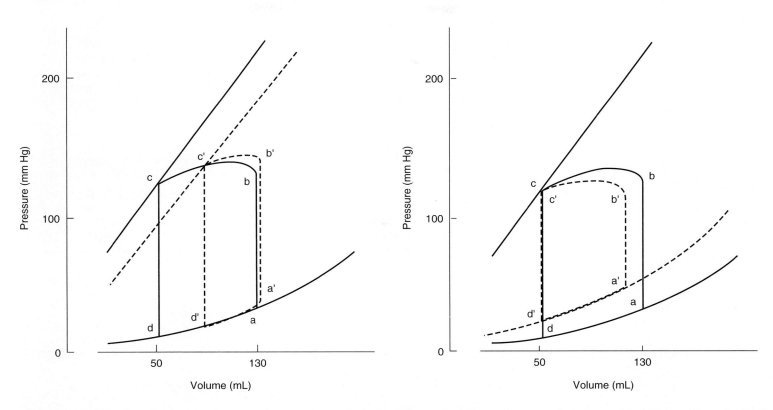

Left: Systolic dysfunction shifts the isovolumic pressure-volume curve to the right. The stroke volume decreases from b-c to b′-c′. **Right:** Diastolic dysfunction shifts the diastolic pressure-volume curve upward and to the left. The stroke volume is reduced from b-c to b′-c′.

Reproduced, with permission, from McPhee SJ, Lingappa VR, Ganong WF [editors]: *Pathophysiology of Disease*, 4th ed. McGraw-Hill, 2003.

VALVULAR LESIONS AND CARDIAC MURMURS

Type of Lesion	Function	Murmur	Possible ECG Changes	Clinical Significance
Aortic Stenosis	Creates high-resistance area that forces left ventricle to generate high pressures to eject blood through narrowed orifice.	Crescendo-decrescendo (diamond-shaped) systolic ejection murmur.	LVH, LBBB.	• Ventricular systolic pressure much higher than systolic pressure in respective artery is pathognomonic. • May lead to LVH and LVF.
Aortic Insufficiency or Regurgitation	Blood flows back into left ventricle during diastole, reducing effective CO.	Diastolic decrescendo, often high-pitched, blowing murmur that begins with A_2	LVH, with narrow, deep Q waves.	• High systolic pressures associated with low diastolic pressures, leading to large pulse pressures (> 100 mm Hg), reflected by water-hammer or Corrigan pulses. • Causes left ventricular dilation, which leads to LVF.
Pulmonary Stenosis	Creates high-resistance area that forces right ventricle to generate high pressures to eject blood through narrowed orifice.	Systolic ejection crescendo-decrescendo murmur, often with harsh quality.	RVH, right atrial abnormality.	• Usually congential, may be acquired with hypertrophic cardiomyopathy. • May lead to RVH and RVF.
Pulmonary Insufficiency or Regurgitation	Blood flows back into right ventricle during diastole, reducing input to lungs.	Diastolic decrescendo, often high-pitched, blowing murmur that begins with pulmonic valve closure (P_2).	RVH.	• Usually associated with pulmonary hypertension. • Causes right ventricular dilation, which leads to RVF.
Mitral Valve Stenosis	Impedes filling of left ventricle, allowing pressure gradient to develop between left atrium and left ventricle during diastole.	• Presystolic or early diastolic crescendo murmur with low-pitched rumble. • Heard on atrial contraction and during rapid passive ventricular filling.	• Left atrial abnormality, atrial fibrillation. • RVH if associated with pulmonary artery hypertension.	May lead to pulmonary edema (high pulmonary venous pressures), left atrial enlargement, or atrial fibrillation.

Mitral Insufficiency or Regurgitation	Allows blood to flow from left atrium to left ventricle during diastole.	Holosystolic murmur of uniform intensity.	Left atrial abnormality, LVH, atrial fibrillation.	• Very high atrial pressures during systole. • Heart chambers dilate to try to compensate for regurgitant blood, which may lead to heart failure.
Mitral Valve Prolapse	May cause regurgitation, allowing blood to flow from left atrium to left ventricle during diastole.	Late systolic murmur, often preceded by nonejection click.	Often normal; may have ST-depression or T-wave changes in inferior leads.	• More common in women. • May be autosomal dominant. • Associated with Marfan syndrome.
Tricuspid Valve Stenosis	Impedes filling of right ventricle, allowing pressure gradient to develop between right atrium and right ventricle during diastole.	• Presystolic or early diastolic crescendo murmur with low-pitched rumble. • Heard on atrial contraction and during rapid passive ventricular filling.	Right atrial abnormality, atrial fibrillation.	• Elevates systemic venous pressure leading to dependent edema. • May produce giant a waves or cannon waves visible as pulsations in distended jugular veins.
Tricuspid Insufficiency or Regurgitation	Allows blood to flow from right atrium to right ventricle during diastole.	Holosystolic murmur of uniform intensity.	• Right atrial abnormality. • Findings related to cause of insufficiency.	• Usually rheumatic etiology. • Caused or simulated by carcinoid syndrome. • Very high atrial pressures during systole. • Heart chambers dilate to try to compensate for regurgitant blood, which may lead to heart failure.

CARDIAC CONTRACTILITY

Concept	Description	Important Points
Preload	• Resistance or pressure increase created during diastole by ventricular filling against which heart must contract in order to eject blood and produce SV. • Initial length of cardiac muscle fibers before contraction, which depends on VEDV. • *Optimum preload*: optimal overlap of thick and thin filaments, at which point systolic pressure is maximum and contraction is strongest.	• Preload increases with: ventricular filling, total blood volume, venous pressure, negative intrathoracic pressure, and CO. • Preload decreases with: increased intrapericardial pressure, decreased ventricular compliance, and standing. • *Diastolic filling beyond optimum preload results in no further increase in developed pressure.*
Afterload	• Resistance or pressure against which ventricles must work to expel cardiac blood. • Created by ventricular ejection during systole as blood is added to aorta faster than it can drain out through capillaries and veins. • Afterload is equal to total peripheral resistance.	• Vessel diameter, elasticity, and mass; tissue mass; and amount of muscle contraction influence afterload. • At constant preload, raising afterload increases systolic pressure until ventricle cannot generate enough force to open aortic valve; ventricular systole then becomes *isometric*, and blood is not ejected.
Positive Inotropy (increased contractility)	• Greater contractile force at constant preload or ventricular volume. • Generation of same force from smaller VEDV. • *Increases SV.* • Increases maximal velocity of muscle fiber shortening, which increases rate of development of ventricular pressure; *velocity of muscle fiber shortening and force developed are inversely related.*	• Sympathetic stimulation increases contractility. • Parasympathetic stimulation decreases contractility. • Anrep effect: increased afterload increases contractility, which helps maintain SV; this is important for increasing CO during exercise. • Increased ventricular volume invokes Frank-Starling law, increasing force of contraction and returning SV toward normal.
Negative Inotropy (decreased contractility)	Decrease in force of contraction at any fiber length or ventricular volume.	• Sympathetic stimulation decreases contractility. • Parasympathetic stimulation increases contractility. • Factors that decrease contractility: cardiac disease, hypoxia, hypercapnia, acidosis, infection, decreased VEDV, and length of cardiac muscle fibers. • Heart failure: damaged heart loses intrinsic inotropy and ability to increase SV, so that CO must be maintained primarily by increasing HR; over time, these compensatory mechanisms also fail.

Frank-Starling Law	• Energy produced by heart when it contracts is proportional to end-diastolic length (initial length) of its muscle fibers.	• Positive inotropy (due to an increase in fiber length or preload) shifts Frank-Starling curve up and to left.
	• End-diastolic length of cardiac muscle fibers is proportional to VEDV or preload.	• Negative inotropy shifts Frank-Starling curve down and to right.
	• Demonstrates relationship between SV and VEDV.	

MYOCARDIAL CONTRACTILITY AND THE FRANK-STARLING CURVE

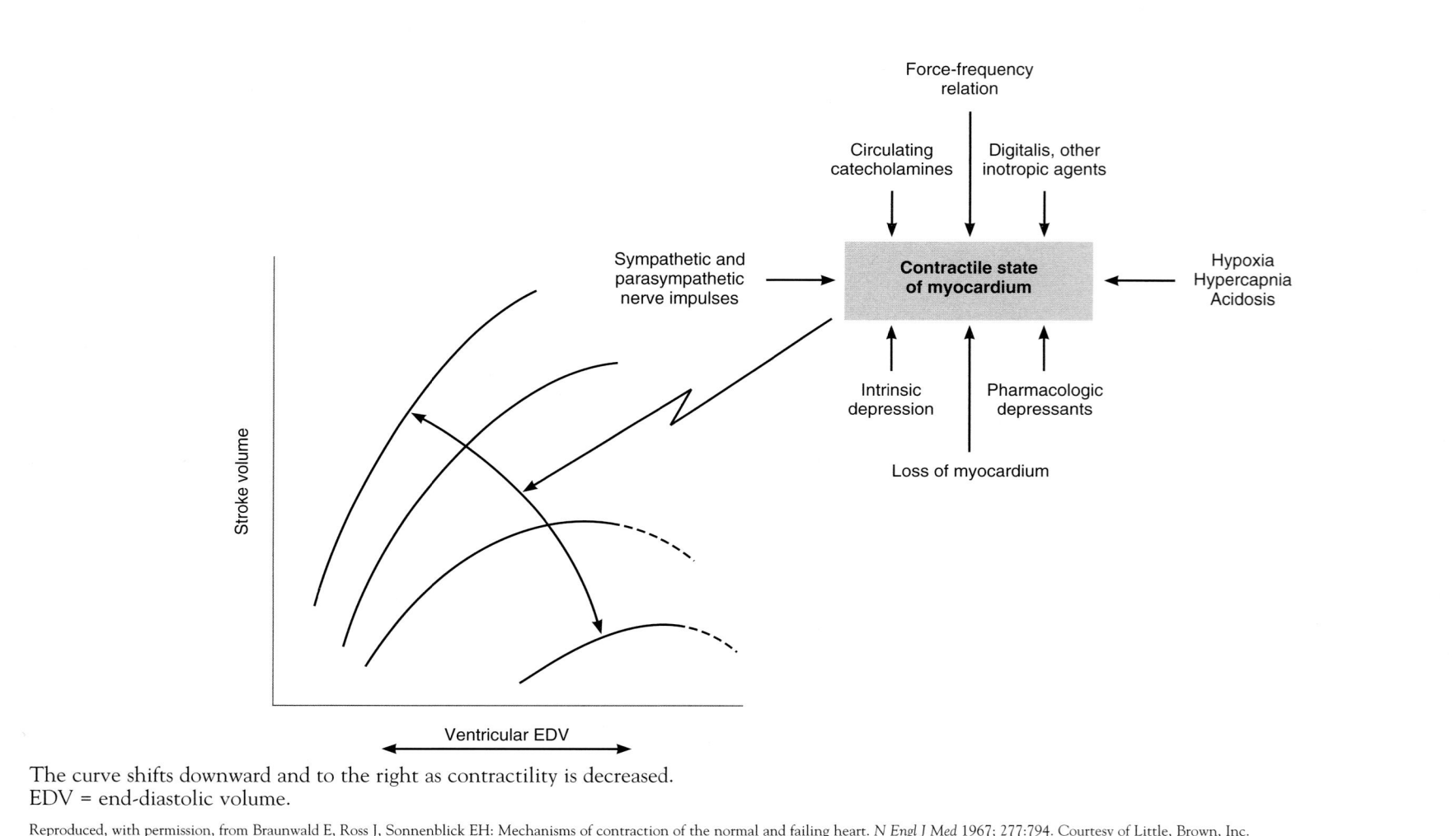

The curve shifts downward and to the right as contractility is decreased.
EDV = end-diastolic volume.

Reproduced, with permission, from Braunwald E, Ross J, Sonnenblick EH: Mechanisms of contraction of the normal and failing heart. *N Engl J Med* 1967; 277:794. Courtesy of Little, Brown, Inc.

SEQUENCE OF EVENTS IN HEART FAILURE

Step No.	Event
1	Damage to heart (eg, chronic hypertension or MI) increases its work load and leads to loss of intrinsic inotropy.
2	• Chronic volume overload, leads to dilation/increased heart volume. • Chronic pressure overload leads to hypertrophy/increased wall thickness.
3	• Dilated, thin-walled ventricle challenged by law of Laplace; fewer myocytes per area to do same amount of work (to increase wall tension in attempt to maintain pressure/force). • This larger ventricle must work harder to generate same SV.
4	• Ability of heart to increase SV is limited. • CO is maintained, primarily increasing HR. • Eventually, compensatory mechanisms fail, and SV, EF, and CO decline.
5[1]	Diastolic dysfunction ("backward failure"): elasticity of ventricle is reduced, hindering cardiac filling during diastole and causing venous congestion.
6[1]	Systolic dysfunction ("forward failure"): ventricular contractions are weakened, and SV, EF, and CO are reduced.
7	• CO is initially insufficient only during exercise. • With disease progression, CO becomes poor at rest as well.
8	Inadequate CO triggers baroreceptor-mediated increases in sympathetic activity.
9	Renal vasoconstriction and activation of renin-angiotensin-aldosterone system occurs, causing Na^+ and H_2O retention (despite increased atrial natriuretic peptide and brain natriuretic peptide).

[1]May occur alternatively.

TYPES OF HEART FAILURE

Type	Description	Signs/Symptoms	Treatment
Right-Sided Heart Failure	Involves mainly right ventricle.	Visceral congestion (liver, spleen, GI tract), peripheral edema, sacral edema, pleural effusion, ascites.	• Treat underlying cause. • Medical therapy: ACE-inhibitors (block angiotensin II), vasodilators (decrease afterload/work of heart), diuretics (reduce fluid overload), positive inotropics (digitalis), nitrates or hydralazine (reduce preload), β-blockers. • Change in lifestyle: low-sodium diet, cessation of tobacco and alcohol, decreased emotional stress.
Left-Sided Heart Failure	Involves mainly left ventricle.	Dyspnea and orthopnea that may progress to pulmonary congestion and edema.	
CHF	• Syndrome in which heart is unable to pump sufficient blood to meet body's O_2 demands. • Passive congestion of organs. • Often starts in left side of heart and progresses to right side of heart.	Fatigue, weakness, dyspnea, orthopnea, pulsus alternans, edema, chronic dry or frothy cough, nocturia, oliguria, palpitations, rapid weight gain, distended neck veins.	
Cor Pulmonale	• Right ventricular enlargement secondary to intrapulmonary disease or pulmonary hypertension. • Most common cause of right ventricular failure.	Same as right ventricular failure.	
High-Output Failure	CO that is inadequate relative to needs of tissue.	Causes: AV shunts, chronic anemia, thiamin deficiency, and thyrotoxicosis.	

IV. Electrical Activity of the Heart

NORMAL ECG WAVES AND COMPLEXES

Waves/Complexes	Cardiac Activity	Important Points
P Wave	Atrial depolarization.	Normally positive (upright) in standard limb leads and inverted in aVR.
QRS Complex	Ventricular depolarization and atrial repolarization from endocardium to epicardium.	Duration (normally 0.06–0.1 s) increased in many cardiac disease states such as ventricular hypertrophy.
		Q wave: negative wave before positive R wave. • Normally absent in V_1 and V_2.
		R wave: positive wave after Q wave. • Possible second positive wave is R′. • rSR′: small, initial R wave; S wave; large, final R wave (eg, RBBB). • If no R wave is present, a completely negative wave is termed QS complex.
		S wave: negative wave following positive R wave.
T Wave	• Ventricular repolarization from epicardium to endocardium. • Midportion of T wave is "vulnerable period" when ventricular myocardium is in various stages of polarization.	• Normally in same direction as QRS complex. • Inverted in many cardiac disease states such as ventricular hypertrophy.
PR Interval	Atrial depolarization and conduction through AV node (includes normal AV conduction delay).	• Measured from onset of P wave to onset of QRS complex. • Duration normally 0.12–0.21 s, depending on HR.
PR Segment	Atrial contraction.	• Isoelectric segment from end of P wave to beginning of QRS complex. • Duration normally 0.1 s.

Continued

NORMAL ECG WAVES AND COMPLEXES (Continued)

Waves/Complexes	Cardiac Activity	Important Points
ST Segment	Ventricular contraction prior to repolarization.	• Isoelectric segment between return of S wave and beginning of T wave. • Elevated or depressed in cardiac ischemia. • Depressed in ventricular hypertrophy.
RR Interval	Duration of cardiac cycle.	• Time between successive QRS complexes. • HR = 60/RR interval in seconds.
QT Interval	Ventricular depolarization plus ventricular repolarization.	• Measured from start of QRS complex to end of T wave. • Duration normally 0.4 s and varies inversely with HR (reflects duration of action potential in ventricular myocardial cells). • Long QT syndrome/torsades de pointes associated with increased incidence of ventricular arrhythmias and sudden death.

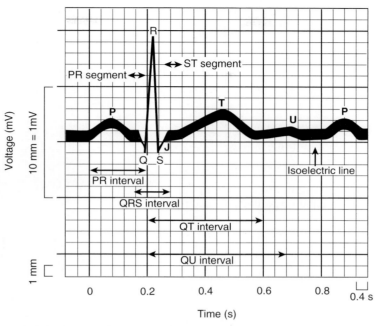

A standard ECG is a recording of electrical activity of the heart. The recording speed is 25 mm/sec, and the amplification is 1 mV (= 1 cm deflection). Each small horizontal division represents 0.04 sec, and each large division 0.2 sec. Each small vertical division represents 0.1 mV.

Reproduced, with permission, from Goldman MJ: *Principles of Clinical Electrocardiography*, 12th ed. Originally published by Appleton & Lange. Copyright © 1986 by The McGraw-Hill Companies, Inc.

ECG LEAD PLACEMENTS AND CORRESPONDING WAVEFORMS

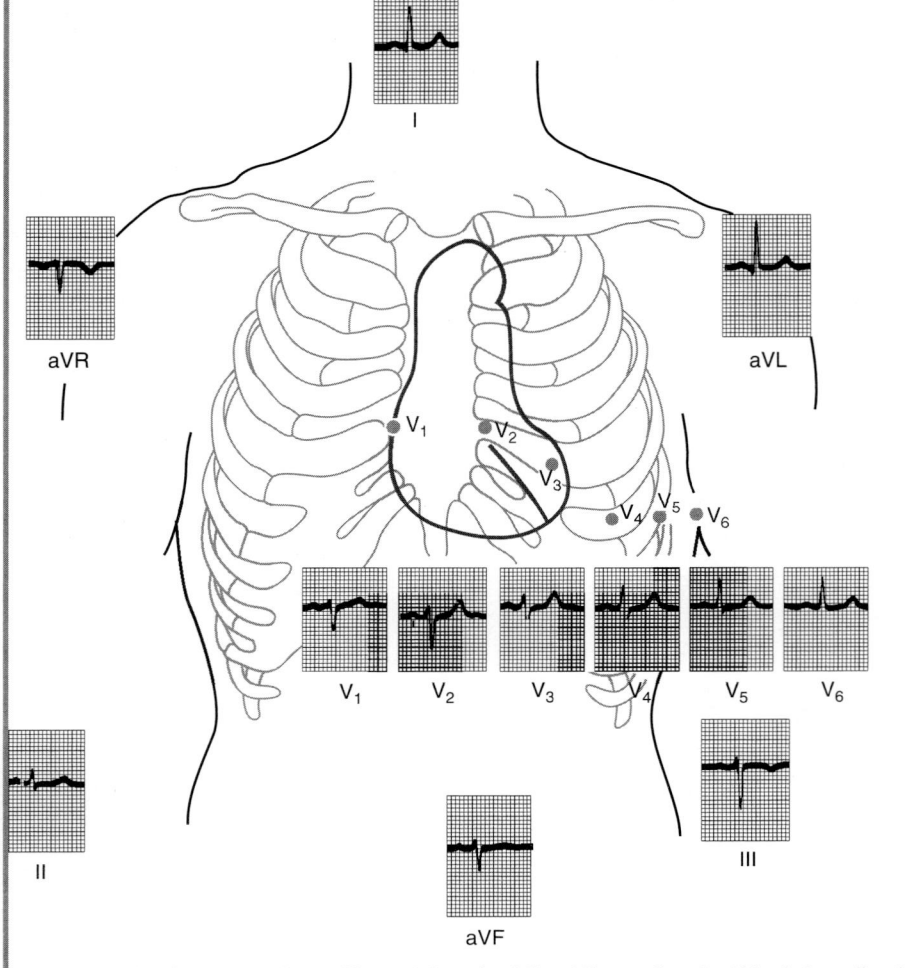

Three bipolar limb leads: measure potential differences between any two of the active limb electrodes.

- Lead I (mV) = (+)LA – (–)RA
- Lead II (mV) = (+)LL – (–)RA
- Lead III (mV) = (+)LL – (–)LA

Six unipolar chest (precordial) leads: measure potential differences as the impulse travels from the right side of the heart to the left side of the heart.

- Right leads: $V_1 – V_3$
- Left leads: $V_4 – V_6$

Three augmented unipolar leads: measure potential differences between one limb and the other two limbs.

- aVR: from right arm; looks at cavities of ventricles (downward deflection)
- aVL: from left arm; looks at ventricles (positive deflection)
- aVF: from left leg; looks at ventricles (positive deflection)

LA = left arm; LL = left leg; RA = right arm.

ECG CHANGES ASSOCIATED WITH ABNORMAL K+ CONCENTRATION

K+ Level	ECG Changes
Hyperkalemia	• Mild hyperkalemia: tall, peaked T waves caused by altered repolarization. • Moderate hyperkalemia: paralysis of atria and prolongation of QRS complexes with disappearance of P waves. • Severe hyperkalemia: may progress to ventricular tachycardia and ventricular fibrillation.
Hypokalemia	• Prolongation of PR interval, prominent U waves, and late T-wave inversion in precordial leads. • If T and U waves merge, apparent QT interval is often prolonged. • If T and U waves are separated, QT interval duration is seen as normal. • Not as rapidly fatal as hyperkalemia.

ECG AXIS DEVIATION

Axis	Description	Causes
Normal	• Between −30° and +90°. • Between 2 and 6 o'clock.	
Right Deviation	• Between +90° and +180°. • To right of +90°. • Between 6 and 9 o'clock.	RVH (eg, secondary to chronic lung disease, pulmonary hypertension, or pulmonary valve stenosis), RBBB.
Left Deviation	• Between −30° and −90°. • To left of −30°. • Between 2 and 12 o'clock.	LVH (eg, secondary to systemic hypertension), LBBB, obesity.
Indeterminate	• Extreme right axis or left axis deviation. • Between −90° and −180°. • Between 9 and 12 o'clock.	• RVH, RBBB. • LVH, LBBB, obesity.

SINUS RHYTHMS

Type of Rhythm	Description	ECG Findings	Clinical Significance
Normal Sinus Rhythm	• HR = 70 bpm at rest. • SA node is pacemaker.	• Each p wave is followed by normal QRS complex. • Normal PR, QT, and RR intervals.	• Electrical system of heart is intact.
Sinus Arrhythmia	• HR is synchronized with respiration. • HR increases during inspiration and decreases during respiration because of reflex inhibition of vagal tone.	• RR interval varies in set pattern. • Remainder of ECG normal.	• Common in healthy individuals.
Sinus Tachycardia	• HR > 100 bpm.	• ECG normal except for increased rate.	• Normal response to physical or emotional stress, fever, hyperthyroidism, and as reflex response to low arterial pressures.
Sinus Bradycardia	• HR < 60 bpm.	• ECG normal except for decreased rate.	• Normally occurs during sleep, commonly seen in endurance athletes, hypothermia, hypothyroidism, inferior MI, or as part of sick sinus syndrome.
Sinus Nodal Reentrant Tachycardia	• HR = 130–140 bpm. • Reentry within sinus node and peri-nodal tissues.	• P waves near normal.	• Accounts for 10% of paroxysmal supraventricular tachycardias. • Vagal activation may slow or stop it. • AV block may occur without affecting tachycardia.

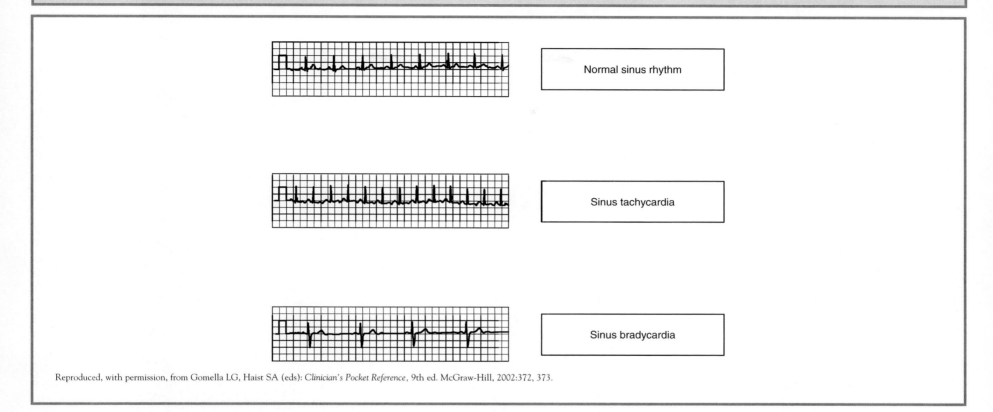

Normal sinus rhythm

Sinus tachycardia

Sinus bradycardia

Reproduced, with permission, from Gomella LG, Haist SA (eds): *Clinician's Pocket Reference*, 9th ed. McGraw-Hill, 2002:372, 373.

ATRIAL RHYTHMS

Type of Rhythm	Description	ECG Findings	Clinical Significance
Atrial Rhythm (atrial arrhythmia)	Generated from ectopic pacemaker.	Abnormal P wave, otherwise normal.	May cause severe ventricular tachycardia and inadequate ventricular filling, resulting in decreased CO and symptoms of heart failure.
Atrial Tachycardia	AV nodal or intra-atrial reentrant activity or automatic atrial ectopic focus causes tachycardia.	• P wave morphology depends on location of ectopic focus. • Irregular rates of 140–220 bpm.	• Associated with overindulgence in caffeine, nicotine, or alcohol, or anxiety attacks. • Stimulating vagal reflex by pressing on eyeball (oculocardiac reflex) or massaging carotid sinus may convert tachycardia and flutter to normal sinus rhythm.
Paroxysmal Atrial Tachycardia	AV nodal (most common) or intra-atrial reentrant activity or automatic atrial ectopic focus causes tachycardia that is associated with some degree of AV block.	• AV nodal reentry: retrograde/inverted P wave buried in QRS and PR < 50% RR interval. • Intra-atrial reentry: positive P wave in II, III, and aVF; PR > 50% RR interval. • Atrial ectopic focus: positive or negative P wave in II, III, and aVF; PR > 50% RR interval.	• May be seen in organic heart disease or in patients taking digitalis. • Other causes: Wolff-Parkinson-White syndrome or sinus node reentry (rare).
Premature Atrial Contractions	• Atrial ectopic site becomes pacemaker for one beat and causes shift in rhythm. • Premature beat discharges SA node, which then repolarizes and fires *after* normal interval.	• Premature P wave, perhaps with abnormal morphology. • Abnormal PR interval.	• Atrial extrasystoles occur normally. • Patient may or may not be aware of occasional irregularity in cardiac rhythm.

| Atrial Flutter | • AV node is unable to transmit all of atrial impulses because of either single ectopic focus or reentry.

• Most commonly, large counterclockwise circus movement in right atrium is present. | • Saw-toothed P waves.

• Atrial rates of 200–350 bpm. | • Paroxysmal and chronic.

• Associated with pulmonary embolism, alcohol, thyrotoxicosis, CAD, and COPD.

• Almost always associated with 2:1 or greater physiologic AV block.

• In adults, AV node cannot conduct more than about 230 bpm (eg, AV block from 4:1 to 3:1 may cause rapid shifts in ventricular rate). |
| Atrial Fibrillation | • Irregular, rapid atrial rate.

• Small portions of atria contract at any one time, while large portions remain refractory (causing irregular, disorganized contractions).

• Ventricular rate is irregularly irregular.

• Only a fraction of atrial impulses that reach AV node are transmitted to ventricles. | • F waves (small, irregular oscillations) at baseline.

• No recognizable P waves.

• RR interval is irregularly irregular.

• Atria beat 300–500 bpm, causing ventricles to beat irregularly at 80–160 bpm. | • Paroxysmal and chronic.

• Associated with pulmonary embolism, alcohol, thyrotoxicosis, CAD, and COPD.

• Associated with AV valve disease that causes enlarged, weak atria and decreased CO.

• Associated with thrombi in atrial appendages, which may be source of pulmonary emboli (right atrium) or systemic emboli (left atrium).

• Therapy includes long-term anticoagulation. |

ECG TRACINGS OF ATRIAL RHYTHMS

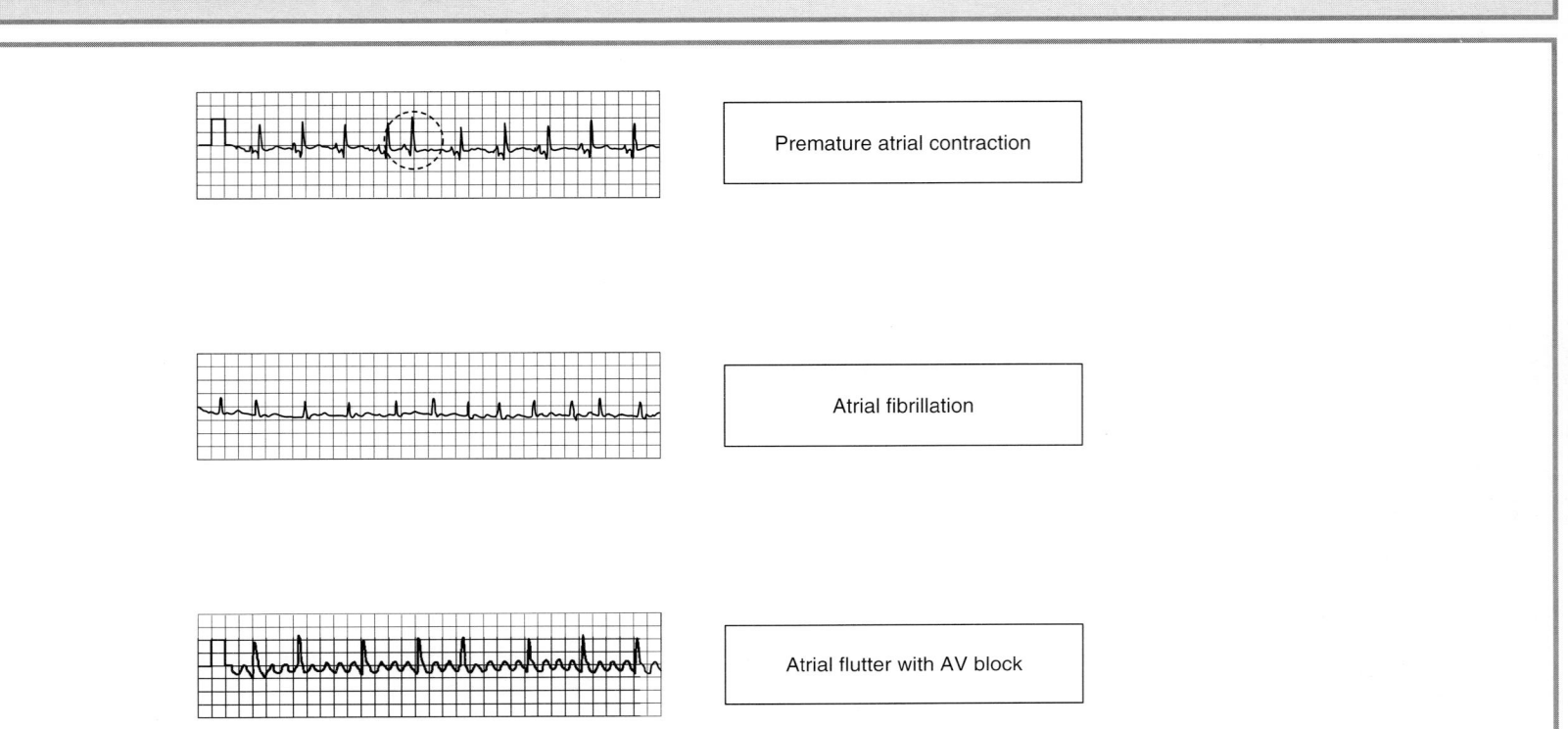

Premature atrial contraction

Atrial fibrillation

Atrial flutter with AV block

Reproduced, with permission, from Gomella LG, Haist SA (eds): *Clinician's Pocket Reference*, 9th ed. McGraw-Hill, 2002:373, 375.

VENTRICULAR RHYTHMS

Type of Rhythm	Description	ECG Findings	Clinical Significance
Paroxysmal Ventricular Tachycardia	• Rapid, regular, repetitive discharge from ectopic ventricular site, usually as result of reentry. • Action potentials travel via slowly conducting ventricular muscle instead of Purkinje fibers, causing prolonged depolarization and asynchrony.	• Wide, bizarre QRS at rapid rate. • P waves are usually indistinguishable, although SA node activity continues independently of ventricles. • Supraventricular tachycardia has His bundle deflection on electrogram, paroxysmal ventricular tachycardia does not.	• Ineffective ventricular contractions result in decreased SV and CO. • Life-threatening if degenerates into ventricular fibrillation. • Associated with CAD, drug toxicity, Swan-Ganz stimulation. • Alterations in vagal tone (carotid sinus massage, Valsalva maneuver) do not affect ventricular tachycardias, because ventricles do not receive any efferent vagal innervation.
Premature Ventricular Contraction	• Premature beats that arise from ventricular myocardium. • Atrial rate is unaltered (no retrograde conduction). • Compensatory pause results in stronger-than-normal beat following premature ventricular contraction. • Does not reset normal rhythm like atrial premature beats. • Does not interrupt regular discharge of SA node.	• Prolonged (> 0.1 s), bizarre QRS with no preceding P wave. • P wave of next normal SA nodal impulse buried in QRS of extrasystole. • T wave usually oppositely directed from QRS. • RR interval of beat preceding premature ventricular contraction and premature ventricular contraction interval together equals two normal cycle lengths.	• May occur in otherwise healthy individuals (usually benign). • Associated with heart disease (ischemia of CAD increases irritability of myocardium), drug toxicity, or Swan-Ganz stimulation. • May produce fibrillation if it occurs during vulnerable period (increases likelihood of reentry).

Continued

VENTRICULAR RHYTHMS (Continued)

Type of Rhythm	Description	ECG Findings	Clinical Significance
Ventricular Fibrillation	• Rapid, irregular, ineffective contractions of small segments of ventricular myocardium. • Due to very rapid discharge of multiple ventricular ectopic foci or circus movement. • Contracting heart looks like "bag of worms."	Undulating waves of varying frequency and amplitude, often precipitated by premature ventricular contractions.	• Absent peripheral pulse. • No CO. • Affected individuals need cardiopulmonary resuscitation. • Most frequent cause of sudden death in patients with MI. • ECG must be used to distinguish ventricular fibrillation from cardiac standstill. • May be caused by electric shock during vulnerable period.
Torsades de Pointes	• Also known as long QT syndrome. • Congenital or acquired ventricular tachyarrhythmia.	• Prolonged QT interval. • Amplitude of QRS complexes vary in a sinusoidal pattern around isoelectric line. • Rate changes from 160 to 280 bpm.	• Associated with antiarrhythmic drugs (quinidine, procainamide, disopyramide, amiodarone); psychoactive drugs (phenothiazine, antidepressants); or K^+ or Mg^{2+} depletion. • Auditory stimuli and physical or psychological stress may provoke arrhythmia. • Patients are at risk for sudden death.

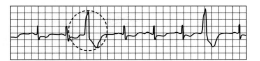

Premature ventricular contraction

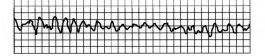

Ventricular tachycardia

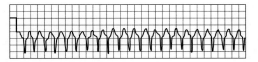

Ventricular fibrillation

Reproduced, with permission, from Gomella LG, Haist SA (eds): *Clinician's Pocket Reference*, 9th ed. McGraw-Hill, 2002:376, 378.

CONDUCTION DISTURBANCES

Type	Description	ECG Findings	Clinical Significance
Blocks at SA Node			
Sinoatrial Exit Block and Sinus Arrest or Pause	Sinus impulse fails to activate atria.	• Sudden, unexpected failure of P wave. • Exit block: sinus impulse generated but not propagated. • Arrest: absent sinus impulse.	• Associated with MI, digitalis toxicity, and degenerative cardiac fibrosis. • Failure of emergence of ectopic pacer causes hemodynamic collapse and syncope. • Symptomatic patient may require pacing.
Sick Sinus Syndrome	• Group of symptoms may include sinus bradycardia, sinus exit block or arrest, and bradycardia-tachycardia syndrome. • Indicates intrinsic defect of SA node. • Often associated with AV nodal abnormalities.	• Alternating atrial flutter and atrial fibrillation with prolonged periods of asystole. • P wave disappears while ectopic pacemaker (usually junctional or ventricular) drives ventricles.	• Seen in elderly and in patients recovering from coronary occlusion. • Symptomatic patients require artificial pacing.

CONDUCTION DISTURBANCES (Continued)

Type	Description	ECG Findings	Clinical Significance
Blocks at AV Node			
First-degree	Conduction disturbance with no effect on ventricles (all atrial impulses reach ventricles).	Slowed conduction through AV node prolongs PR interval beyond 0.21 s.	Associated with increased vagal tone and many systemic diseases.
Second-degree	AV node fails to transmit all atrial impulses. • 2:1–a ventricular beat following every second atrial beat. • 3:1–a ventricular beat following every third atrial beat.	Wenckebach (Mobitz type I): • Progressive lengthening of PR interval until one impulse fails to be transmitted (ventricular beat is dropped). • PR interval after each dropped beat is normal or slightly prolonged. Periodic (Mobitz type II): • Occasional conduction failure. • Resulting atrial-to-ventricular rate is, for example, 6:5 or 8:7. • PR interval is constant. Constant: • Higher degree of block. • Atrial-to-ventricular rate is constant small-number ratio (eg, 2:1 or 3:1).	Associated with organic heart disease.
Third-degree (complete)	• AV node conduction is completely interrupted. • Atria and ventricles beat at independent rates (idioventricular rhythm).	• If pacemaker is remaining nodal tissue, HR is 45 bpm. • If block is infranodal and pacemaker is bundle of His or ventricle, maximal HR is 35 bpm. • May be periods of asystole until an ectopic ventricular focus begins firing.	Associated with organic heart disease, septal MI.

Continued

CONDUCTION DISTURBANCES (Continued)

Type	Description	ECG Findings	Clinical Significance
Bundle Branch Block			
Right	Delayed activation of right ventricle.	• Wide QRS (duration > 0.12 s), large R′, inverted ST interval and T wave (ie, they are opposite to QRS) in V_1 and V_2. • Right axis deviation. • Incomplete RBBB has RR′ but normal duration of QRS (0.08–0.10 s).	• Occurs secondary to chronic heart and pulmonary disease. • May occur acutely as consequence of pulmonary embolism. • Because initial ventricular activation is normal, *acute MI can be diagnosed in presence of RBBB.*
Left	• Changes sequence of left ventricular depolarization cause delayed activation of left ventricle. • Includes left fascicular block or hemiblock, left anterior-superior fascicular block, and left posterior-inferior fascicular block. • Bifascicular = RBBB + left anterior or left posterior block.	• Wide QRS (duration > 0.12 s), large R′ with slur or notch between RR′ in V_5 and V_6. • Inverted ST interval and T wave (ie, they are opposite to QRS). • All types of LBBB have left axis deviation except left posterior-inferior fascicular block, which has right axis deviation.	• Rare in absence of organic heart disease. • Because initial ventricular activation is abnormal, *cannot diagnose acute MI in presence of LBBB.* • Left anterior-superior fascicular block is more common than posterior-inferior fascicular block. • Posterior-inferior fascicular block is usually associated with RBBB.
Wolff-Parkinson-White Syndrome			
	• Aberrant conduction pathway (bundle of Kent) between atria and ventricles that parallels normal AV junction structures. • *Normal delay between atrial and ventricular activation is decreased or eliminated.* • Reentrant rhythm.	• Shortened PR interval, usually less than 0.1 s. • Widened QRS complex with slurred initial upstroke (delta wave or PJ interval).	• Aberrant pathway predisposes to premature atrial tachycardia because of reentry phenomenon. • Fast conduction causes decreased ventricular filling and CO. • Adenosine and Ca^{2+} blockers suppress conduction through AV node, but do not effect bypass tract; surgical ablation can destroy it.

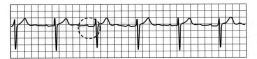

First-degree AV block

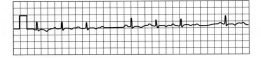

Second-degree AV block,
Mobitz type I (Wenckebach)

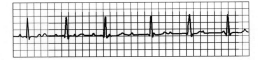

Third-degree AV block,
(complete heart block)

Reproduced, with permission, from Gomella LG, Haist SA (eds): *Clinician's Pocket Reference*, 9th ed. McGraw-Hill, 2002:379, 380.

ECG TRACINGS OF BUNDLE BRANCH BLOCK

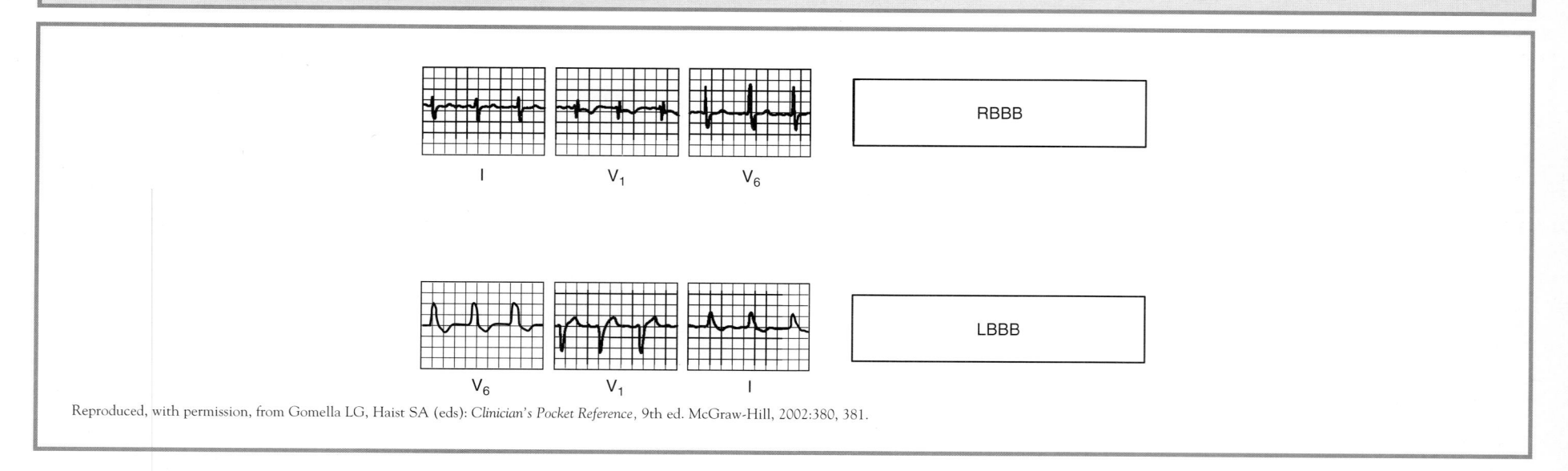

Reproduced, with permission, from Gomella LG, Haist SA (eds): *Clinician's Pocket Reference*, 9th ed. McGraw-Hill, 2002:380, 381.

V. Cardiovascular Regulation

> ## EFFECTS OF LOCAL AND HORMONAL FACTORS ON CARDIOVASCULAR REGULATION

Factor	Effect
Local Factors	
Adenosine	Constricts systemic vasculature.
Carbon Dioxide	Systemic increases in Pa_{CO_2} stimulate sympathetic nervous system, which increases HR, cardiac contractility, and CO; this compensates for direct depressant effect of increased Pa_{CO_2} on heart.
Endothelin-1	Relaxes vascular smooth muscle via cGMP and aids in angiogenesis.
Histamine	Dilates myocardial vasculature.
Lactate	Increases capillary permeability.
Nitric Oxide (endothelium-derived relaxing factor) and Prostacyclin	• Dilate systemic vasculature and inhibit platelet aggregation. • Aspirin shifts production balance between thromboxane A_2 and prostacyclin in favor of prostacyclin. • Prolonged aspirin administration reduces clot formation and helps prevent MI and stroke.
Oxygen	• Moderate degrees of hypoxia stimulate sympathetic nervous system, which increases HR, cardiac contractility, and CO. • Severe degrees of hypoxia depress cardiovascular system.
pH, Osmolality, Heat Produced by Increased Metabolism	Decreased pH, increased osmolality, and increased heat dilate systemic vasculature.
Serotonin and Vessel Injury	Constrict systemic vasculature and have positive inotropic and chronotropic effects.
Thromboxane A_2	Constricts systemic vasculature and promotes platelet aggregation.

Continued

EFFECTS OF LOCAL AND HORMONAL FACTORS ON CARDIOVASCULAR REGULATION (Continued)

Factor	Effect
Hormonal Factors	
Angiotensin II	Constricts systemic vasculature and causes fluid retention, resulting in elevated blood pressure.
Atrial Natriuretic Peptide	Constricts systemic vasculature.
Epinephrine	Constricts systemic vasculature.
Glucagon	Positive chronotropic effect.
Insulin	Dilates systemic vasculature.
Kinins (eg, bradykinin) and Substance P	Dilate systemic vasculature, natriuresis.
Norepinephrine	Constricts systemic vasculature and stimulates aldosterone.
Vasoactive Intestinal Polypeptide	Constricts vasculature in skeletal muscles and liver.
Vasopressin	Constricts systemic vasculature and increases systemic vascular resistance.

NERVOUS REGULATION OF THE CARDIOVASCULAR SYSTEM

Location	Mechanism	Function
Heart	Parasympathetic cholinergic (vagal) stimulation via muscarinic receptors.	• Decreases HR via bilateral innervation. • Right vagus nerve predominantly affects SA node by decreasing firing rate (maintains HR of about 70 bpm). • Left vagus nerve predominantly affects AV node by slowing conduction velocity, prolonging refractory periods, and promoting AV block. • Overly strong vagal stimulation may cause sinus arrest and lead to asystole; activation of ectopic pacemaker or vagal escape allows recovery. • *In healthy, resting people, inhibitory parasympathetic effects predominate over facilitatory sympathetic effect.*
	Sympathetic noradrenergic stimulation via β_1-receptors.	• Increases HR at SA node (positive chronotropic effect). • Increases conduction rate and impulse transmission at AV node. • Increases force of contraction (positive inotropic effect). • Increases automaticity of ectopic sites. • Inhibits tonic vagal stimulation.
Resistance Vessels		• Tonic vasoconstriction, which regulates tissue blood flow and arterial pressure. • Increased vasoconstriction lowers blood flow and raises arterial pressure.
Venous Capacitance Vessels		• Varies volume of blood stored in veins. • Increased venoconstriction increases stored blood and accompanies rises in blood pressure.
Resistance Vessels of Skeletal Muscles	Sympathetic cholinergic stimulation.	Vasodilation which increases blood flow to contracting muscle, resulting in decreased muscle O_2 consumption.
Heart	Ventricular sensory receptor stimulation.	Decreases HR and peripheral vascular resistance.

NERVOUS REGULATION OF THE CARDIOVASCULAR SYSTEM (Continued)

Location	Mechanism	Function
Lungs	Pulmonary stretch receptors via vagal afferents.	Inflation of lungs or decreased intrathoracic pressure causes vasodilation, decreased blood pressure, and reflex increase in HR.
Carotid Sinus and Aortic Arch	Baroreceptor and chemoreceptor stimulation.	• Bradycardia, decreased blood pressure, decreased CO, and vasodilation in response to increased blood pressure. • Main effect is to increase rate and depth of respiration with secondary vagal inhibition and increased HR in response to decreased blood pressure. • Primary reflex of vagal stimulation and decreased HR occurs in absence of respiratory response.

REFLEX MECHANISMS OF THE CARDIOVASCULAR SYSTEM

Reflex	Location	Effect
Somatosympathetic	Resistance vessels.	• Pressor response to somatic afferent nerve stimulation. • Pain and exercising muscles cause increased arterial pressure.
Baroreceptor	Buffer nerves (cranial nerves IX and X) in carotid sinus and aortic arch.	• Increased arterial blood pressure increases discharge from baroreceptor nerve fibers, causing bradycardia, decreased blood pressure, decreased CO, and vasodilation. • Decreased blood pressure has opposite effect.
	• Type A receptors discharge in atrial systole. • Type B receptors discharge late in diastole.	Increased venous return increases discharge from atrial baroreceptor nerve fibers, causing decreased blood pressure, vasodilation, and increased HR.
Bainbridge	Heart.	• Rapid infusion of blood or saline produces increase in HR if initial HR is low. • Competes with baroreceptor-mediated decrease in HR produced by volume expansion.
Bezold-Jarisch (Coronary Chemoreflex)	Heart.	In experimental animals, injection of serotonin, capsaicin, and related drugs into coronary arteries supplying left ventricle (not atria or right ventricle) causes apnea followed by rapid breathing, hypotension, and bradycardia.
Pulmonary Chemoreflex	Pulmonary artery.	Injection of serotonin, capsaicin, and related drugs into pulmonary artery produces apnea followed by rapid breathing, hypotension, and bradycardia.
Cushing	Sympathetic nervous system.	• Increased intracranial pressure causes systemic vasoconstriction and increased systemic arterial pressure (vasomotor area stimulated by local hypoxia and hypercapnia caused by decreased blood supply). • Higher blood pressure causes reflex decrease in HR via arterial baroreceptors. • Helps maintain cerebral blood flow in presence of high intracranial pressure.

PATHWAY OF BARORECEPTOR REFLEX

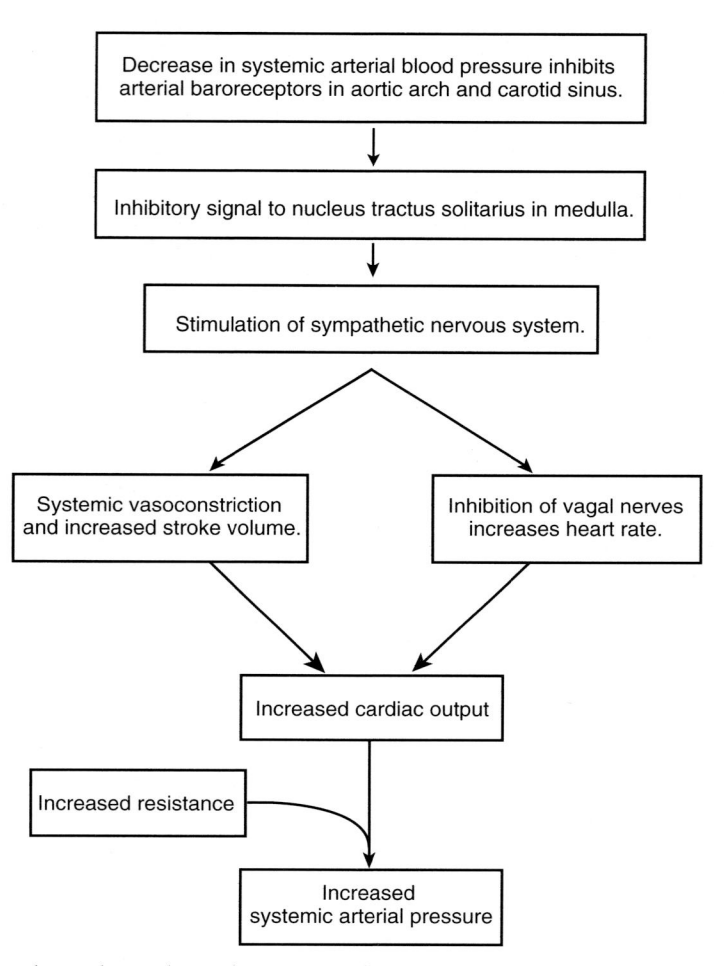

The baroreceptor reflex, a negative feedback loop, plays a key role in short-term adjustments to blood pressure and HR. It responds to abrupt changes in CO, blood volume and pressure, and peripheral resistance. For example, it operates during exercise or when moving from a sitting to a standing position to maintain cardiovascular stability.

CARDIOVASCULAR RESPONSE TO STRESS: EXERCISE

Change Due to Exercise	Body's Response	Effect
Activation of sympathetic nervous system.	Increased HR and contractility.	• Increased CO, SV, and venous return. • Increased blood flow to brain, heart, and active skeletal muscle.
	Peripheral vasoconstriction and increased peripheral resistance (eg, inactive muscle, viscera, and skin).	Maintenance of blood pressure.
Increased CO and arterial pressure.	Stimulation of baroreceptor reflex.	• Compensatory vasodilatation. • Decreased blood pressure and HR.
Activation of muscle reflexes.	Vasoactive metabolites accumulate in active muscles.	• Dilation of resistance vessels causing up to 30-fold increase in blood flow. • Decreased SVR decreases afterload, enabling heart to pump more effectively. • Vessel compression by skeletal and respiratory muscles aids in venous return to heart.
Increased blood flow to muscles.	Increased capillary recruitment.	Increased exchange of water, gases, and solutes with net movement into active muscle and increased lymph flow.
• High concentrations of CO_2 and lactic acid. • Increased temperature of contracting muscle.	• Right shift in O_2-dissociation curve. • Affinity of hemoglobin for O_2 decreases.	• More effective removal of O_2 from blood. • Partial pressures of arterial O_2 and CO_2 remain normal.
Vascular pressure changes.	Systolic pressure increases more than diastolic pressure.	• Increased pulse pressure. • Balance of increased CO and decreased SVR results in only small increase in mean blood pressure.

CARDIOVASCULAR RESPONSE TO STRESS: SHOCK

Type of Shock	Cause	Selected Signs and Symptoms	Subtypes	Compensatory Responses	Important Points
Hypovolemic	Low blood volume.	Diaphoresis, hypotension, tachycardia, agitation that may progress to coma.	• Septic. • Hemorrhagic. • Dehydration.	• Vasopressin and stimulation of renin-angiotensin-aldosterone and sympathetic nervous systems help maintain arterial pressure. • Decreased capillary pressure helps maintain blood volume. • Chemoreceptor stimulation activates respiratory system, which assists in venous return and promotes vasoconstriction.	• Compensated shock: compensatory mechanisms are able to maintain blood pressure. • Decompensated shock: compensatory mechanisms fail, and blood pressure falls. • Acute respiratory distress syndrome (ARDS) is possible late complication of shock that can be fatal. • Incidence of cardiogenic shock in patients with MI is 10%. • Obstructive shock caused by extracardiac mechanical obstruction to cardiovascular flow (eg, pulmonary embolism, cardiac tamponade, tension pneumothorax); not same as cardiogenic shock.
Cardiogenic	Reduced CO (eg, from severe CHF, MI, arrhythmias, other cardiomyopathy).	Same as those of hypovolemic shock, plus pulmonary, visceral, and extremity congestion.	None		
Vasogenic	Excessive vasodilation due to neural reflexes (eg, nervous system trauma); toxic substances (eg, drug overdose); or endocrine failure.	Loss of consciousness.	• Neurogenic. • Anaphylactic.		

VI. Circulation in Special Regions

ORGANIZATION OF SPECIAL CIRCULATIONS

Vessels	Coronary	Cerebral	Splanchnic
Arteries	• Coronary arteries receive 5% of CO *during diastole*. • Hemoglobin releases 50% of its arterial O_2 content to myocardium and 25% to rest of body. • Major coronary arteries travel in epicardium and send penetrating branches to myocardium, where they form arcades. • Coronary arteries are end arteries, but anastomoses can become functional in presence of occlusion. • Right coronary artery predominates in 50% of persons.	• Brain receives 20% of CO. • Two carotid arteries form circle of Willis. • Two vertebral arteries form basilar artery. • Circulations of each carotid artery stay separate.	Splanchnic organs receive 30% of CO via celiac, superior and inferior mesenteric arteries. Intestines: • Series of parallel circulations that include branches of superior and inferior mesenteric arteries and extensive system of anastomoses. • Blood flow to mucosa is greater than that to remainder of intestinal wall. Liver: • Receives 15% of CO. • Largest reservoir for blood in splanchnic circulation (25–30% of liver volume is blood). • Blood flow in venous and hepatic arterial systems varies reciprocally, with decreased flow in one prompting increased flow in other.
Veins	• Coronary sinus drains left ventricle. • Anterior coronary veins drain right ventricle. • Right coronary-luminal vessels carry larger portion of blood than left coronary-luminal vessels.	• Venous drainage is primarily via internal jugular vein. • Blood-brain barrier helps maintain constancy of neuron environment.	• Blood from intestines, pancreas, and spleen drains via hepatic portal vein. • Hepatic portal vein and hepatic artery converge on sinusoids in liver, which drain as follows: central lobular veins → hepatic vein → inferior vena cava.

REGULATION OF SPECIAL CIRCULATIONS

Type of Regulation	Coronary	Cerebral	Splanchnic
Autoregulation	With stable metabolic rate, blood flow remains relatively constant despite fluctuations in coronary perfusion pressure.	• Works for arterial pressures 80–180 mm Hg. • Blood pressure < 80 mm Hg causes decreased cerebral blood flow and syncope (reactive hyperemia.) • Blood pressure > 180 mm Hg causes increased permeability of blood-brain barrier, leading to cerebral edema.	• Hepatic arterial system has ability to autoregulate. • Portal venous system does not autoregulate, so with any increase in blood flow or pressure, resistance remains same or decreases.
Neural	• Sympathetic stimulation increases myocardial metabolic activity, which leads to dilation of coronary vessels and increased coronary blood flow. • Central vagal stimulation also causes vasodilation of coronary vessels.	• Increased neural activity in one area is associated with increased blood flow in that area (total cerebral blood flow remains constant). • Ischemia and increased intracranial pressure stimulates vagal outflow (causing bradycardia and decreased respiration) and Cushing reflex.	• Sympathetic α-receptor stimulation constricts mesenteric arterioles and capacitance vessels. • Sympathetic β-receptor stimulation causes vasodilation. • In liver, sympathetic via α-receptor stimulation constricts presinusoidal resistance vessels in portal venous and hepatic systems.
Local and Metabolic	• Increased metabolic activity decreases coronary resistance and increases coronary blood flow. • Hypoxia stimulates release of vasodilators (adenosine, CO_2, H^+, K^+, lactate, nitric oxide, prostaglandins), provokes reactive hyperemia, and O_2 supply is increased.	• *[CO_2] is major controller of cerebral blood flow.* • Decreased $PaCO_2$ (hyperventilation) causes cerebral vasoconstriction and decreased blood flow. • Cerebral circulation stops when intracranial pressure is greater than arterial pressure.	• Functional hyperemia: food ingestion and absorption increases intestinal blood flow. • Gastrin and cholecystokinin increase intestinal blood flow.

FETAL CIRCULATION

Structure	Pathway of Blood Flow
Atria	• Inferior vena cava to right atrium. • Most blood flows through foramen ovale to left atrium, and remainder flows through right ventricle. • Crista dividens divides output from right atrium. • Left atrium receives deoxygenated blood from lungs via pulmonary vein. • Well-oxygenated blood flow: left atrium → left ventricle → ascending aorta → head, heart, and upper body.
Ventricles	• *Two ventricles function in parallel due to presence of foramen ovale and ductus arteriosus.* • Right ventricle receives deoxygenated blood from heart and upper body via superior vena cava. • Poorly oxygenated blood flow: right ventricle → pulmonary artery → ductus arteriosus → aorta → lower body and viscera. • Small amount of blood flow from right ventricle goes to lungs.
Aorta	• From aorta, 50% of blood flows through umbilical artery to placenta for reoxygenation. • 50% flows to lower body and viscera.
Lungs	High resistance in collapsed fetal lungs and pulmonary arterial pressure that is higher than pressure in aorta discourage pulmonary blood flow.
Liver	• 50% of O_2-rich blood from placenta to umbilical vein flows through portal system to inferior vena cava. • 50% flows through ductus venosus to inferior vena cava. • Inferior vena cava also receives poorly oxygenated blood from lower body.

CHANGES IN FETAL CIRCULATION AFTER BIRTH

Major Change	Step No.	Effect
Closure of Umbilical Vessels	1	SVR and pressure in left atrium and ventricles increase.
	2	*Ductus venosus closes*, forcing all blood entering liver to pass through hepatic sinusoids, which causes immediate drop in blood pressure and flow in inferior vena cava and right atrium.
	3	Asphyxia and cooling of body activate respiratory center.
Lung Aeration	4	Pulmonary vascular resistance decreases, which causes increased blood flow through pulmonary system and left atrium.
	5	Pressure in left atrium rises above that in right atrium, forcing foramen ovale to close.
	6	Flow through ductus arteriosus reverses: flow of venous blood is now right-to-left and oxygenation of systemic arterial blood is improved.
High PaO_2 of Arterial Blood	7	*Ductus arteriosus constricts.*
	8	Aerated lungs release bradykinin which aids in complete closure (may take up to 2 days).
	9	"Heart murmur of newborn" may be heard due to turbulent blood flow through partially open ductus arteriosus.
		(Prostaglandin E_1 production in premature infants keeps ductus arteriosus open; indomethacin helps it close.)

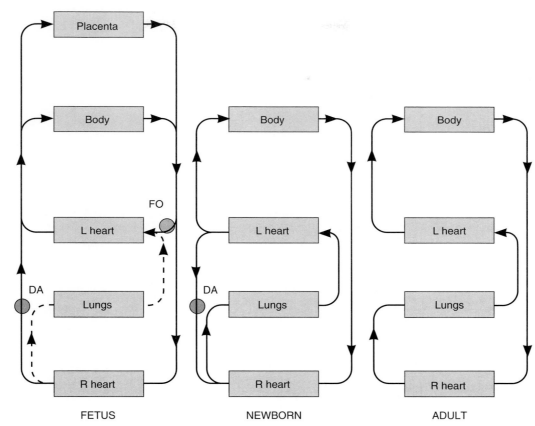

FETUS   NEWBORN   ADULT

DA = ductus arteriosus; FO = foramen ovale.

Modified, with permission, from Born GVR et al: Changes in the heart and lungs at birth. *Cold Spring Harbor Symp Quant Biol* 1954;19:102.

CHAPTER 4
RESPIRATORY SYSTEM

ABBREVIATIONS

ARDS = adult respiratory distress syndrome

COPD = chronic obstructive pulmonary disease

ERV = expiratory reserve volume

DPG = 2,3-diphosphoglycerate

FEV$_1$ = forced expiratory volume in 1 second

FEV$_{1\%}$ = ratio of FEV$_1$ to FVC

FIO$_2$ = fractional concentration of oxygen in inspired gas

FRC = functional residual capacity

FVC = forced vital capacity

Hgb = hemoglobin

IC = inspiratory capacity

IRV = inspiratory reserve volume

NO = nitric oxide

P$_{50}$ = oxygen tension that produces 50% saturation of hemoglobin with oxygen

PA = alveolar pressure

PBS = pressure at body surface

PCW = transthoracic pressure

PL = transpulmonary pressure

PRS = transrespiratory pressure

PaCO$_2$ = arterial CO$_2$ tension

PaO$_2$ = arterial O$_2$ tension

PACO$_2$ = alveolar CO$_2$ tension

PAO$_2$ = alveolar O$_2$ tension

PCO$_2$ = partial pressure of CO$_2$

PEEP = positive end-expiratory pressure

PO$_2$ = partial pressure of O$_2$

PPL = interpleural pressure

RBC = red blood cell

RV = residual volume

TLC = total lung capacity

TV = tidal volume

VA = alveolar dead space

$\dot{V}$A = alveolar ventilation

VC = vital capacity

$\dot{V}$D = dead space ventilation

V/Q = ventilation-perfusion (ratio)

VD = anatomic dead space

VDS = physiologic dead space

$\dot{V}$D = minute ventilation

TERMS TO LEARN

Acclimatization	Increased altitude tolerance over a period of time.
Atelectasis	Failure of part of the lung to expand due to collapsed alveoli.
Compliance	Distensibility; change in volume of a structure for each unit change in pressure ($C = \Delta V/\Delta P$); indicates how easily a structure can be stretched or inflated.
Cyanotic Congenital Heart Disease	Congenital anatomic abnormality (eg, interatrial septal defect) creates a right-to-left shunt, allowing large amounts of unoxygenated venous blood to bypass pulmonary capillaries and dilute oxygenated blood in systemic arteries; this leads to low O_2 saturation of hemoglobin.
DPG (2,3-Diphosphoglycerate)	Organic phosphate that predominates in RBCs and decreases O_2 affinity of Hgb; [DPG] falls with low pH and rises in anemia, chronic hypoxemia, and at high altitudes.
Elastance	Retractive (recoil) force generated by the distention of a structure; inversely related to compliance.
Expiration (Exhalation)	*Passive breathing of air out of lungs via elastic recoil of lungs and chest wall*; recoil generated by inspiratory lung expansion. During stress, when inspiration is increased, active contraction of expiratory muscles is required.
Hypoxemia	Presence in blood of an abnormally low concentration of O_2.
Inspiration (Inhalation)	Negative pressure breathing; an active breathing of air into lungs produced by contraction of muscles of inspiration.
Mixed Venous Hemoglobin Saturation	O_2 level in pulmonary venous blood; mixed venous O_2 tension (PVO_2) = 40 mm Hg when whole body Hgb saturation is 75%.
Obstructive Airway Disease	Processes that *impair expiration*, leading to trapping of air in lungs and overinflation; thoracic cage may become *barrel-shaped*, and *diaphragm may flatten*. Examples include asthma, chronic bronchitis, and emphysema.
Partial Pressure (of a Gas)	Pressure exerted by any one gas in a mixture of gases; equals fraction of that gas multiplied by total pressure. For example, PO_2 is 760 mm Hg (atmospheric pressure) $\times$ 0.21 (% of O_2 in dry air) = 160 mm Hg.
PEEP (Positive End-Expiratory Pressure)	Pressure often applied at end of expiration to keep alveoli open and improve oxygenation in mechanical ventilation.
Respiratory Exchange Ratio	Ratio of O_2 consumption to CO_2 production at any given time; at steady state, this ratio equals 0.8; 80 molecules of CO_2 are exhaled for every 100 molecules of O_2 taken up from alveoli into pulmonary capillary blood.

Respiratory Quotient	Ratio of CO_2 production to O_2 consumption; at equilibrium, this quotient varies depending on fuel. For example, it is 0.7 for lipids, 1.0 for carbohydrates, and 0.85 for amino acids.
Restrictive Airway Disease	Diseases involving processes that *impair inspiration* → underinflation (eg, pneumonia, pulmonary fibrosis, congestive heart failure); decreased lung volume and compliance and decreased chest wall compliance. Elevated abdominal pressure interferes with descent of diaphragm.
Surfactant	Complex substance *produced by type II alveolar cells* that lines alveolar surface and has multiple functions. It *decreases surface tension, increasing lung compliance* and decreasing work of respiration; increases alveolar radius, reducing transmural pressure required to maintain alveolar inflation (per Law of Laplace); reduces pulmonary capillary filtration, preventing pulmonary edema; *promotes alveolar stability*; and *prevents alveolar collapse (atelectasis) at end-expiration*.
Venous Admixture	Venous blood that returns to lungs without passing air-filled alveoli and mixes with oxygenated blood from the lung, decreasing systemic PaO_2 (eg, normal fetal circulation, anatomic and physiologic shunts [V/Q mismatch]); venous admixture from < 1% of cardiac output is normal.

I. Introduction

PULMONARY DISEASE

Disorder	Description	Signs/Symptoms	Treatment	Important Points
Asthma (COPD)	Reversible airway obstruction (inflammation, bronchoconstriction, mucus plugging) in response to extrinsic or intrinsic stimuli (eg, allergens, exercise, cold air, aspirin).	Coughing, wheezing, shortness of breath.	Bronchodilators and corticosteroids.	• Findings include normal lung compliance, increased FRC, and prolonged expiratory phase. • Hyperinflation: flattened, inefficient diaphragm.
ARDS	• Response to severe insult to lung tissue. • Early exudative and later fibroproliferative stage.	Respiratory failure	Mechanical ventilation.	• Mortality is 20–30%. • In survivors, permanent lung injury can result.
Cystic Fibrosis (COPD)	• Congenital recessive disorder involving chromosome 7. • Cl⁻ channels are abnormal. • Airway mucus thick and inspissated, leading to obstruction.	• Delayed passage of meconium (due to ileus) in newborns. • Cough and frequent lung infections. • In sweat glands, defective transport of Na^+ and Cl^-, leading to high sweat content of these electrolytes.	• Chest physical therapy, bronchodilator. • Antibiotics to treat frequent lung infections. • Avoid β-blockers.	• Chronic pancreatitis occurs in both sexes (abnormal function of pancreatic ducts). • Men also have inspissated secretions in sperm ducts, which may obstruct passage of spermatozoa, leading to infertility.
Emphysema (COPD)	Long-term destruction of alveoli cause: • Increased physiologic dead space. • Loss of lung elasticity and increased compliance. • Air trapping and hyperinflation.	• Cough, increased work of breathing, and hypoxia. • May lead to hypercapnia and respiratory failure.	• May require corticosteroids and bronchodilators. • Antibiotics treat frequent lung infections.	• Affected individuals develop barrel chest and flattened diaphragm. • Most common cause is heavy smoking. • 2% cases are due to congenital deficiency of active α_1-antitrypsin.

Pulmonary Edema	Left-sided heart failure causes fluid to back up into pulmonary tissue.	Shortness of breath, orthopnea, decreased breath sounds, rales.	Diuretics.	Patients have feeling of suffocation.
Pulmonary Hypertension	• Sustained elevation in pulmonary artery pressure that may lead to right-sided heart failure. • Etiology is unknown or secondary to COPD or other pulmonary disease, inhalation of cocaine, or appetite suppressant drugs (dexfenfluramine).	Progression from mild to severe shortness of breath with eventual hypoxemia.	• Treat COPD and systemic hypertension. • Prostacyclin causes vasodilation and vascular remodeling.	Resection of > 60% of total lung mass may lead to pulmonary hypertension.

SELECTED GAS LAWS

Law	Explanation	Equation
Boyle Law	• For ideal gas, there is indirect relationship between pressure and volume, if temperature and amount remain constant. • If volume of structure containing constant number of gas molecules is increased, pressure will decrease. • If volume of structure containing constant number of gas molecules is decreased, pressure will increase.	$P_1V_1 = P_2V_2$ • P = pressure of ideal gas. • V = volume of ideal gas.
Charles Law	• For ideal gas, there is direct relationship between volume and absolute temperature, if pressure and amount remain constant. • If volume of structure containing constant number of gas molecules is increased, temperature will increase. • If volume of structure containing constant number of gas molecules is decreased, temperature will decrease.	$V_1T_2 = V_2T_1$ • V = volume of ideal gas. • T = temperature of ideal gas.
Dalton Law	Total pressure of a gas mixture equals sum of partial pressures of all gases present.	$P_{total} = P_1 + P_2 + P_3 + \ldots + P_N$ • P = pressure. • N = total number of gases in mixture.
Fick Law of Diffusion	• Large surface area and small distance between alveolar gas and pulmonary capillary blood normally allow rapid equilibration. • Pulmonary edema or increased thickness of interstitium increases diffusion distance and slows diffusion.	$V_{O_2} = D_{O_2}A(P_{AO_2} - P_{VO_2})/\Delta X$ • V_{O_2} = volumetric rate of O_2 transfer. • A = area for exchange. • D_{O_2} = diffusion coefficient for O_2. • ΔX = length of diffusion pathway.

☞ Remember the names of the gas laws in alphabetical order and key words in reverse alphabetical order:

Boyle's	Volume
Charles's	Temperature
Dalton's	Partial pressure
Fick's	Diffusion

II. Mechanics of Breathing and Gas Exchange

LUNG VOLUMES AND CAPACITIES

Lung Volumes/Capacities	Definition/Equation	Normal Value (L)
TV	Volume of gas inspired or expired with each breath during normal quiet breathing.	0.5
IRV	Additional volume that can be inspired above TV.	3.
ERV	Volume of gas that can be forcefully expired after normal expiration.	1.0.
RV	Volume of gas that remains in lungs after maximal expiration.	1–1.2 (air left in lungs after maximal expiratory effort).
TLC	• Volume of gas in lungs after maximal inspiration. • TLC = TV + IRV + ERV + RV.	5–6.
VC	Maximal volume of gas that can be expired after maximal inspiration.	4–5.
IC	• Maximal volume that can be inspired after normal expiration. • IC = TV + IRV.	3.5.
FRC	• Volume of gas that remains in lungs at end of normal expiration that allows oxygenation of blood between breaths. • FRC = RV + ERV.	1.8–2.2 (40% of maximal lung volume).

LUNG VOLUMES AND RELATED MEASUREMENTS

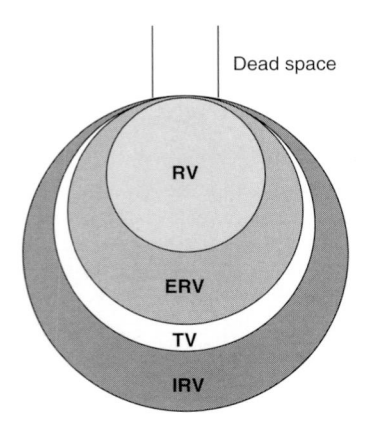

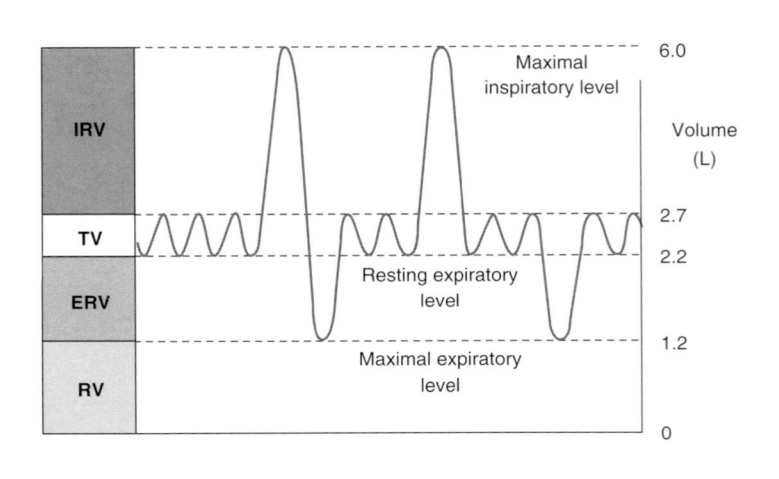

		Volume (L)		
		Men	Women	
Vital capacity	IRV	3.3	1.9	Inspiratory capacity
	TV	0.5	0.5	
	ERV	1.0	0.7	Functional residual capacity
	RV	1.2	1.1	
Total lung capacity		6.0	4.2	

Respiratory minute volume (rest): 6 L/min

Alveolar ventilation (rest): 4.2 L/min

Maximal voluntary ventilation (BTPS): 125–170 L/min

Timed vital capacity: 83% of total in 1 s; 97% in 3 s

Work of quiet breathing: 0.5 kg-m/min

Maximal work of breathing: 10 kg-m/breath

IRV, inspiratory reserve volume, TV, tidal volume; ERV, expiratory reserve volume; RV, residual volume.

Modified, with permission, from Ganong WF: *Review of Medical Physiology*, 21st ed. McGraw-Hill, 2003:655.

LUNG VENTILATION

Feature	Description	Normal Values and Formulas
Types of Dead Space		
Anatomic Dead Space (V_D)	• Volume of inspired air that does not participate in gas exchange. • In healthy people, V_D equals total dead space (ie, anatomic dead space = physiologic dead space.	• 0.15 L (2 mL/kg of body weight). • $V_D = V_{DS} - V_A$
Alveolar Dead Space (V_A)	• Volume of gas in an alveolus that is ventilated but not perfused. • In healthy people, there is no alveolar dead space.	• $V_A = V_{DS} - V_D$.
Physiologic Dead Space (V_{DS})	• Volume of gas not equilibrating with blood. • Wasted ventilation. • Increase in physiologic dead space lowers P_{CO_2} in mixed expired gas.	• Usually 30% of V_T. • $V_{DS} = V_D + V_A$.
Types of Ventilation		
Minute Ventilation ($\dot{V}_E$)	• Volume of air inspired or expired per minute. • *Always > $\dot{V}_A$.* • *$\dot{V}_E$ increases linearly with V_T until half of VC is reached.* • Higher levels of ventilation then occur by increases in respiratory frequency with little change in V_T (inefficient breathing that results in more wasted ventilation).	• 6 L/min. • $\dot{V}_E = V_T \times f.$[1]
Alveolar Ventilation ($\dot{V}_A$)	• Volume of air that enters and leaves alveoli each minute. • Always < $\dot{V}_E$.	• 4.2 L/min. • $\dot{V}_A = (V_T - V_D) \times f.$[1] • $\dot{V}_A = (\dot{V}_E - \dot{V}_D)$.
Dead Space Ventilation ($\dot{V}_D$)	Part of $\dot{V}_E$ that fails to reach area of lungs involved in gas exchange.	• 2.25 L/min. • $\dot{V}_D = V_D \times f.$[1] • $\dot{V}_D = \dot{V}_E - \dot{V}_A$.

Continued

LUNG VENTILATION (Continued)

Feature	Description	Normal Values and Formulas
Alveolar Tension		
Alveolar O_2 Tension (P_{AO_2})	• Inspired O_2 is continually removed from alveoli by diffusion into pulmonary capillary blood.	• 100 mm Hg.
	• Alveolar gas equation shows P_{ACO_2} affected by P_{ACO_2}, fraction of inspired O_2, and barometric pressure.	• $P_{AO_2} = P_{IO_2} - P_{ACO_2}/R + [(P_{ACO_2})(F_{IO_2})(1 - R/R)]$.
Alveolar CO_2 Tension (P_{ACO_2})	• Alveolar and arterial P_{CO_2} are essentially equal because of high diffusibility of CO_2; O_2 has no direct effect.	• 40 mm Hg. • $P_{ACO_2} = (\dot{V}_{CO_2} \times K)/\dot{V}_A$
	• *Alveolar ventilation equation shows P_{ACO_2} controls alveolar ventilation;* when ventilation increases, P_{ACO_2} decreases; when ventilation decreases, P_{ACO_2} increases.	• $\dot{V}_{CO_2}$ = rate of CO_2 production. • K = constant.

[1] f = frequency, or number of breaths per minute.

SELECTED STRUCTURES THAT AFFECT LUNG FUNCTION

Structure	Description	Function	Clinical Significance
Alveolus	Blind-ended air sac at termination of air passage.	• Exchange of O_2 and CO_2. • *Type II alveolar epithelial cells secrete surfactant.*	*Surfactant aids in decreasing alveolar surface tension, preventing collapse of alveoli and increasing lung compliance.*
Visceral Pleura	External lining of lung.		
Pleural Space	Space between visceral and parietal pleura that contains pleural fluid.	Pleural fluid acts as lubricant and aids in adherence between visceral and parietal pleural membranes.	• Intrapleural pressure is subatmospheric. • If chest wall is opened (eg, pneumothorax), lungs collapse. • If lungs lose their elasticity, chest expands and becomes barrel-shaped.
Parietal Pleura	Internal lining of thoracic cavity.		
Diaphragm	• Dome-shaped sheet of muscle that separates thoracic and abdominal cavities. • Innervated by phrenic nerves (C3–C5).	• Inspiratory muscle. • Contraction causes dome to descend, lifting ribs and expanding volume of thoracic cavity.	• Transection of spinal cord above C3 is fatal without artificial respiration. • Injury below C5 allows quadriplegics to continue to breathe independently (using diaphragm for inspiration and passive expiration).
External Intercostal Muscles	Outermost muscles between ribs.	• Inspiratory muscles. • Contraction causes dome to descend, lifting ribs and expanding volume of thoracic cavity.	Used in normal, passive breathing.
Accessory Muscles of Breathing	• Neck muscles (eg, sternocleidomastoids, scalenes). • Activated when inspiratory airflow is limited or respiratory demand is increased (eg, respiratory failure, exercise).	• Inspiratory muscles. • Contraction lifts clavicles and sternum, elevating ribs and expanding thoracic cavity.	• Used when breathing is voluntary (stress, exercise). • Their use results in increased respiratory rate and increased (negative) pleural pressure.

Continued

SELECTED STRUCTURES THAT AFFECT LUNG FUNCTION (Continued)

Structure	Description	Function	Clinical Significance
Rectus Abdominus	Muscle originating from lower ribs posteriorly that inserts on upper ribs anteriorly.	• Expiratory muscle. • Contraction lowers ribs and compresses abdominal contents, lifting diaphragm and decreasing volume of thoracic cavity.	• Expiration is normally a passive process resulting from elastic recoil of lungs and chest wall. • Expiratory muscles are used when breathing is active and voluntary (eg, stress, exercise), resulting in increased respiratory rate and increased (negative) pleural pressure. • Muscle contraction produces an expiratory force that compresses respiratory gas and increases alveolar pressure, aiding expiration.
Internal Intercostal Muscles	Muscles between ribs, underneath external intercostals.	• Expiratory muscles. • Contraction lowers ribs and decreases thoracic volume.	

Pathway of air movement: nasal passages → pharynx → trachea → bronchi → bronchioles → terminal bronchioles → respiratory bronchioles → alveolar ducts → alveoli.

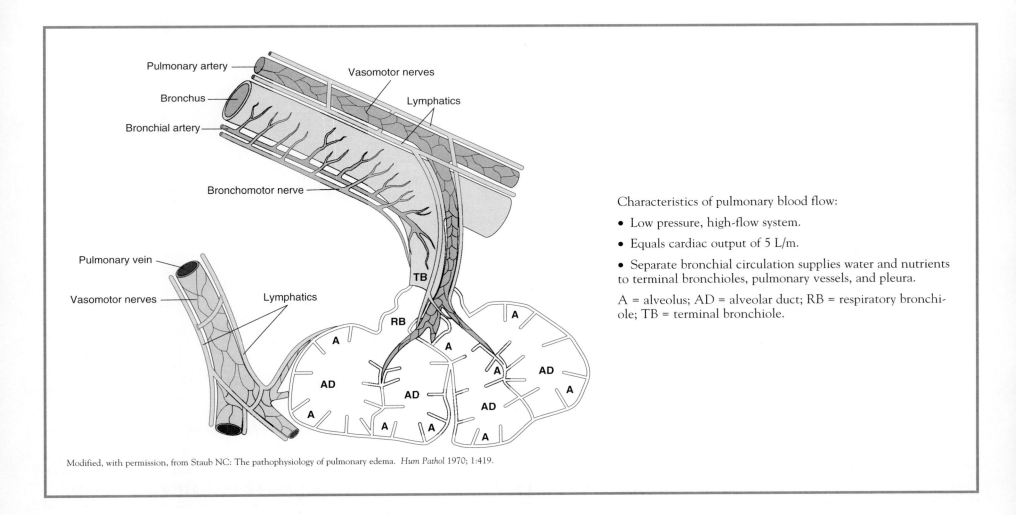

Characteristics of pulmonary blood flow:

- Low pressure, high-flow system.
- Equals cardiac output of 5 L/m.
- Separate bronchial circulation supplies water and nutrients to terminal bronchioles, pulmonary vessels, and pleura.

A = alveolus; AD = alveolar duct; RB = respiratory bronchiole; TB = terminal bronchiole.

Modified, with permission, from Staub NC: The pathophysiology of pulmonary edema. *Hum Pathol* 1970; 1:419.

RESPIRATORY DEFENSE

Factors	Defense Function
Respiratory Passages	Humidify and cool or warm inspired air so it is close to body temperature when it reaches alveoli.
Nostril Hair	• Prevents larger (>10 µm) foreign matter from reaching alveoli. • Particles 2–10 µm in size initiate reflex bronchoconstriction and coughing.
Bronchial Secretions	Contain secretory immunoglobulins (IgA) and other substances that help resist infections and maintain integrity of mucosa.
Epithelia	• Epithelia of paranasal sinuses make bacteriostatic NO. • Pulmonary epithelia release prostaglandin E_2.
Cilia	• Keep foreign matter away from lungs. (Particles < 2 µm reach alveoli and are ingested by macrophages.) • Located in epithelia from anterior third of nose to beginning of respiratory bronchioles.
Pulmonary Alveolar Macrophages	• Ingest inhaled bacteria and small particles. • Help process inhaled antigens for immunologic attack. • Secrete substances that attract granulocytes to lungs. • Cause release of lysosomal enzymes and inflammation when stimulated by irritants (eg, cigarette smoke, silica, asbestos).

FACTORS AFFECTING PULMONARY TRANSMURAL PRESSURES

Pressure	Description/Equation	Clinical Significance
Transmural pressure is driving force that determines airflow.		
Alveolar (PA)	• Transairway pressure. • Pressure gradient between alveoli and atmosphere, which is responsible for rate of gas flow into or out of lungs.	• Because PA is negative during inspiration and positive during expiration, direction of gas flow reverses. • When PA is 0 (atmospheric pressure), gas flow is 0. • When pressure difference between alveoli and atmosphere is greatest, rate of gas flow is highest.
Interpleural (PPL)	• Inspiratory force of chest wall increases lung volume and opposes elastic recoil force of distended lungs. • Opposing forces are equal but in opposite directions, generating a negative interpleural pressure.	• With relaxed respiratory muscles and open airways, PPL = −5 cm H_2O, and lungs have 2–2.5 L of gas. • Can be estimated by measuring intrathoracic esophageal pressure (relaxed esophagus).
	During inspiration, lung volume increases, PPL becomes progressively more negative.	Change in PPL from start to end of inspiration is used to calculate dynamic lung compliance.
	During expiration, PPL returns to resting level.	PPL can become positive with forced expiration.
Transpulmonary (PL)	• Transmural pressure across lungs. • PL = PA − PPL.	• Determines lung volume. • Pulmonary equilibrium volume < 10% of maximum lung volume.
Transthoracic (PCW)	• Transmural pressure across chest wall. • PCW = PPL − PBS. • PBS = pressure at body surface (normally atmospheric pressure).	• Equilibrium volume of chest wall is 80% of maximum. • At lung volumes less than chest wall equilibrium, PCW is negative (PPL< PBS) as chest wall is trying to reach equilibrium.
Transrespiratory (PRS)	• Transmural pressure across entire respiratory system. • PRS = PA − PBS.	• Relaxation pressure curve equals sigmoid-shaped curve of respiratory system pressure versus volume. • Results from summation of elastic properties of lungs and chest wall (PRS = PL + PCW).

FACTORS AFFECTING PULMONARY COMPLIANCE

Factor	Description/Equation	Clinical Significance
Lung Compliance	$\Delta V_L/\Delta P_L$ • Normal = 0.2 L/cm H_2O at FRC.	• *Restrictive lung disease* (tuberculosis, silicosis) produced by scarring or fibrosis of lungs and/or destruction of functional lung tissue *causes decreased compliance*. • *Emphysema and aging* are both associated with loss of alveoli and decreased retractive forces in lungs, *causing increased compliance*. • Preservation of alveolar tissue in asthma allows lung compliance to be closer to normal.
Specific Compliance	• Compliance adjusted for volume: $\Delta V/\Delta P \times V$. • Measures absolute distensibility of a structure.	After pneumonectomy, lung volume and compliance are decreased by one half while specific compliance stays same.
Alveolar Surface Tension	Elastance force attributed to Law of Laplace ($P_L = 2T/r$) that *increases tendency of lungs to deflate*. • T = tension. • r = radius.	• Surfactant decreases surface tension in lungs. • In respiratory distress syndrome of premature infants, key defect is failure of type II alveolar epithelial cells to secrete adequate amount of surfactant. • Inflation of lungs requires increased work. • Alveoli collapse during deflation because surface tension does not decrease, leading to respiratory fatigue and failure. • Treat with exogenous surfactant and PEEP .
	Low surface tension is important to maintain alveolar stability as lung volume decreases toward FRC.	Recoil forces of air-filled lungs exceed those of fluid-filled lungs.

FACTORS AFFECTING PULMONARY RESISTANCE

Factor	Description	Clinical Significance
Airway Resistance	• Determined by rate of gas flow (velocity of gas molecules multiplied by cross-sectional area) and diameter of airways. • *Highest resistance to flow is in intermediate-sized bronchi.*	• From trachea to alveolar ducts, total cross-sectional area of airways progressively increases. • Velocity of airflow decreases rapidly. • In trachea and main bronchi, airflow is turbulent (noisy). • In small airways, airflow is laminar and silent.
	• *Airway radius is most important determinant of resistance (Poiseuille law).* • *Smaller airway means higher resistance for any flow rate.*	• COPD (emphysema, asthma, bronchitis) narrows small airways, leading to high airway resistance. • Patients with COPD must generate higher inspiratory and expiratory pressures.
Neural Control of Airway Diameter	*Sympathetic stimulation by circulating adrenergic substances (epinephrine, isoproterenol) leads to bronchodilation via β_2-receptors (decreased airway resistance).*	β-blockers are contraindicated in asthma.
	Vagal (cholinergic) stimulation leads to bronchoconstriction and increased mucous formation (increased airway resistance).	• Cholinergic activity is major component of asthma. • Systemic or nebulized anticholinergics may block this effect.
	Noncholinergic excitatory mediators (substance P, neurokinins) cause bronchoconstriction, mucous secretion, and increased vascular permeability.	These compounds are involved in pathogenesis of asthma.
	Vasoactive intestinal peptide and other nonadrenergic mediators relax smooth muscle and inhibit mucous production.	

VARIATION IN VENTILATION CAUSED BY CHANGES IN AIRWAY RESISTANCE OR COMPLIANCE

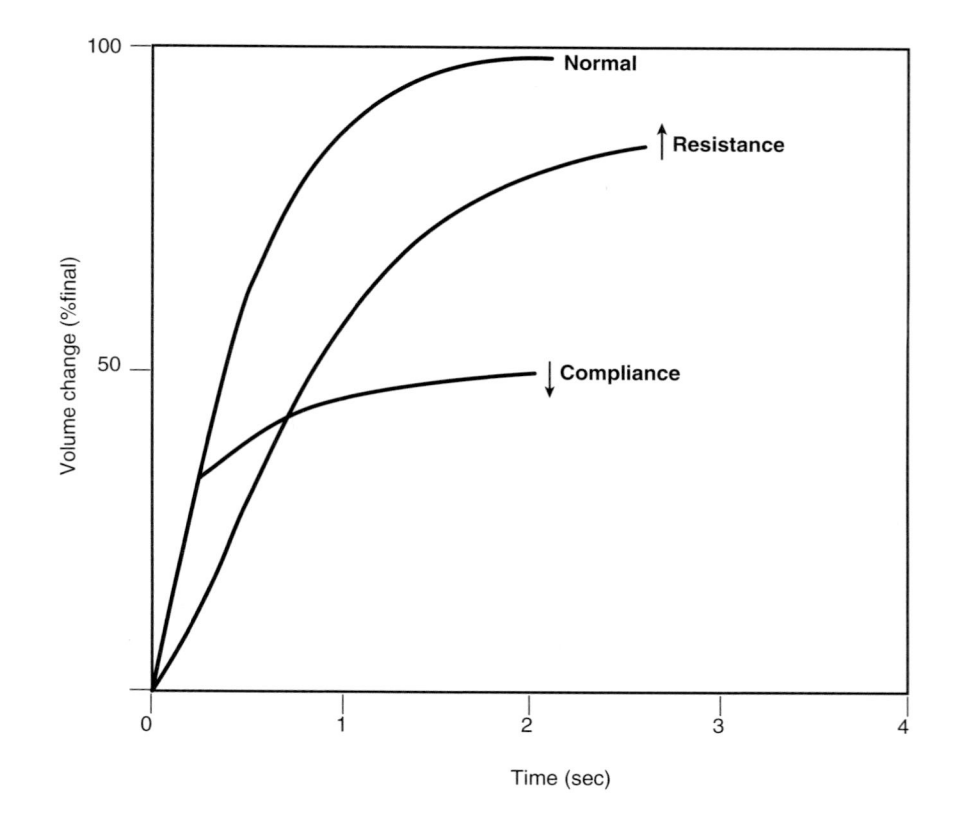

Normally, ventilation reaches 97% of its equilibrium volume during a 2-second normal inspiration. When resistance is increased, the equilibrium volume is lower; the lung is underventilated relative to its FRC volume. With decreased compliance, the lung fills as fast as it would normally, but because it is stiffer, it is also underventilated.

Modified, with permission, from Berne RM, Levy MN: *Principles of Physiology*, 3rd ed. Mosby: 2000:330.

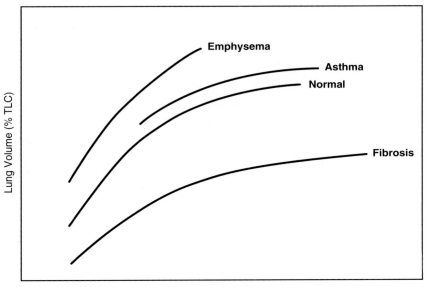

Pressure-volume loops demonstrate change in lung volume plotted against transpulmonary pressure. The linear part of the curve demonstrates that breathing is effort independent

- Regardless of effort, maximal expiratory flow at given volume cannot be exceeded

- Additional increases in effort to raise driving pressure diminishes the increases in expiratory flow

Shifts in the curve indicate lung compliance.

- Shift of curve up and to the left indicates increased compliance (eg, obstructive lung disease)

- Shift of curve down and to the right indicates decreased compliance (eg, restrictive lung disease)

Modified, with permission, from Berne RM, Levy MN: *Principles of Physiology*, 3rd ed. Mosby: 2000:315.

STATIC AND DYNAMIC PRESSURE-VOLUME LOOPS

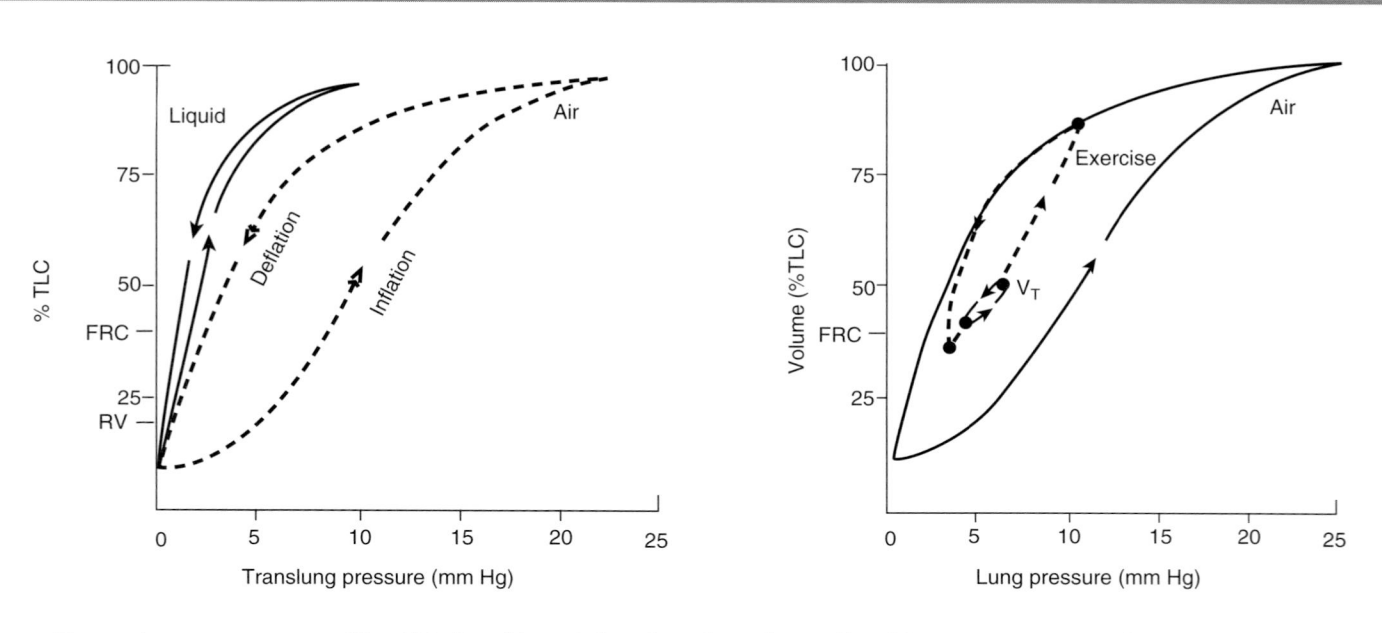

- Transpulmonary pressure of liquid-inflated lung is less than that of air-inflated lung at any given volume.
- In air-inflated lung, compliance is less during inflation than during deflation (higher pressure is required at any given volume).
- Demonstrates how surfactant decreases surface tension in the lungs.
- During normal tidal breathing, there is not much change in lung volume or transmural pressure.
- The slope of the line joining the points of no flow (end-inspiration and end-expiration) is used to calculate dynamic lung compliance.

Modified, with permission, from Berne RM, Levy MN: *Principles of Physiology*, 3rd ed. Mosby: 2000:317, 319.

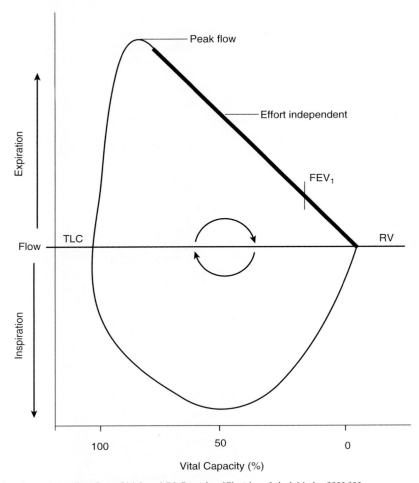

Peak flow

Effort independent

FEV_1

Expiration

Inspiration

Flow

TLC

RV

100

50

0

Vital Capacity (%)

Modified, with permission, from Berne RM, Levy MN: *Principles of Physiology*, 3rd ed. Mosby: 2000:320.

The small central loop represents normal tidal breathing, and the large loop represents a maximal forced inspiration from RV to TLC, followed by a maximal forced expiration back to RV. The most important information is contained in the expiratory curve. The thickened line is independent of effort, and the effort-independent velocity is a function of airway collapsibility, or dynamic compression.

PULMONARY FUNCTION TESTS

Test	Description	Purpose	Information Provided
VC	• Maximal volume of gas that can be expired after maximal inspiration. • Most commonly performed pulmonary function test.	Evaluates size of lungs.	Both reduced TLC of restrictive disease and increased RV of obstructive disease decrease VC.
FVC	• Volume expired with maximal force. • Move from TLC to RV. • Normal value: > 80% of predicted.	Evaluates resistance properties of airways and strength of expiratory muscles.	Decreased FVC is consistent with obstructive pulmonary disease.
FEV_1	• Maximal volume expired in first second of FVC. • Timed VC. • Varies inversely as function of airway resistance and directly as function of maximal expiratory pressure. • Normal value: 3 L.	Most commonly used screening test for airway disease.	*FEV_1 reduced in obstructive airway disease or weakness of expiratory muscles* (low flow rates with high airway resistance).
	• $FEV_{1\%}$ = FEV_1/FVC (ie, percent of VC expired in 1 second). • Normal value: > 80% of predicted.		*FEV_1 increased in restrictive airway disease* (low VC with high flow rates, symmetrically reduced FEV_1 and FVC [normal FEV_1:FVC ratio]).
Maximal Expiratory Pressure	Highest pressure that can be generated during expiration through device with closed airway.	Determines whether cause of low expiratory flow rate is increased airway resistance or weakness of expiratory muscles.	• Patients with high airway resistance can generate normal expiratory pressures of 100 cm H_2O. • Patients with expiratory muscle weakness generate lower expiratory pressure.

Maximal Voluntary Ventilation	• Maximum breathing capacity. • Largest volume of gas that can be moved into and out of lungs in 1 minute by voluntary effort. • Normal value: 125–170 L/min.	Determines highest rate of ventilation for any condition.	• Compare results to predicted values based on age, height, and sex. • Results vary with degree of cooperation.

OBSTRUCTIVE VERSUS RESTRICTIVE LUNG DISEASE

Disease Type	Description	Resistance	FVC	FEV$_1$	FEV$_1$%	Examples
Obstructive	• Processes that impair expiration result in trapping air in lungs, leading to overinflation. • Thoracic cage may become barrel-shaped and diaphragm may flatten even during expiration, leading to impaired movement and shortness of breath.	↑	↓	↓	< 80% of predicted.	Asthma, chronic bronchitis, emphysema.
Restrictive	• Processes that impair inspiration lead to underinflation, decreased lung volume and compliance, decreased chest wall compliance. • Elevated abdominal pressure interferes with descent of diaphragm.	↓	↓	↓	> 80% of predicted.	Pneumonia, pulmonary fibrosis, congestive heart failure.

III. Gas Diffusion and Transport

RESPIRATORY GAS DIFFUSION

Factor	Description	Normal Values, Formulas, Examples	Clinical Significance/Important Points
Diffusing Capacity	Diffusing capacity of lung for given gas is directly proportional to surface area of alveolar-capillary membrane and inversely proportional to its thickness.	$D_L = \dot{V}/(P_A - P_C)$ • V = volume of gas absorbed by lungs per minute. • $P_A - P_C$ = partial pressure gradient between alveoli and capillaries.	Exercise increases diffusing capacity: it increases blood flow, increasing pulmonary capillary recruitment and surface area for gas exchange. Lung disease decreases diffusing capacity: • Emphysema destroys alveoli, *reducing* exchange *surface area*. • Interstitial lung disease and pulmonary edema *increase diffusion distance*. • Ventilation-perfusion mismatch *reduces partial pressure gradient*.
Perfusion-limited Gas Exchange	Gas exchange is limited by amount of blood flowing through pulmonary capillaries.	Normal gas transfer is perfusion-limited.	• Equilibration between alveolar gas and pulmonary capillary blood takes place. • Afterward, O_2 transfer stops until capillary blood is replaced by unsaturated venous blood.
Diffusion-limited Gas Exchange	Gas exchange is not limited by blood flowing through pulmonary capillaries.	• CO exchange is diffusion-limited. • $D_{L_{CO}}$ is used to evaluate diffusion capacity of respiratory system. • $D_{L_{CO}} = \dot{V}_{CO}/P_{A_{CO}}$. • NORMAL $D_{L_{CO}}$ = 25 mL/min per mm Hg at rest and increases during exercise.	• Equilibration does not take place between alveolar and pulmonary capillary blood. • Increasing diffusion gradient by raising F_{IO_2} improves conditions. • Diffusion-limited gas exchange causes arterial hypoxia; some diseases reduce rate of O_2 transfer or decrease P_{AO_2} causing decreased rate of diffusion.

Diffusion of O_2	• CO_2 continuously diffuses out of alveoli into blood stream (composition of alveolar gas remains relatively constant).	• Pathway: alveolar P_{O_2} (100 mm Hg) → plasma → pulmonary capillary alveolar P_{O_2} (40 mm Hg).	Most effective mechanism for improving O_2 delivery is to decrease diffusion path length by recruiting more functional alveoli.
		• Initial partial pressure difference = 60 mm Hg.	
Diffusion of CO_2	• CO_2 continuously diffuses into alveoli from blood stream	• Pathway: pulmonary capillary P_{CO_2} (46 mm Hg) → plasma → alveolar P_{CO_2} (40 mm Hg).	$D_{L_{CO}} > D_{O_2}$ explains why CO_2 retention is not problem in alveolar fibrosis even though reduction in D_{O_2} is severe.
	• *Diffusion of CO_2 across alveolar-capillary barrier is 20 times faster than that of O_2 (CO_2 is more soluble in H_2O).*	• Initial partial pressure difference = 6 mm Hg.	

O₂ AND CO₂ TRANSPORT BETWEEN THE LUNGS AND THE SYSTEMIC CIRCULATION

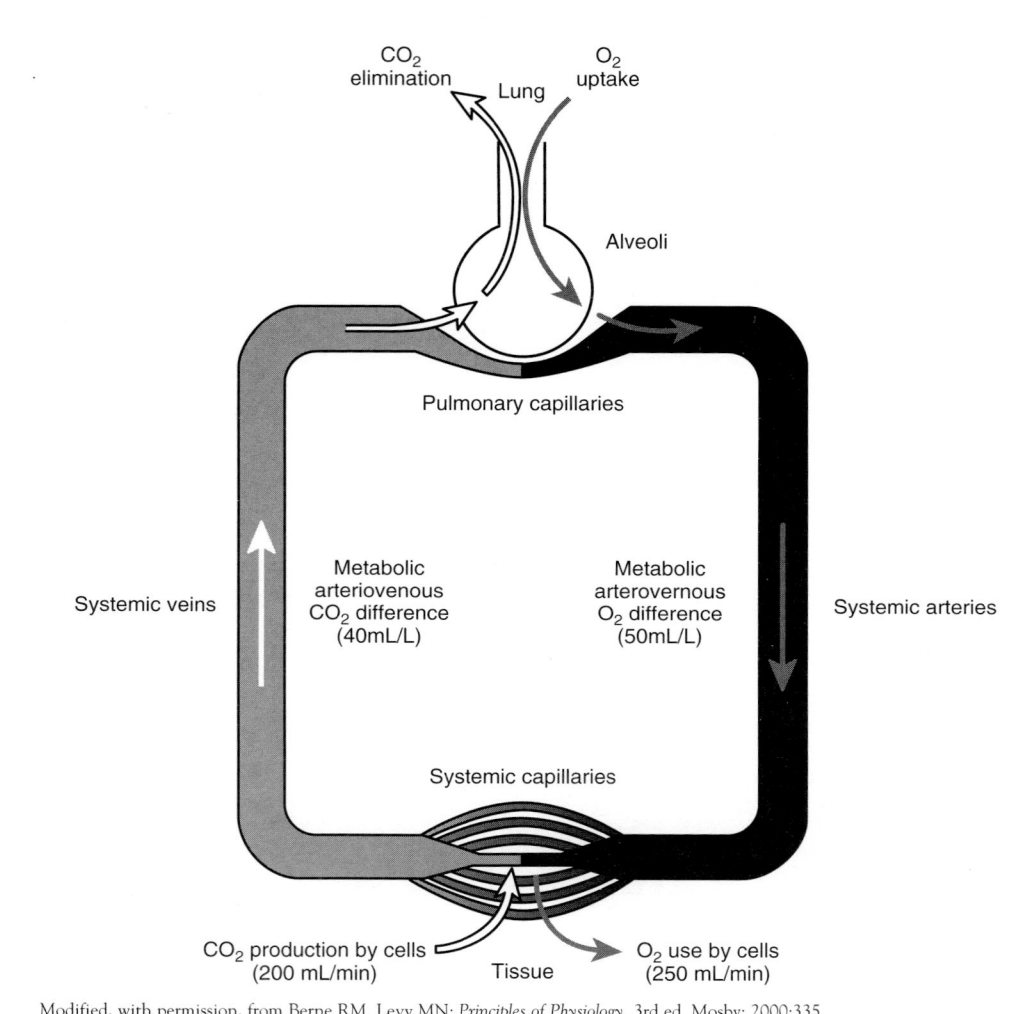

The systemic arterial blood transports O_2 from the lungs to the tissue capillaries. The systemic venous blood transports CO_2 from tissue capillaries to lungs.

Modified, with permission, from Berne RM, Levy MN: *Principles of Physiology*, 3rd ed. Mosby: 2000:335.

IMPORTANT CONCEPTS IN O_2 TRANSPORT

Properties	Description	Normal Value	Influencing Factors
P_{50}	• PO_2 that produces 50% saturation of Hgb with O_2. • Inversely related to Hgb affinity. • Decreased P_{50} means increased Hgb affinity (ie, O_2 combines more readily with Hgb). • Increased P_{50} means decreased Hgb affinity (ie, Hgb releases O_2 more readily to tissues). • Hgb saturation (%) = [(O_2 content – dissolved O_2)/O_2 capacity] × 100.	27 mm Hg (arterial blood).	• Bohr effect: increased PCO_2 → decreased blood pH → increased P_{50}. • Deoxyhemoglobin.
O_2 Capacity	• Maximal amount O_2 that can be carried in blood by Hgb. • Hgb concentration × 1.34 ml O_2/g.	20 mL/dL.	Hgb levels (normal Hgb concentration is 12–15 g/dL).
O_2 Content	• Total volume of O_2 carried in blood. • $HgbO_2$ + dissolved O_2.	• Hgb carries 98.5%. • 1.5% dissolved in plasma.	Amount of O_2 dissolved depends on O_2 tension in blood.
Mixed Venous O_2 Content	Weighted average of blood flow and O_2 consumption throughout body.	150 mL (75% Hgb saturation).	• State of activity (eg, rest versus exercise). • Activity affects vasoconstriction, vasodilation, and O_2 consumption.
O_2 Delivery	• Amount of O_2 presented to tissues per minute. • Arterial O_2 content × cardiac output.	1 L/min.	• Decreased arterial O_2 content. • Decreased cardiac output.
O_2 Reserves	"Stored" O_2 in body that provides about 5 minutes of basal O_2 consumption.		• Severe cold exposure. • Recovery without permanent brain damage is possible after 1 hour because O_2 demand in this state is drastically reduced.

OXYHEMOGLOBIN DISSOCIATION CURVE

Portion of Curve	Interpretation
Sigmoid	• O_2 affinity for Hgb varies as P_{O_2} varies. • More O_2 bound indicates higher affinity of Hgb for each subsequent O_2 molecule. • Quantity of O_2 taken up in lungs is maximized even at lower-than-normal P_{AO_2}. • Quantity released in systemic capillaries is substantial at relatively high P_{O_2}.
Steep Portion	• Dissociation (unloading) zone. • Occurs at P_{O_2} < 60 mm Hg. • Allows Hgb to release large amounts of O_2 in response to relatively small changes in P_{O_2}. • Keeps P_{O_2} in capillary blood high so diffusion gradient for O_2 is maintained. • P_{O_2} in tissues is very low (metabolism consumes O_2), causing O_2 to diffuse from blood to tissue.
Plateau	• Association (loading) zone. • Occurs at P_{O_2} > 60 mm Hg. • Provides margin of safety, allowing P_{AO_2} to be reduced substantially while maintaining high Hgb saturation. • Example: arterial Hgb saturation remains adequate despite lower P_{aO_2} at high altitudes or in mild pulmonary disease.

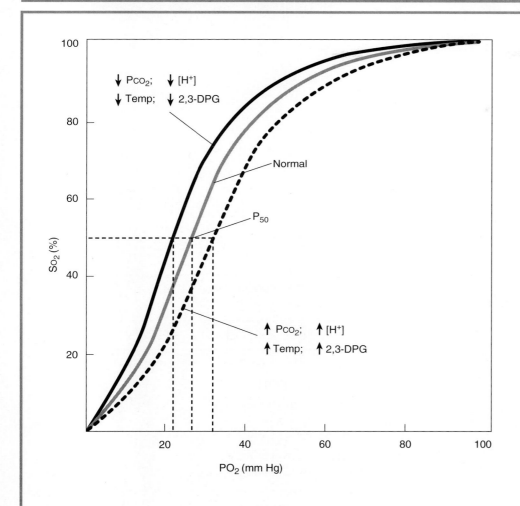

Normal Values at 37 °C: pH, 7.4; P_{CO_2}, 40 mm Hg; [2,3-DPG], 15 μmol/g of Hgb.

Left shift:

- Indicates increase in O_2 affinity (O_2 remains bound to Hgb).

- CO and fetal Hgb cause left shift.

- Fetal Hgb has higher affinity for Hgb and is not affected by 2,3-DPG.

Right shift:

- Indicates decrease in O_2 affinity (increase in release of O_2 to tissues)

- All factors that cause right shift increase 2,3-DPG, such as increased altitude and temperature, exercise, and the Bohr effect (increased P_{CO_2}, decreased pH, increased P_{50}).

Modified, with permission, from Berne RM, Levy MN: *Principles of Physiology*, 3rd ed. Mosby: 2000:335.

CO$_2$ TRANSPORT IN BLOOD

Form of CO$_2$	Description	Amount (%)
HCO$_3^-$	• In RBCs, carbonic anhydrase reacts with H$_2$O to form carbonic acid, which dissociates into HCO$_3^-$ and H$^+$. • Most CO$_2$ carried in plasma as HCO$_3^-$. Chloride shift • As HCO$_3^-$ diffuses out of RBCs, 70% enters plasma. • Excess leaves RBCs in exchange for Cl$^-$.	60
Carbamino Compounds	CO$_2$ that combines with NH$_3$ groups on blood proteins, especially Hgb.	30
Dissolved	CO$_2$ is 20 times more soluble in blood than O$_2$, so more CO$_2$ than O$_2$ is in simple solution at equal partial pressures.	10

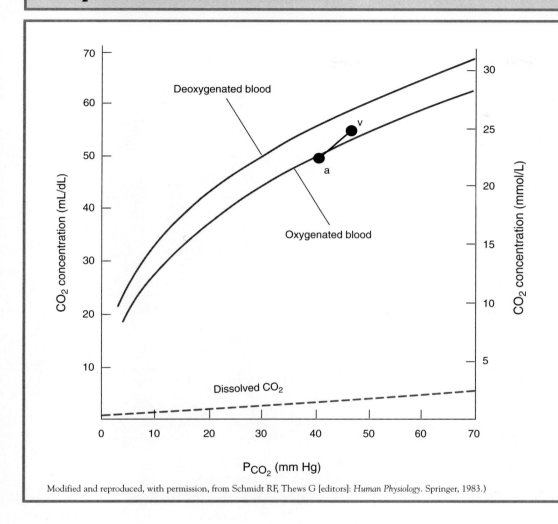

Left shift of curve demonstrates the Haldane effect.

- Binding of O_2 to Hgb reduces its affinity for CO_2.
- Venous blood carries more CO_2 than arterial blood.

Arterial point (a) and venous point (v) indicate the total CO_2 content in arterial blood and venous blood, respectively.

Modified and reproduced, with permission, from Schmidt RF, Thews G [editors]: *Human Physiology.* Springer, 1983.)

ABNORMAL GAS LEVELS

Condition	Description	Etiology	Results	Important Points
O_2 Toxicity	Abnormally high $[O_2]$ in blood.	Overoxygenation from external source.	After 8 hours, respiratory passages become irritated, with possible bronchopulmonary dysplasia.	Risk of damage much worse in pediatric population than adult population.
Hypercapnia	Abnormally high $[CO_2]$ in blood.	Hypoventilation.	Eventual central nervous system depression with confusion, coma, and eventual death.	Bicarbonate levels are elevated, in an attempt to correct for respiratory acidosis.
Hypocapnia	Abnormally low $[CO_2]$ in blood.	Hyperventilation.	Decreased cerebral blood flow, leading to dizziness and paresthesias.	Can develop low plasma calcium (may develop carpal-pedal spasms and Chvostek sign).
CO Poisoning	Abnormally high $[CO]$ in blood.	From external source (fire, machinery).	• Hemoglobin molecules unable to pick up oxygen. • Mild poisoning results in headache and nausea. • Once 70–80% of Hgb converted to carboxyhemoglobin (cherry-red color), death occurs.	Affinity of Hgb for CO is 200 times that of O_2.
Asphyxia (apnea)	No air movement.	Airway obstruction (eg, foreign body, drowning).	• Immediate hypercapnia and hypoxia. • Stimulation of violent respiratory efforts. • Blood pressure and heart rate rise sharply.	• Respiratory efforts eventually cease, with subsequent drop in blood pressure and heart rate. • Asystole in 4–5 minutes.

IV. Ventilation, Perfusion, and Gas Exchange

ZONES OF LUNG PERFUSION

Zone	Degree of Blood Flow	Description	Clinical Significance
Perfusion zones of lung depend on relationships among pulmonary arterial, venous, and alveolar pressures.			
1	Any region with no blood flow.	• Arterial pressure < alveolar pressure. • Capillaries are collapsed.	Does not exist in normal lungs.
2	Gradient increases from apex to base of lungs.	• Arterial pressure > alveolar pressure > venous pressure. • Alveolar pressure > venous outflow pressure, leading to compression of capillaries or venules exposed to alveolar pressure.	• Waterfall effect: arterial-alveolar gradient is driving force for blood flow. • Changes in downstream (venous) pressure do not alter blood flow.
3	Blood flow increases from apex to base of lungs.	• Arterial pressure > venous pressure > alveolar pressure. • Distention and recruitment of all vessels because of increased hydrostatic pressure, leading to decreased resistance to blood flow.	During exercise, there is distention of zone 3 and 4 vessels because of slight increase in arterial pressure.
4	Region of reduced blood flow.	Exists when pulmonary venous pressure is abnormally high (eg, left ventricular failure) or when pulmonary edema produces accumulation of fluid around blood vessels (vascular cuffing).	Vascular cuffing increases vascular resistance and reduces local blood flow.

EFFECT OF INTRAPLEURAL PRESSURES ON VENTILATION

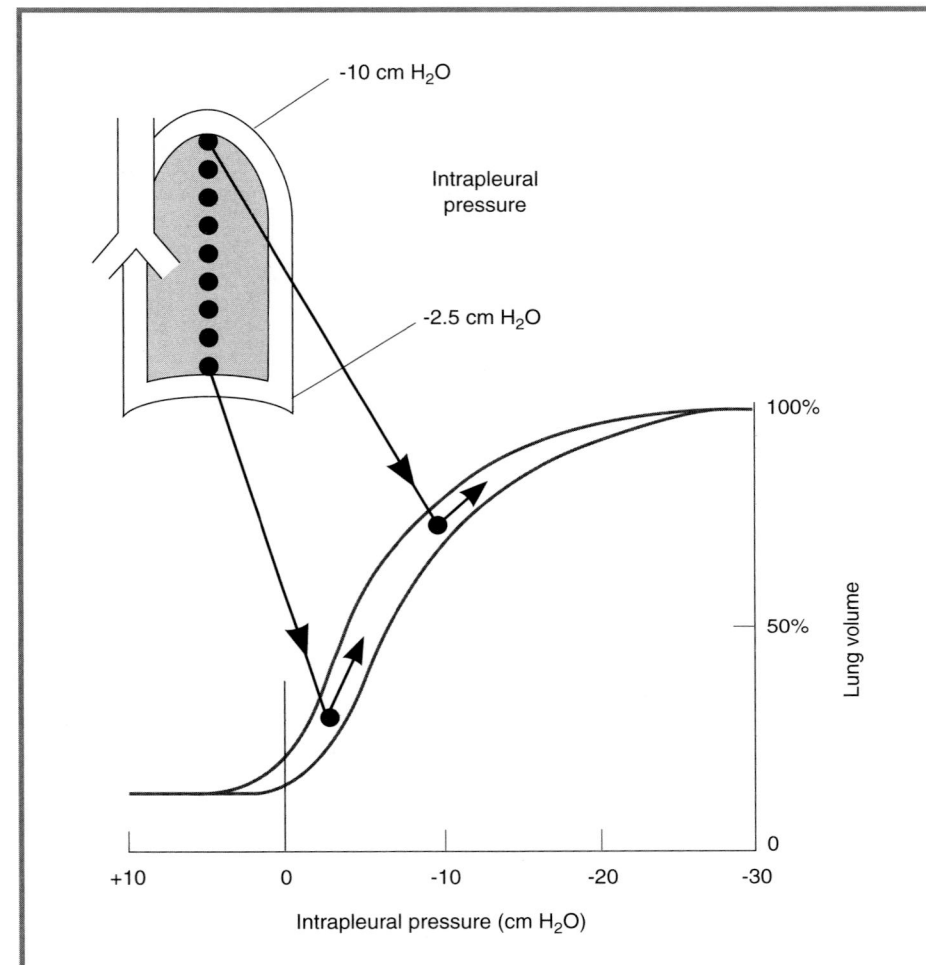

From the apex to the base of upright lung:

- Transpulmonary pressure increases.
- Intrapleural pressure increases.
- Blood flow increases.
- Ventilation increases.
- V/Q ratio decreases (relative change in blood flow from apex to base > relative change in ventilation).

Reproduced, with permission, from West JR: *Ventilation/Blood Flow and Gas Exchange*, 3rd ed. Blackwell, 1977.

FACTORS THAT AFFECT PULMONARY BLOOD FLOW

Factors	Mechanism	Effects
Sympathetic Nervous System	Stimulation of vascular smooth muscle via α-adrenergic catecholamines.	Vasoconstriction.
	Stimulation of vascular smooth muscle via β-adrenergic catecholamines.	Vasodilation.
Humoral Factors	Angiotensin II, arachidonic acid metabolites, endothelin, and thromboxane A_2 affect vascular smooth muscle.	Vasoconstriction.
	Atrial natriuretic peptide, bradykinin, histamine, NO, prostacyclin, and vasopressin affect vascular smooth muscle.	Vasodilation.
Partial Pressures of Arterial Gases	Increased PaO_2.	Vasodilation
	Increased $PaCO_2$.	Vasoconstriction.
Gravity	• Upright, upper lungs are above heart and bases are at or below it. • This results in a pressure gradient in pulmonary arteries from top to bottom of lungs.	Pressure gradient in pulmonary arteries results in increase in pulmonary blood flow from apices to bases.
Hydrostatic Pressure	• Hydrostatic pressure near lung bases > apices. • Increased hydrostatic pressure favors net outward filtration of capillaries	• "Leaky lung." • Most filtrate returned to circulation as lymph.
Hypoxic Pulmonary Vasoconstriction	• Alveolar hypoxia, hypercapnia, and acidosis produce pulmonary vasoconstriction and systemic vasodilation. • Increases pulmonary vascular resistance in hypoxic areas, shifting blood flow to better ventilated regions.	• Balances ventilation and perfusion. • Pulmonary hypertension may develop.
Changes in Lung Volume	• Alter pulmonary vascular resistance. • Resistance is minimal when volume is close to FRC and increases at both higher and lower lung volumes. • Large extra-alveolar vessels are dilated at high lung volumes and constrict with inspiration. • Small alveolar vessels (pulmonary capillaries) are compressed by enlarged alveoli at high lung volumes (does not vary with breathing).	• Decreased resistance to blood flow. • During inspiration, capillary vascular resistance increases while larger vessels dilate, increasing their contained blood volume.

FACTORS INFLUENCING THE DISTRIBUTION OF VENTILATION

Influencing Factors	Description	Important Points
PL	Pressure difference from pulmonary artery to left atrium (Ppa − Pla).	• Pulmonary vascular resistance equals transpulmonary pressure/flow. • At normal resting cardiac output (Q) of 5 L/min, pulmonary vascular resistance = (Ppa − Pla)/Q, or (14 − 8)/5 = 1.2 mm Hg/(L/min).
	In vertical lung, PPL increases from −10 cm H_2O at apex to −2 cm H_2O at base.	Changes in PPL alter PL, resulting in variation in regional lung volume, with high inflation and low compliance at apex and low inflation and high compliance at base.
	Hydrostatic pressure difference in vertical lung between apex and base is 7.5–10 cm H_2O.	VT in vertical lung greatest at base at start inspiration with linear reduction from base to apex.
Volume	With constant compliance, each alveolus receives air in proportion to its volume.	Maldistribution of ventilation is rare in healthy individuals.
	Regional maldistribution of ventilation is increased by reducing end-expiratory volume to RV or by inspiring to TLC.	Increased regional maldistribution is normal part of aging. Lung becomes more compliant or distensible.
	• Rate of acinar volume change = resistance × compliance = time constant. • Example: percentage of passively exhaled air requires constant amount of time, regardless of starting volume.	In diseased lungs, unequal time constants in different areas of lung lead to differences in regional alveolar ventilation and Po_2.
	Increased time constant because of high airway resistance.	• Decreased rate of acinar filling and emptying, leading to underventilation. • Example: obstructive lung disease; with rapid breathing, lungs do not deflate to FRC, and alveolar pressure remains positive at end-expiration (intrinsic PEEP).
	Decreased time constant because of low compliance.	Stiff lungs lead to rapid but small volume changes, resulting in underventilation (eg, pulmonary fibrosis).

Airway Closure	• Occurs when regional transpulmonary pressure is reduced to critical level.	Early airway closure alters alveolar ventilation and increases work of breathing (high pressures must be developed to reopen closed airways).
	• P_{PL} exceeds atmospheric pressure.	Examples:
		• Inflammation, excess mucus, and bronchial smooth muscle contraction leading to narrowed airway and early closure.
		• Chronic lung disease leading to loss of elastic recoil, resulting in decreased P_{PL} and early airway closure.

VENTILATION-PERFUSION MISMATCH

V/Q Ratio	Description	Clinical Significance
Normal (1)	Most efficient gas exchange: • P_{AO_2} = 100 mm Hg. • P_{ACO_2} = 40 mm Hg. • $P_{aO_2} - P_{AO_2}$ gradient < 20 mm Hg.	• In healthy lungs, V/Q ratio is not uniformly distributed. • V/Q ratio normally varies from 0.6 at base to 0.3 at apex. • *Hypoxic vasoconstriction in hypoventilated units is single most effective mechanism for shifting flow away from underventilated units.*
Low (< 1)	• Reduced alveolar ventilation relative to perfusion. • P_{O_2} in alveolus falls and P_{CO_2} rises. • Less O_2 is delivered and less CO_2 is expired.	
	Physiologic shunt: V/Q > 0 but < 1. • Affected area of lung has low P_{AO_2}, leading to blood with low P_{O_2} and low Hgb saturation. • Mixture of this blood with that from better ventilated areas causes decrease in overall arterial O_2 tension and content. • There is no abnormal connection between arterial and venous systems.	• Normally, small part of cardiac output goes through pulmonary vasculature without contacting alveolar air. • 100% O_2 in patient with significant physiologic shunt (V/Q mismatch) raises P_{aO_2} above 500 mm Hg. • Associated with pulmonary edema and pneumonia.

Continued

VENTILATION-PERFUSION MISMATCH (Continued)

V/Q Ratio	Description	Clinical Significance
Low (< 1) (Continued)	Anatomic shunt: V/Q = 0. • Mixture of true venous blood with oxygenated blood. • Blood flow bypasses lungs and goes through anatomic channel (eg, fistula) from pulmonary artery to vein. • Nonventilated area of lung causes rapid decrease in P_{AO_2} until it equals P_{O_2} in mixed venous blood, resulting in no further gas exchange. • *Normal individuals have anatomic shunt of < 5% of cardiac output.*	• Endotracheal tube in mainstem bronchus leads to underventilation of opposite lung with normal flow, producing low V/Q, decreased O_2 saturation. and absent breath sounds. • 100% O_2 in patient with significant anatomic shunt does not raise P_{aO_2} above 500 mm Hg because shunted blood is never exposed to high P_{AO_2}. • Associated with ventricular septal defect.
High (> 1)	• Reduced perfusion relative to ventilation. • P_{CO_2} falls, and P_{O_2} rises. • Less CO_2 is delivered and less O_2 enters blood. • Alveolar and capillary P_{O_2} are high but O_2 uptake is minimal. • No blood flow to area of lung (V/Q = ∞), which means no gas exchange (ventilation of alveolar dead space).	• Associated with pulmonary emboli. • Endotracheal tube in mainstem bronchus produces high V/Q in ipsilateral lung (causes overventilation and increased airway pressure).

V. Control of Breathing

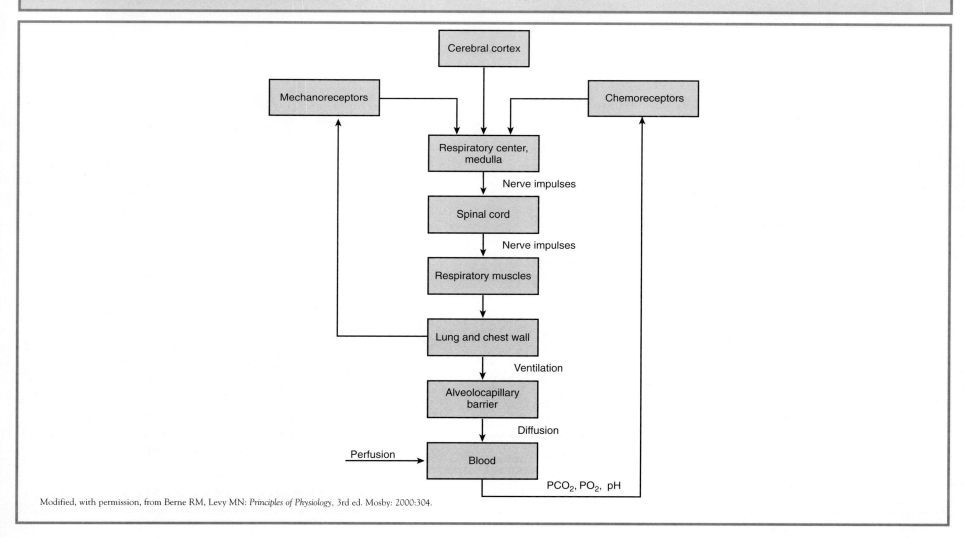

Modified, with permission, from Berne RM, Levy MN: *Principles of Physiology,* 3rd ed. Mosby: 2000:304.

CHEMICAL CONTROL OF BREATHING

Factor	Increased	Decreased	Important Points
Pa_{CO_2}	• *Causes cerebral vasodilation (can cause cerebral edema).* • Increased blood flow washes CO_2 from tissues, reducing ventilatory drive.	No stimulation of ventilation by hypoxia until $Pa_{O_2} < 60$ mm Hg.	Hypercapnia results in inverse relationship between ventilation and Pa_{O_2}.
H^+	Stimulates peripheral chemoreceptors, leading to increased ventilatory drive, which results in decreased Pa_{CO_2}.	Results in depressed ventilation and rise in Pa_{CO_2}, thus raising H^+ (metabolic alkalosis with compensatory respiratory acidosis).	Increased H^+ in CSF suppresses ventilatory drive.
Pa_{O_2}	• *Patients with hypercapnia given 100% O_2 may have blunted response to high CO_2 levels, leading to CO_2 narcosis.* • *Treat by decreasing O_2 supply to stimulate ventilation.*	*Enhanced sensitivity of CO_2-induced ventilation.*	• Respiratory depressants (ethanol, benzodiazepines) decrease alveolar ventilation, leading to increased Pa_{O_2} and decreased Pa_{O_2}. • If alveolar-arterial gradient is normal, gas exchange abnormality is caused by only respiratory depressant. • If gradient is increased, other factors such as V/Q mismatch or diffusion abnormality from aspiration must be evaluated.

THE FOUR MAJOR TYPES OF pH ABNORMALITIES

Abnormality	Example	Compensatory Mechanism	pH
Metabolic Acidosis	Diabetic ketoacidosis.	Hyperventilation $\rightarrow$ decreased $PaCO_2$ and $[H^+]$ $\rightarrow$ respiratory alkalosis.	Mild acidosis.
Metabolic Alkalosis	Protracted vomiting $\rightarrow$ loss of HCl.	Hypoventilation $\rightarrow$ increased $PaCO_2$ and $[H^+]$ $\rightarrow$ respiratory acidosis.	Mild alkalosis.
Respiratory Acidosis	Hypoventilation not secondary to decreased $[H^+]$.	Increased PCO_2 and $[H^+]$ $\rightarrow$ metabolic alkalosis.	Mild acidosis.
Respiratory Alkalosis	Hyperventilation not secondary to increased $[H^+]$.	Decreased PCO_2 and $[H^+]$ $\rightarrow$ metabolic acidosis.	Mild alkalosis.

CENTRAL NERVOUS SYSTEM CONTROL OF BREATHING

Area of Brain	Function	Clinical Significance
Thalamus and Cerebral Cortex	• Volitional control of breathing. • Modify rate and depth of respiration in relation to volitional motor activities of chest wall and diaphragm.	Pathways for volitional control travel via corticospinal tract, bypassing medulla.
Pontine Respiratory Group	• Outflow from this region enhances inspiration. • Receives signals from lung stretch receptors, which inhibit dorsal medulla until inspiration ends and expiration begins. • Inhibited by vagus nerve.	• Trauma to pons or vagotomy causes apneustic breathing (long inspiration with breath holding and short exhalations). • For transections rostral to pons, normal automatic respirations are maintained.

Continued

CENTRAL NERVOUS SYSTEM CONTROL OF BREATHING (Continued)

Area of Brain	Function	Clinical Significance
Dorsal Respiratory Group	• Automatic, involuntary breathing. • Initial processing of afferent feedback from airways and peripheral chemoreceptors. • Provides inspiratory stimuli to phrenic motor neurons.	Goal is to keep Pa_{CO_2} and PA_{CO_2} near 40 mm Hg. Ondine curse: • Automatic control lost without loss of voluntary control. • Patients have bulbar poliomyelitis or disease processes that compress medulla.
Ventral Respiratory Group	• Automatic, involuntary breathing. • Provides connections to cranial motor neurons, bulbospinal axons to phrenic and intercostal respiratory motor neurons.	*Transection of brainstem below medulla stops respiration.*
Reticular Activating System	• *Increases respiratory drive.* • Influences brainstem control by affecting state of alertness.	Activity decreases during sleep, leading to decreased respiratory drive and minute ventilation, which results in increased P_{CO_2}.

VI. Respiratory Response to Stress

HYPOXIA

Type of Hypoxia	Cause(s)	Po$_2$ Level	Hgb Level
Anemic	Insufficient hemoglobin to carry O$_2$.	Normal.	Low.
Arterial	Insufficient arterial oxygenation.	Low.	Normal.
Histotoxic	Inactivation of enzymes by toxins (eg, cyanide).	Normal.	Normal.
Ischemic	Inadequate blood flow to provide required O$_2$.	Normal.	Normal.
Stagnant	Slow circulation. • Causes kidney and heart damage during shock. • Causes liver and brain damage during congestive heart failure. • If prolonged, leads to ARDS.	Low.	Normal.

CYANOSIS

Etiology	Description	Clinical Significance
Appears when capillary blood contains more than 5 g/dL deoxyhemoglobin.	Bluish color to nail beds, lips, mucous membranes, and earlobes resulting from inadequate amount of O$_2$ in blood.	• *Cyanosis is not a reliable sign of hypoxia.* • Skin pigmentation or poor lighting may mask cyanosis. • Polycythemia and high levels of methemoglobin are associated with cyanosis without hypoxia. • Conditions associated with hypoxia without cyanosis: histotoxic hypoxia (normal blood gas), CO poisoning (cherry red color hides cyanosis), and anemia (low hemoglobin).

EFFECTS OF EXTREME STRESS ON VENTILATION

Situation	Conditions	Body's Response
Exercise	Increased O_2 demand, increased CO_2 production lead to buildup of O_2 debt and metabolic lactic acidosis.	• Increased ventilation (provide more O_2, remove more CO_2, buffer lactic acidosis). • Hyperventilation, leading to compensatory respiratory alkalosis. • Respiratory rate does not return to basal levels until O_2 debt is paid.
High Altitude	Decreased barometric pressure and Po_2.	• Neurologic signs indicate hypoxia, which may result in loss of consciousness. • Chronic mountain sickness is intolerance to high altitudes, which leads to ventilatory depression, severe polycythemia, and pulmonary and cerebral edema.
Drowning	Suffocation by immersion in water.	• Gasp of water triggers laryngospasm leading to death from asphyxia without any water in lungs. • Relaxation of glottis allows fluid to enter lungs, where it is absorbed and dilutes plasma, leading to intravascular hemolysis.
Decompression Sickness	Too rapid ascent from deep water.	• Nitrogen diffuses into lungs along pressure gradient. • If ascent is too rapid, nitrogen escapes in tissues (forms bubbles), leading to joint pain, paresthesias, occlusion of blood flow to brain or spinal cord, and death.

PHYSIOLOGIC RESPONSES IN ACCLIMATIZATION

System	Response
Renal	• *Erythropoietin secretion increases*, resulting in increased RBCs after 2–3 days in low barometric pressure. • Excretion of Na^+ reduces plasma bicarbonate which raises blood H^+.
Nervous	• Bicarbonate is decreased in brain interstitial fluid. • Small amounts of anaerobic metabolism may occur in hypoxic brain allowing lactate ions to replace bicarbonate ions.
Cardiovascular	Stimulation of peripheral chemoreceptors (carotid bodies) increases ventilation and reduces Pa_{CO_2} and H^+.
Hematologic	2,3-DPG increases in RBCs, decreasing affinity of O_2 for Hgb.
Pulmonary	• Respiratory alkalosis in response to decreased P_{CO_2} as well as decreased O_2. • Rate and depth of breathing increase.

SLEEP APNEA

Type	Respiratory Effort?	Etiology	Physical Signs and Symptoms	Important Points
Obstructive	• Yes. • Pleural pressure cycles but air flow does not.	• Relaxation of oropharyngeal muscles causes temporary obstruction.	• Snoring, headaches, fatigue, daytime sleepiness. • If prolonged, incidence of pulmonary hypertension, myocardial infarction, cerebrovascular accident, and heart failure may increase.	• Occurs at any age. • Most common during rapid-eye movement sleep, when muscles are most hypotonic. • Arousal response changes stage of sleep and allows activation of upper airway muscles and end of apnea. • Treatment is surgery or external ventilatory support.
Central	• No. • All breathing ceases because of transient decreases in respiratory drive.	• Congestive heart failure. • Neurologic disorders that affect the brainstem or respiratory control centers.	• No attempt to breathe, no air flow, no change in pleural pressure.	• Biot breathing (see Abnormal Respiratory Patterns). • Periodic breathing is a type of central apnea. • Treat primary disorder. • External ventilatory support may help.

ABNORMAL RESPIRATORY PATTERNS

Type	Etiology	Breathing Pattern
Cheyne-Stokes Respiration	• Brain depression due to disease, drug overdose, hypoxia, or heart failure. • May occur in otherwise healthy individuals in transition from wakefulness to sleep.	Periodic, with cycles of hypoapnea or apnea alternating with hyperapnea.
Biot Breathing	Brain damage—increased intracranial pressure (eg, meningitis).	Periods of normal breathing interrupted by sudden periods of apnea.
Kussmaul Respiration	Compensatory response to metabolic acidosis (eg, diabetic ketoacidosis).	Rapid, deep breathing in attempt to produce compensatory respiratory alkalosis.

PNEUMOTHORAX

Type	Description	Need for Treatment
Open	• Open connection between pleural cavity and outside world. • Lung collapses due to lack of negative pressure. • Air moves in and out of pleural cavity with inspiration and expiration.	Urgent but not immediate.
Closed	• Fixed amount of air in pleural cavity, which does not increase or decrease with inspiration or expiration. • Due to physical space air takes up in cavity, lung is not able to expand fully. • Air in pleural cavity will be resorbed.	Urgency dependent on size of pneumothorax.
Tension	• "One-way valve:" air enters pleural cavity during inspiration but is unable to exit during expiration. • Causes rapid collapse of lung, hypoxia, and shock due to rapid compression of great veins.	Immediate.

CHAPTER 5

GASTROINTESTINAL SYSTEM

ABBREVIATIONS

ACh = acetylcholine

cAMP = cyclic adenosine monophosphate

CCK = cholecystokinin

CNS = central nervous system

GI = gastrointestinal

GIP = gastric inhibitory peptide

LES = lower esophageal sphincter

MMC = migrating myoelectric complex

NSAID = nonsteroidal anti-inflammatory drug

UES = upper esophageal sphincter

VIP = vasoactive intestinal polypeptide

VLDL = very low density lipoprotein

Absorption	Process by which molecules are transported through GI tract epithelial cells into blood or lymph.
Amylopectin	Plant starch that is the major source of carbohydrate in most human diets; branched polymer of glucose units, with α-1,4 chains and branch points formed by α-1,6 glycosidic links.
Bile Salts	Sodium and potassium salts of bile acids.
Celiac Disease (gluten enteropathy)	Disease characterized by reduction of absorptive surface area in small intestinal villi and malabsorption of carbohydrates, proteins, and lipids in which patients mount an immune response against a component of gluten (a major wheat protein).
Cellulose	β-1,4-linked glucose polymer; cellulose and other molecules with these links remain undigested because intestinal enzymes cannot hydrolyze β-glycosidic links.
Cholecystagogues	Substances that promote gallbladder emptying (eg, CCK, gastrin).
Choleretics	Substances that enhance bile acid secretion.
Conjugated Bile Acids	Bile salts conjugated to glycine or taurine (catalyzed by glucuronyl transferase). At neutral pH, conjugated bile acids are more water soluble than unconjugated bile acids.
Digestion	Process by which ingested molecules are cleaved into smaller ones via reactions catalyzed by enzymes that can then be absorbed from GI tract lumen.
Endocrine Pancreas	Cells in islets of Langerhans (< 2% of pancreas volume) that secrete insulin, glucagon, somatostatin, and pancreatic polypeptide.
Exocrine Pancreas	Acinar cells that produce digestive enzymes for food metabolism such as α-amylase, lipases, and proteases.
Glycogen	Animal starch; sucrose and lactose are the principal dietary disaccharides, and glucose and fructose are the principal monosaccharides.
Hemochromatosis	Syndrome caused by hemosiderosis (overload of iron deposits) and characterized by pigmentation of skin, pancreatic damage ("bronze diabetes"), cirrhosis, gonadal atrophy, and a high incidence of hepatic cancer.
Jaundice (icterus)	Yellow color imparted to skin, sclera, and mucous membranes when free or conjugated bilirubin accumulates in blood (eg, hemolytic anemia, bile duct obstruction).

Continued

Micelles	Cylindrical disks formed by bile salts that help keep cholesterol and lipids in solution and aid in their transportation to brush border epithelial cells for intestinal absorption.
Steatorrhea	Fatty, bulky, clay-colored stool due to impaired digestion and absorption of fat.
Swallowing Center	Central integrating area for swallowing in medulla and lower pons. Sensory impulses from pharynx are transmitted to medulla; motor impulses from swallowing center travel to pharynx and upper esophagus via vagal motor nerves.
VIPomas	Tumors of VIP-secreting cells that cause watery diarrhea syndrome and pancreatic cholera.
Xerostomia	Dry mouth, possibly due to lack of functional salivary glands. Lack of saliva results in absence of protective secretory immunoglobulins and basic pH, causing increased dental caries and infections of the buccal mucosa.
Zollinger-Ellison Syndrome	Gastrinoma; these pancreatic, gastric, or duodenal tumors cause hypersecretion of gastric acid, causing severe upper GI tract ulcers. Treatment involves surgical resection of tumor and proton-pump inhibitors.

I. Anatomy

MICROANATOMY OF THE STOMACH, INTESTINE, AND COLON

Key Cell Types	Location	Function
(Columnar) Surface Epithelial	Gastric mucosa.	• Secrete mucus and alkaline fluid. • *Mucus and* HCO_3^- *together* protect surface epithelial cells from mechanical injury and gastric acid by maintaining surface at near-neutral pH.
Chief (peptic)	Fundus and body of stomach.	• Secrete lipase. • Secrete pepsinogens that are rapidly converted to pepsins at low pH. • Pepsins are proteases that function optimally at pH ≤ 3. • Neutral pH irreversibly inactivates pepsins.
Enterochromaffin	Throughout intestine.	Secrete hormones and serotonin.
Enterochromaffin-like	Gastric mucosa.	• Synthesize and store histamine when stimulated by ACh or gastrin. • Histamine stimulates HCl secretion by parietal cells.
G	Pyloric region of stomach.	Secrete gastrin.
Goblet	Stomach, small intestine, and colon.	Secrete mucus.
Mucous Neck	Cardiac glandular region below LES and pylorus.	Secrete mucus.
Paneth	Crypts of Lieberkühn of small intestine.	Endocrine cells.
Parietal (oxyntic or acid-secreting)	Fundus and body of stomach.	Secrete HCl and intrinsic factor.
Peyer Patches	Throughout intestine.	Lymphatic tissue.

HCL SECRETION BY PARIETAL CELLS IN THE STOMACH

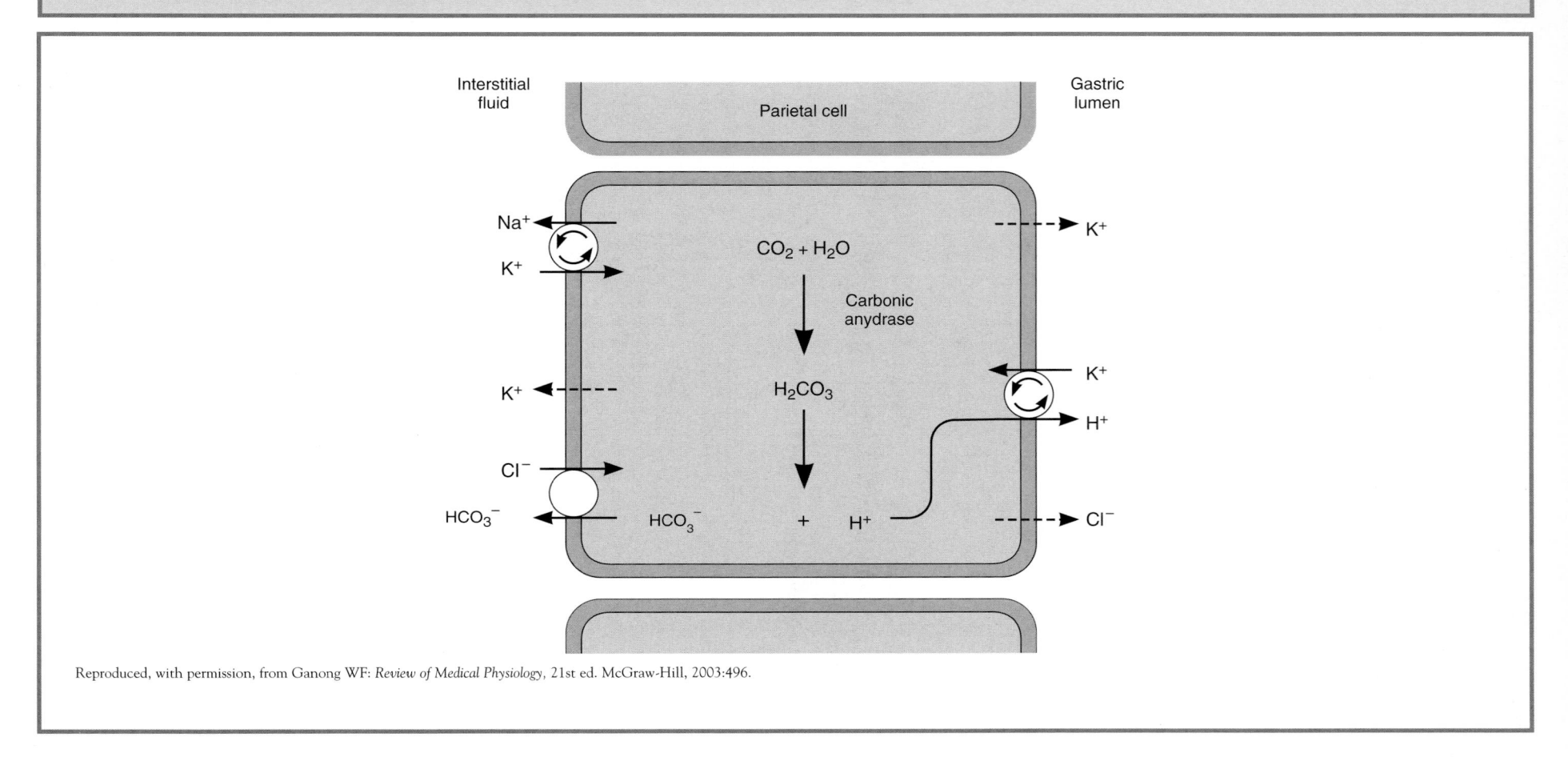

Reproduced, with permission, from Ganong WF: *Review of Medical Physiology*, 21st ed. McGraw-Hill, 2003:496.

MICROANATOMY OF THE INTESTINAL WALLS

Structure[1]	Description
Epithelium	• Single layer of specialized cells that lines lumen. • Varies greatly from one part of GI tract to another.
Lamina Propria	Loose connective tissue containing collagen, elastin, glands, lymph, and capillaries.
Muscularis Mucosae	• Thin, innermost layer of intestinal smooth muscle. • Contractions form characteristic folds and ridges.
Submucosa	Loose connective tissue containing collagen, elastin, glands, larger nerve trunks, and blood vessels.
Muscularis Externa	• Two layers of smooth muscle cells: inner circular and outer longitudinal. • Contractions mix and circulate luminal contents and propel them along GI tract.
Meissner (Submucosal) Plexus	Dense network of nerve cells in submucosa between circular and longitudinal muscle layers.
Enteric Nervous System/Intramural Plexus	• Neural network of GI tract, including submucosal and myenteric plexuses. • Integrates motor and secretory activities. • If GI tract sympathetic and parasympathetic nerves are cut, many motor and secretory activities continue via enteric nervous system.
Serosa/Adventitia	• Outermost layer. • Connective tissue covered with layer of squamous mesothelial cells.

[1]Described from inside to outside.

LAYERS OF THE GASTROINTESTINAL TRACT

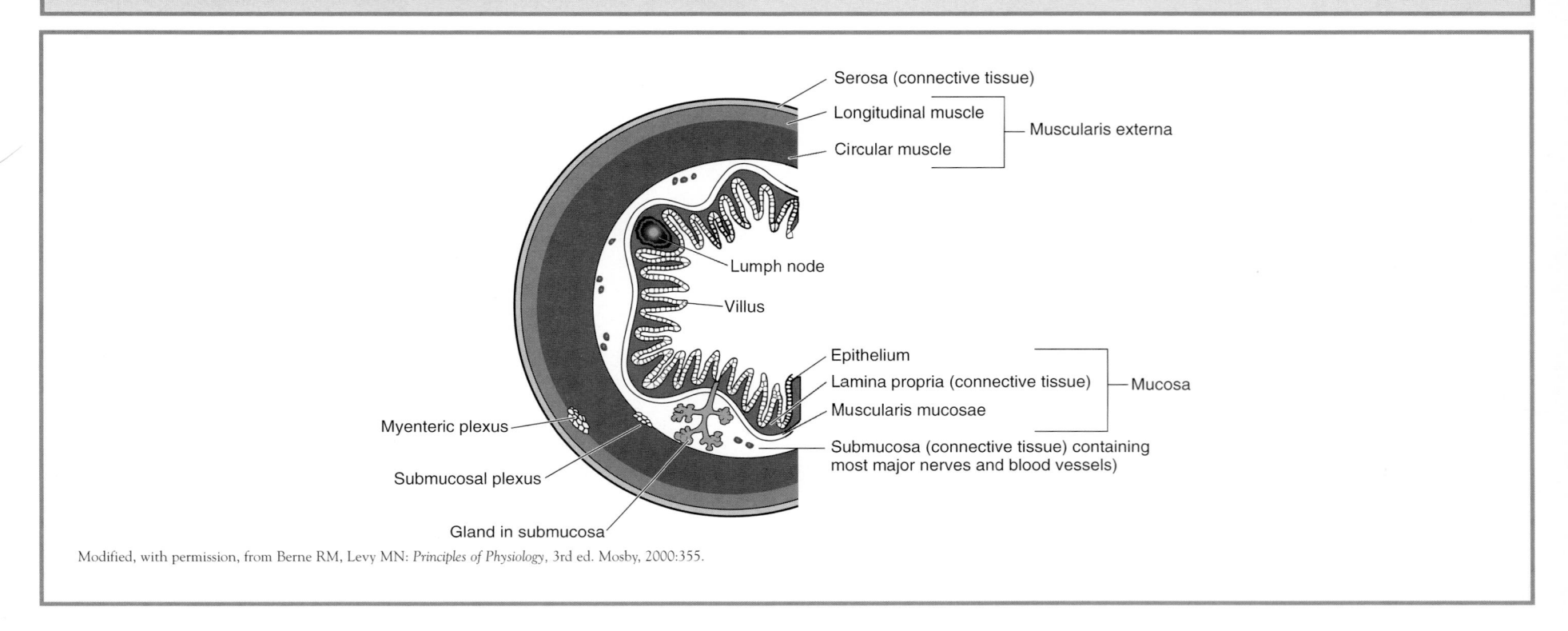

Modified, with permission, from Berne RM, Levy MN: *Principles of Physiology*, 3rd ed. Mosby, 2000:355.

GROSS ANATOMY OF THE GASTROINTESTINAL TRACT

Structure	Description	Function
Esophagus	• Upper one third is striated muscle, lower one third is smooth muscle, middle one third consists of both smooth and striated muscle. • Innervated by vagus nerve. • Includes LES.	• Moves food from pharynx to stomach. • LES separates acidic environment of stomach from esophagus.
Stomach	Upper *fundus* and central *body:* • Thin muscularis externa. • Contracts weakly and food stays unmixed. • Volume can increase up to 1.5 L without great increase in gastric pressure.	Reservoir for food. Contents form layers based on density. • Liquids are emptied rapidly. • Larger particles are retained for longer periods. • Fats form oily top layer and are emptied later.
	Lower antrum: • Thick muscularis externa (thickness increases toward pylorus). • Strong contractions fragment food.	Fragments and mixes food with gastric secretions that acidify and hydrolyze contents, forming chyme.
	Gastric contractions/slow waves: • 3/min. • Start in middle of body (pacemaker zone) and travel toward pylorus, increasing in force and velocity as they approach gastroduodenal junction.	Fasting state: • 90-min quiescence followed by MMC. • MMC is intense cycle of contractions that periodically sweeps from stomach to terminal ileum.
	• Pylorus is sphincter at gastroduodenal junction that separates antrum from duodenal bulb. • Gastric mucosa is resistant to acid but damaged by bile. • Duodenal mucosa is resistant to bile but damaged by acid.	• Gastric contents emptied into duodenum at controlled rate. • Too-rapid gastric emptying leads to duodenal ulcers. • Regurgitation of duodenal contents leads to gastric ulcers.

Continued

GROSS ANATOMY OF THE GASTROINTESTINAL TRACT (Continued)

Structure	Description	Function
Small Intestine	• Three quarters of human GI tract. • Chyme traverses in 2–4 hours.	Digestion and absorption: • Mixes chyme with digestive secretions.
	Duodenum: • First 5%. • 10–12 slow waves/min. • No mesentery. • As antrum contracts, duodenum relaxes.	• Brings chyme into contact with absorptive surface of microvilli. • Propels chyme toward colon.
	Jejunum: • Middle 40%. • 8–9 slow waves/min.	Duodenum also receives pancreatic exocrine secretions and bile from liver via sphincter of Oddi.
	Ileum: • Last 55%. • 8–9 slow waves/min.	
Colon	• Ileocecal sphincter separates terminal ileum from cecum (first part of colon) and is normally closed. • Parts: cecum, ascending colon, transverse colon, descending colon, sigmoid colon, rectum, and anal canal. • Longitudinal muscle layer of muscularis externa is concentrated into bands called taenia coli. • Circular muscle layer is concentrated into haustra. • Anal canal is kept closed by internal and external anal sphincters. • Internal anal sphincter is smooth muscle; external anal sphincter is striated muscle.	• Peristalsis in terminal ileum relaxes sphincter, and chyme slowly enters cecum, allowing colon to absorb most salts and water. • Contractions mix chyme and circulate it across mucosal surface of colon at rate of 5–10 cm/h. • Contractions contribute to back-and-forth mixing of luminal contents. • No further digestion except that performed by bacteria present. • Ions, water, vitamins, and minerals produced by bacteria are absorbed.

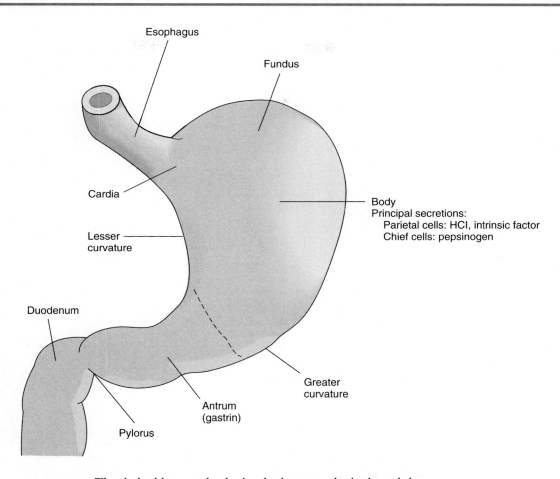

The dashed line marks the border between the body and the antrum.

Modified, with permission, from Ganong WF: *Review of Medical Physiology*, 21st ed. McGraw-Hill, 2003:495.

II. Gastrointestinal Motility

REGULATION OF GASTROINTESTINAL TRACT ACTIVITY

Types of Control	Nervous System	Pathway/Description	Function
Intrinsic: Direct Control	Enteric.	Myenteric and submucosal plexuses connect afferent sensory fibers (from mechanoreceptors and chemoreceptors) with efferent neurons to smooth muscle and secretory cells, creating *local reflex arcs entirely within GI tract.*	• Coordinates GI activities in absence of extrinsic innervation. • Basic electrical rhythm of small intestine is independent of extrinsic innervation.
		Afferent fibers from myenteric and submucosal plexuses also send fibers to CNS, creating central reflex arcs for fine motor control.	*Localized mechanical or chemical stimulation of intestinal mucosa causes contraction above and relaxation below point of stimulation.*
		Stimulatory secretomotor neurons.	Release ACh and VIP onto glands, epithelial cells, and submucous blood vessels.
Extrinsic: Modulatory Control	Sympathetic.	Prevertebral and paravertebral ganglia send postganglionic, adrenergic fibers to celiac, superior, and inferior mesenteric and hypogastric plexuses and then to GI tract. • Superior mesenteric plexus innervates proximal colon. • Inferior mesenteric and superior hypogastric plexuses innervates distal colon. • Inferior hypogastric plexus innervates rectum and anal canal.	*Excitation inhibits motility and secretion,* and increases constriction of pyloric sphincter.
	Parasympathetic	• Vagus nerve innervates from proximal colon to level of transverse colon. • Pelvic nerves from sacral spinal cord innervate distal colon (descending, sigmoid, rectum, anus). • Preganglionic, cholinergic fibers terminate on ganglion cells in intramural plexuses. • Ganglion cells directly innervate smooth muscle and secretory cells.	• *Excitation stimulates motility and secretion.* • Excitatory cholinergic vagal fibers constrict pyloric sphincter, and inhibitory vagal fibers relax it.

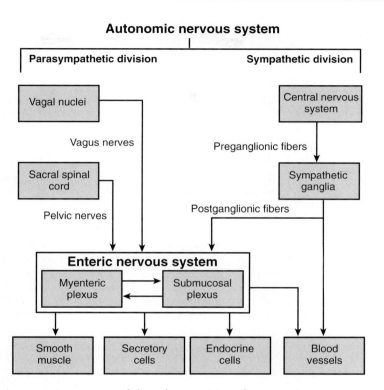

Autonomic nerves modulate the activities of enteric system neurons.

Modified, with permission, from Costa M, Furness JB: *Br Med Bull* 38:247, 1982.

ELECTROPHYSIOLOGY IN GASTROINTESTINAL MOTILITY

Types of Contractions	Description	Functions and Important Points
Slow Waves	• Basis of electrical rhythm of GI tract, initiated by *interstitial cells of Cajal*. • Triphasic wave generated by interstitial cells between longitudinal and circular layers of muscularis externa. • Creates oscillations of resting membrane potential that cause muscle contraction. • Frequency varies from 3/min in stomach to 12/min in duodenum. • Gap junctions enable rapid conduction of slow waves throughout GI tract.	• One or more action potentials may be triggered during peak of slow wave, causing stronger contraction of smooth muscle and major mixing and propulsive movements. • Amplitude and frequency modulated by intrinsic (enteric) and extrinsic (autonomic nervous system) nerves and circulating hormones. • *Sympathetic stimulation decreases amplitude*. • *Parasympathetic stimulation increases amplitude*. • ACh and gastrin stimulate gastric contractility by increasing amplitude and duration of plateau phase of gastric slow wave; norepinephrine has opposite effect.
Segmentation	Closely spaced, rhythmic contractions of circular muscle that divide intestine into small segments and contribute to mixing of chyme.	• Mixes contents more than propels them. • *Low rate of chyme propulsion allows time for digestion and absorption*. • In proximal colon, antipropulsive patterns (reverse peristalsis) retain chyme to facilitate absorption of water and salts.
Peristalsis	• Progressive contraction of successive sections of circular smooth muscle. • Small intestine contracts behind food bolus and relaxes ahead of it.	• Moves intestinal contents in orthograde direction. • Law of intestine: small intestinal contractions propel food bolus orthograde, with integration via enteric nervous system.
MMC	*Intense cycle of contractions that sweeps from stomach to terminal ileum every 90 minutes during fasting state*.	• "Housekeeper of small intestine." • *Inhibits migration of colonic bacteria into terminal ileum and empties contents into colon*.
Mass Movement	Wave of contraction resembling a peristaltic wave that occurs one to three times daily.	Pushes contents of a significant length of colon orthograde.

GASTROINTESTINAL REFLEXES

Reflex	Description	Mechanism
Swallowing	Transfer of food from mouth to esophagus.	Tongue voluntarily forces good bolus into pharynx.
		Swallowing reflex stimulated by pharynx:
		• Epiglottis closes larynx, and soft palate closes nasal passages to prevent reflux of food.
		• UES and LES relax in turn to allow passage of food bolus; they constrict once bolus has passed.
		• Food bolus moves down esophagus by gravity and peristalsis.
Gastroileal	Reflex interaction between stomach and terminal ileum.	Elevated secretory and motor functions of stomach increase motility of terminal ileum and accelerate movement of contents through ileocecal sphincter.
Enterogastric	Inhibitory signals sent from the small intestine to the stomach, slowing gastric secretions and motility.	Products of protein digestion and acid in duodenum and duodenal distention initiate decrease in gastric motility.
Intestinointestinal	Distention or irritation in one segment of intestine inhibits activity in other parts of intestine.	Overdistention of one segment of intestine relaxes smooth muscle in rest of intestine.
Gastrocolic	Food entering empty stomach stimulates intestinal and colonic activity.	Food entering stomach causes reflex increase in motility of colon, frequency of mass movements, and desire to defecate.
Colonocolonic	Distention of one part of colon reflexly relaxes other segments of colon.	• Reflex is mediated by enteric nervous system, modulated by sympathetic fibers. • Coordination of rectum and anal canal important for defecation.
Defecation	Evacuation of feces through rectum and anus.	• Urge to defecate: mass movement fills rectum, causing reflex relaxation of internal anal sphincter and reflex constriction of external anal sphincter. • Evacuation: deep breath, downward movement of diaphragm, closed glottis, contractions of respiratory and abdominal wall muscles, all lead to elevation of intrathoracic and intra-abdominal pressures, which force feces through relaxed internal and external sphincters.

Continued

Reflex	Description	Mechanism
Defecation (Continued)	• Process involves both reflex and voluntary actions. • External anal sphincter innervated by somatic motor fibers via pudendal nerves, which allow it to be controlled reflexively and voluntarily. • Efferent pathways are cholinergic parasympathetic fibers in pelvic nerves (sacral cord is integrating center). • Sympathetic innervation plays no significant role in normal defecation.	
Vomiting	• Reflex expulsion of gastric contents from GI tract via mouth (wave of reverse peristalsis). • Area of control is vomiting center or chemoreceptor trigger zone, located on blood side of blood-brain barrier on floor of fourth ventricle in medulla (in area postrema).	• Forced inspiration against closed glottis decreases intrathoracic pressure. • Lowering of diaphragm and abdominal muscle contraction increase intra-abdominal pressure and drive gastric contents into esophagus, aided by reflex relaxation of UES and stomach. • Entry of vomitus into trachea prevented by approximation of vocal cords, closure of glottis, and inhibition of respiration.

DISORDERS OF GASTROINTESTINAL TRACT MOTILITY

Disorder	Description	Clinical Manifestation(s)	Treatment
Achalasia	Deficient myenteric plexus of distal esophagus results in increased resting LES tone and incomplete relaxation on swallowing.	Accumulation of food in esophagus, which becomes massively dilated.	Pneumatic dilation, myotomy, or botulinum toxin injection.
Blind Loop Syndrome	• Stasis of small intestinal contents leading to bacterial overgrowth. • Stasis usually develops after surgically created blind loops of bowel.	Loss of appetite, nausea, macrocytic anemia, malabsorption of vitamin B_{12}, steatorrhea.	Antibiotics for bacterial overgrowth, vitamin supplementation, surgical repair if needed.
Dumping Syndrome	• Emptying of gastric contents into small intestine faster than can be processed. • Emptying usually occurs after vagotomy.	Diarrhea.	Meals of reduced size and increased frequency.
Gastroesophageal Reflux Disease	Reflux of acidic gastric contents into lower esophagus.	Heartburn; esophagitis; possible ulceration, scarring, and stricture of esophagus.	Medications to decrease acid production, surgery (Nissen fundoplication).
Hirschsprung Disease (Congenital Megacolon)	• Congenital absence of enteric neurons from colon. • Reflex relaxation cannot occur.	Functional obstruction of distal colon and dilation of colon proximal to obstruction.	Removal of abnormal segment of colon.
Paralytic (Adynamic) Ileus	• Decreased intestinal motility due to smooth muscle inhibition. • Occurs as result of peritoneal irritation (eg, abdominal surgery, trauma, infection).	Nausea, vomiting, abdominal distention.	Removal of cause of peritoneal irritation and time. • After abdominal surgery, intestinal peristalsis returns first (6–8 hours). • Gastric peristalsis returns next, and colonic activity returns last (in 2–3 days).

III. Gastrointestinal Secretions

GASTROINTESTINAL HORMONES

Hormone	Location	Stimulated by	Effects on Body
CCK	Upper small intestine.	Amino acids, peptides, fatty acids.	• Stimulates gallbladder contraction and secretion of pancreatic enzymes and insulin. • Enhances action of secretin in stimulating pancreatic bicarbonate secretion and delaying gastric emptying. • Increases contraction of pyloric sphincter. • Stimulates release of glucagon. • Initiates satiety (aided by insulin and leptin).
GIP	Upper small intestine.	Duodenal amino acids, glucose, free fatty acids.	• Inhibits gastric acid secretion, motility, and emptying. • Stimulates insulin secretion by pancreas in presence of hyperglycemia.
Gastrin	Antrum of stomach.	Amino acids, peptides, gastric distention, vagal discharge.	• Stimulates parietal cells to secrete HCl. • Stimulates pepsin secretion. • Stimulates GI mucosal growth and motility. • Relaxes pyloric sphincter. • Stimulates secretion of insulin and other pancreatic enzymes.
Motilin	Stomach, small intestine, colon.	HCO_3^-.	• Produces smooth muscle contraction in stomach and intestine. • Is major regulator of MMC.
Neurotensin	Ileum.	Fatty acids.	• Inhibits motility of stomach and small intestine. • Stimulates colonic peristalsis. • Stimulates pancreatic bicarbonate production.

Pepsin	Stomach.	Acid.	Helps digest proteins.
Secretin	Upper small intestine.	Amino acids, peptides, acid.	• Increases secretion of bicarbonate, pepsin, and bile. • Decreases gastric acid secretion. • Increases contraction of pyloric sphincter and inhibits gastric emptying. • Stimulates pancreatic secretion of insulin and HCO_3^-. • Participates in negative feedback loop with HCO_3^- to inhibit its own secretion.
Somatostatin	Stomach, pancreas.	Gastrin, acid.	• Inhibits secretion of gastrin, CCK, VIP, GIP, secretin, and motilin. • Inhibits pancreatic exocrine function, gastric acid secretion, and gallbladder contraction. • Inhibits absorption of glucose, amino acids, and triglycerides. • Acts as a growth hormone–inhibiting hormone.
Substance P	Small intestine.		Increases motility of small intestine.
VIP	GI tract nerves.		• Inhibits gastric acid secretion. • Relaxes intestinal smooth muscle, including sphincters. • Stimulates intestinal secretion of electrolytes and water. • Increases pancreatic release of HCO_3^- and insulin. • Increases release of glucose from liver.

FEATURES OF SALIVARY AND GASTRIC ACID SECRETIONS

Secretion	Production	Characteristics	Function	Regulation
Saliva	• Produced by submaxillary and sublingual glands (mixed serous and mucous glands). • Produced by parotid glands (largest and entirely serous). • Serous acinar cells release salivary amylase. • Mucous acinar cells secrete mucins into saliva.	• pH during resting state is slightly acidic, and primary secretion is isotonic to plasma. • During active secretion, excretory ducts remove Na^+ and Cl^- and add K^+ and HCO_3^- to primary secretion, making pH near 8 and saliva hypotonic to plasma.	• Lubricates food for swallowing. • Facilitates speaking. • Salivary amylase digests starch into oligosaccharide molecules. • Amylase active at pH 4–11, optimal at pH 7, and stops at pH < 4. • Pancreatic α-amylase digests starch in small intestine.	• Hormonal: increases in ACh, norepinephrine, substance P, and VIP produce increased salivary amylase and flow of saliva. • Sympathetic nervous system activation (via superior cervical ganglion): transiently stimulates salivary secretions and constricts glandular blood vessels. • Parasympathetic nervous system activation (via preganglionic facial and glossopharyngeal nerves): increases secretion of salivary amylase and mucins, and stimulates glandular blood flow, growth, and metabolism. • Interruption of parasympathetic stimulation causes glandular atrophy.
Gastric Acid	• Produced in fundus and body of stomach. • HCl produced by parietal cells.	• During resting state (empty stomach), HCl secreted at low basal rate. • During active state (food present), maximum HCl secretion is 10 times basal rate.	• Digestion of protein through activation of pepsinogens. • Destruction of microorganisms.	• ACh via muscarinic receptors and gastrin via CCK-gastrin receptors increase Ca^{2+}, which increases H^+ secretion. • Histamine via H_2 receptors increases cAMP, which increases H^+ secretion. Self-regulation: • In early gastric emptying with chyme pH > 3, gastric acid secretion is stimulated. • In late gastric emptying with chyme pH < 3, gastric acid secretion is inhibited.

REGULATION OF GASTRIC EMPTYING

Duodenal Contents	Mechanism
Hypertonic Solutions	Duodenum releases unidentified hormone that decreases rate of gastric emptying and HCl secretion by parietal cells.
pH < 3.5	Duodenum releases secretin and bulbogastrone. • Secretin decreases rate of gastric emptying by inhibiting antral contractions and stimulating contraction of pyloric sphincter via neural reflex, which means that acid is not dumped into duodenum more rapidly than it can be neutralized by pancreatic and duodenal secretions. • Secretin also inhibits gastrin and secretion of HCl by parietal cells. • Bulbogastrone also inhibits gastrin and secretion of HCl by parietal cells.
Amino Acids and Peptides	Gastrin released from G cells in antrum and duodenum increases strength of antral contractions and constriction of pyloric sphincter, which decreases rate of gastric emptying.
Fatty Acids/Monoglycerides (products of fat digestion)	• Duodenum and jejunum release CCK and gastric inhibitory peptide, which decreases rate of gastric emptying and inhibits HCl secretion by parietal cells via local nervous reflex. • Fat is not emptied into duodenum at rate faster than that at which it can be emulsified by bile acids and lecithin of bile.

INHIBITION OF GASTRIC EMPTYING BY DUODENAL STIMULI

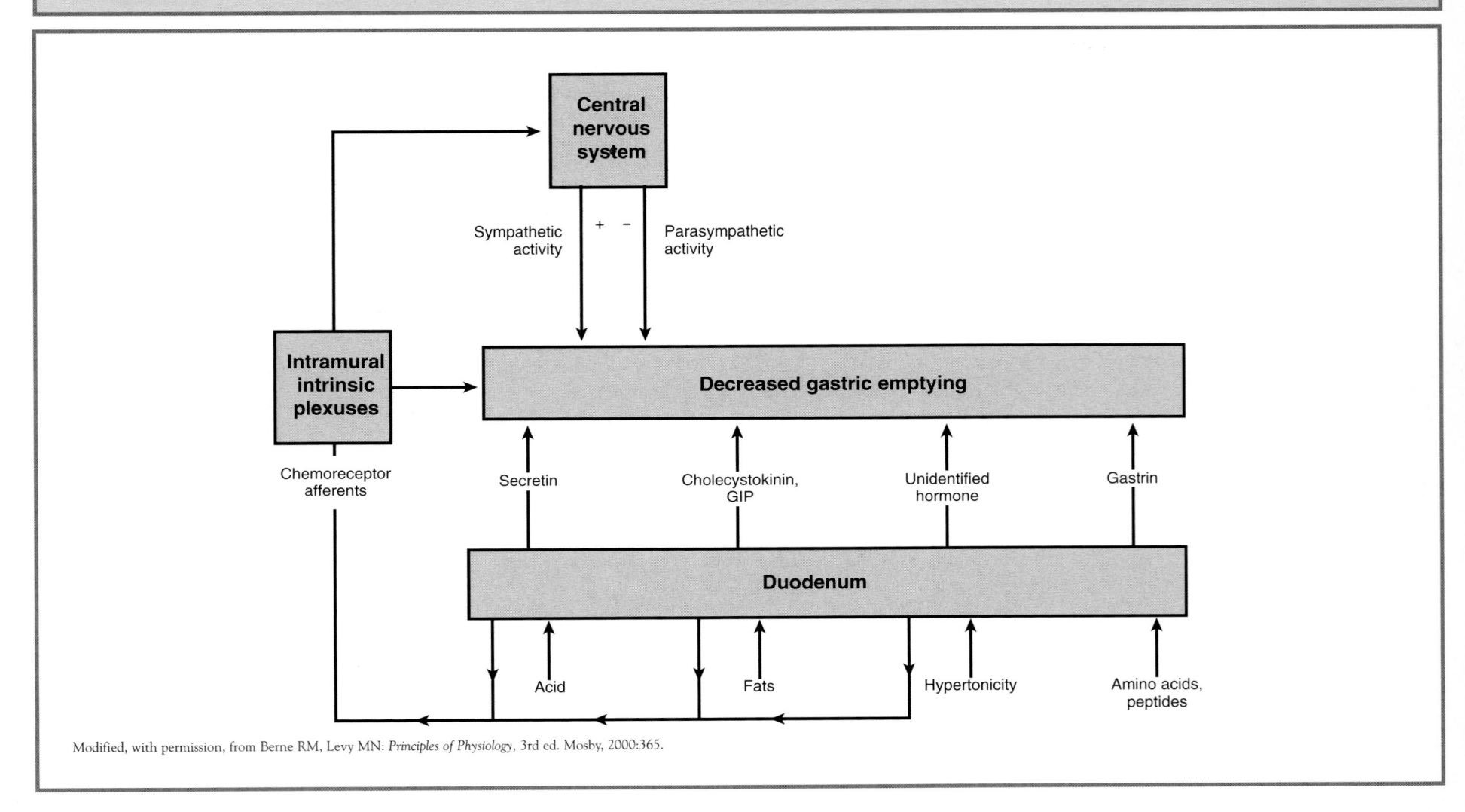

Modified, with permission, from Berne RM, Levy MN: *Principles of Physiology,* 3rd ed. Mosby, 2000:365.

PEPTIC ULCER DISEASE

Ulcer Type	Etiology	Treatment
Gastric	• Caused by decreased effectiveness of gastric mucosal barrier. • Failure of barrier leads to decreased pH at mucosal surface, which inhibits further HCl secretion. • Long-term treatment with NSAIDs *that* decrease rate of mucous and HCO_3^- secretion, and α-agonists (epinephrine) that decrease HCO_3^- secretion. • Both agents may damage mucosal surface, leading to inhibition of further HCl secretion. *Helicobacter pylori infection.*	• Proton-pump inhibitors (omeprazole, lansoprazole, rabeprazole) are often used as first-line treatment; they work by irreversible inhibition of H^+-K^+-ATPase. • H_2-receptor blockers (cimetidine, ranitidine, famotidine) are used to treat non-ulcer dyspepsia; they decrease HCl secretion by decreasing response to elevated gastrin (gastrin stimulates histamine release). • H_2-receptor blockers not as effective in Zollinger-Ellison syndrome; proton-pump inhibitors are current drugs of choice for this disorder. • *H. pylori* in presence of ulcers is treated with antibiotics and drug to suppress HCl secretion (makes *H. pylori* more sensitive to antibiotics). • Proton-pump inhibitors or H_2-receptor antagonists without antibiotics decreases quantity of *H. pylori* and helps ulcer heal; ulcers recur when H_2-blockers are stopped. • Prostaglandins enhance secretion of mucus and HCO_3^- and help protect gastric epithelial surface; therefore, those with ulcers should stop use of NSAIDs.
Duodenal	Often caused by hypersecretion of gastric acid as result of decreased sensitivity of mechanisms that inhibit HCl secretion. Zollinger-Ellison syndrome: gastrin-secreting tumors cause high gastrin levels, which lead to increased secretion of HCl and formation of duodenal ulcers. *H. pylori* infection.	

STRUCTURE, FUNCTION, AND REGULATION OF THE EXOCRINE PANCREAS

Structure	Description	Function	Regulation
Acinar Cells	Polygonal cells organized into lobules that surround blind-ended ducts.	Secrete enzyme component of pancreatic juice, which is important for food digestion.	• Parasympathetic vagal fibers, ACh, CCK, gastrin, substance P, secretin and VIP stimulate pancreatic juice secretion.
Duct System	Drainage pathway: intercalated ducts → acini → intralobular ducts → single extralobular duct from one lobule → larger ducts that converge into a main duct that enters duodenum with common bile duct.	Ductular epithelial cells secrete aqueous component of pancreatic juice.	• CCK stimulates secretion of pancreatic enzymes. • Secretin stimulates secretion of aqueous component. • Sympathetic stimulation from celiac and superior mesenteric plexuses inhibits pancreatic blood flow and enzyme secretion.

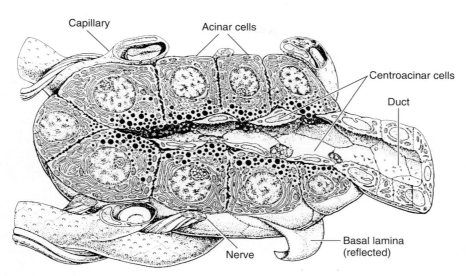

Reproduced, with permission, from Krstic RV: *Die Gewebe des Menschen und der Säaugetiere*. Springer, 1978.

COMPONENTS OF PANCREATIC JUICE

Component	Description	Mechanism of Action/Function
Aqueous	• Rich in HCO_3^-. • Secretion stimulated by secretin.	Neutralizes duodenal contents.
Enzyme	α-amylase (pancreatic amylase) secreted in active form.	Digests carbohydrates; cleaves starch molecules into oligosaccharides.
	Lipases: triacylglycerol hydrolase, cholesterol ester hydrolase, phospholipase A_2.	Digest lipids.
	Proteases are secreted in inactive zymogen forms: trypsinogen, chymotrypsinogen, and procarboxypeptidase.	• Enteropeptidase (also known as enterokinase) from duodenal mucosa initiates activation of trypsinogen, synthesizing trypsin. • Trypsin then activates trypsinogen (autocatalytic reaction), chymotrypsinogen, and procarboxypeptidase.
	Trypsin inhibitor.	Prevents premature activation of proteolytic enzymes in pancreatic ducts.
	Secretion stimulated by CCK.	
	Absence of pancreatic juice causes malabsorption of carbohydrates, fats, and proteins.	
Ions	Na^+, K^+, Cl^-, HCO_3^-.	• Aqueous component is initially hypertonic, with high HCO_3^-. • As pancreatic juice flows down ducts, equilibration with H_2O and HCO_3^- exchange for Cl^- makes it isotonic with plasma.

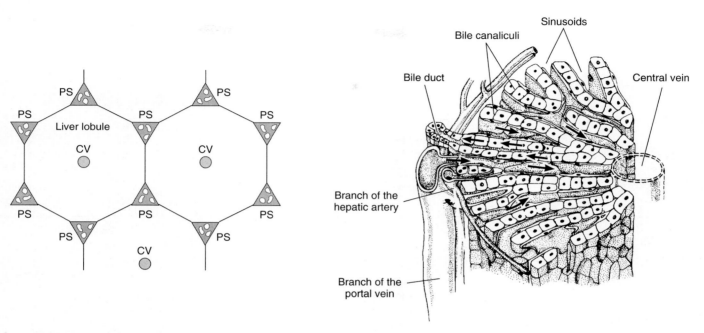

The hepatic lobule is organized around a central vein. Blood from portal vein and hepatic artery enters sinusoids at lobule periphery and flows toward center. Hepatocytes are in direct contact with sinusoidal blood via fenestrations between endothelial cells lining sinusoids, enabling liver to effectively clear blood of various compounds. Kupffer cells act as hepatic macrophages. Biliary canaliculi lie between adjacent hepatocytes and drain into bile ducts at periphery of lobule.

Reproduced, with permission, from Fawcett DW: *Bloom and Fawcett, A Textbook of Histology*, 11th ed. Saunders, 1986.

FUNCTIONS OF THE LIVER

Function	Example(s)	Clinical Significance
Metabolism of Carbohydrates, Lipids, Proteins, and Other Substances	Glycogenolysis and gluconeogenesis.	• Body's response to low blood glucose.
	Oxidation of fatty acids, producing ketone bodies (acetoacetate, β-hydroxybutyrate, and acetone).	• In diabetes, β-oxidation of fatty acids is a major energy source for body. • Levels of ketone bodies in urine and blood indicate severity of diabetic acidosis.
	Synthesizes and secretes VLDL.	VLDL is converted to other types of lipoproteins, which serve as major sources of cholesterol and triglycerides for other body tissues.
	Deaminates amino acids, leading to formation of ammonia.	• Most tissues cannot metabolize ammonia. • Liver converts ammonia to urea, preventing ammonia toxicity.
	Synthesis of nonessential amino acids and major plasma proteins.	Includes albumins, fibrinogens, globulins, lipoproteins, and blood clotting factors.
Storage of Glycogen, Vitamins, and Minerals	Glycogen storage.	Body's response to high blood glucose.
	Storage of vitamins A, D, vitamin B_{12}, and iron.	Most important storage site for iron next to hemoglobin.
Inactivation or Excretion of Hormones, Drugs, and Toxins	• Liver converts these substances into inactive forms by conjugating them with glucuronic acid or its sulfate in smooth endoplasmic reticulum. • Substances are then excreted in bile or by kidneys.	Liver helps rid body of toxic substances.

COMPONENTS OF BILE

Component	Metabolism/Functions
Bile Acids	• Bile salts (conjugated bile acids) emulsify duodenal fats into fatty acids and glycerol for easier digestion by pancreatic lipase. • Bile acids form micelles with products of lipid digestion, leading to enhanced epithelial cell absorption of lipids. • Drugs that inhibit reabsorption of bile acids in ileum promote synthesis of new bile acids from cholesterol and are used to lower level of cholesterol in blood.
Cholesterol	• Bile excretion via feces is major route of cholesterol excretion. • If more cholesterol is present in bile than can be solubilized in micelles, cholesterol gallstones are formed.
Phospholipids	• Lecithin and cholesterol are insoluble in water but dissolve in bile acid micelles. • Lecithin increases amount of cholesterol that can be solubilized in micelles.
Bile Pigments	Formed from porphyrin catabolism: • Senescent red blood cells are degraded in reticuloendothelial system. • Heme is converted to bilirubin. • Most biliverdin is converted to bilirubin. • Hepatocytes remove bilirubin from blood in sinusoids and conjugate it with glucuronic acid. • Conjugated bilirubin (bilirubin glucuronides) is soluble and is secreted into bile. Major component of bile pigment gallstones is insoluble calcium salt of unconjugated bilirubin. • Liver disease is associated with high levels of unconjugated bilirubin and increased likelihood of bile pigment stones.

BILE PATHWAY

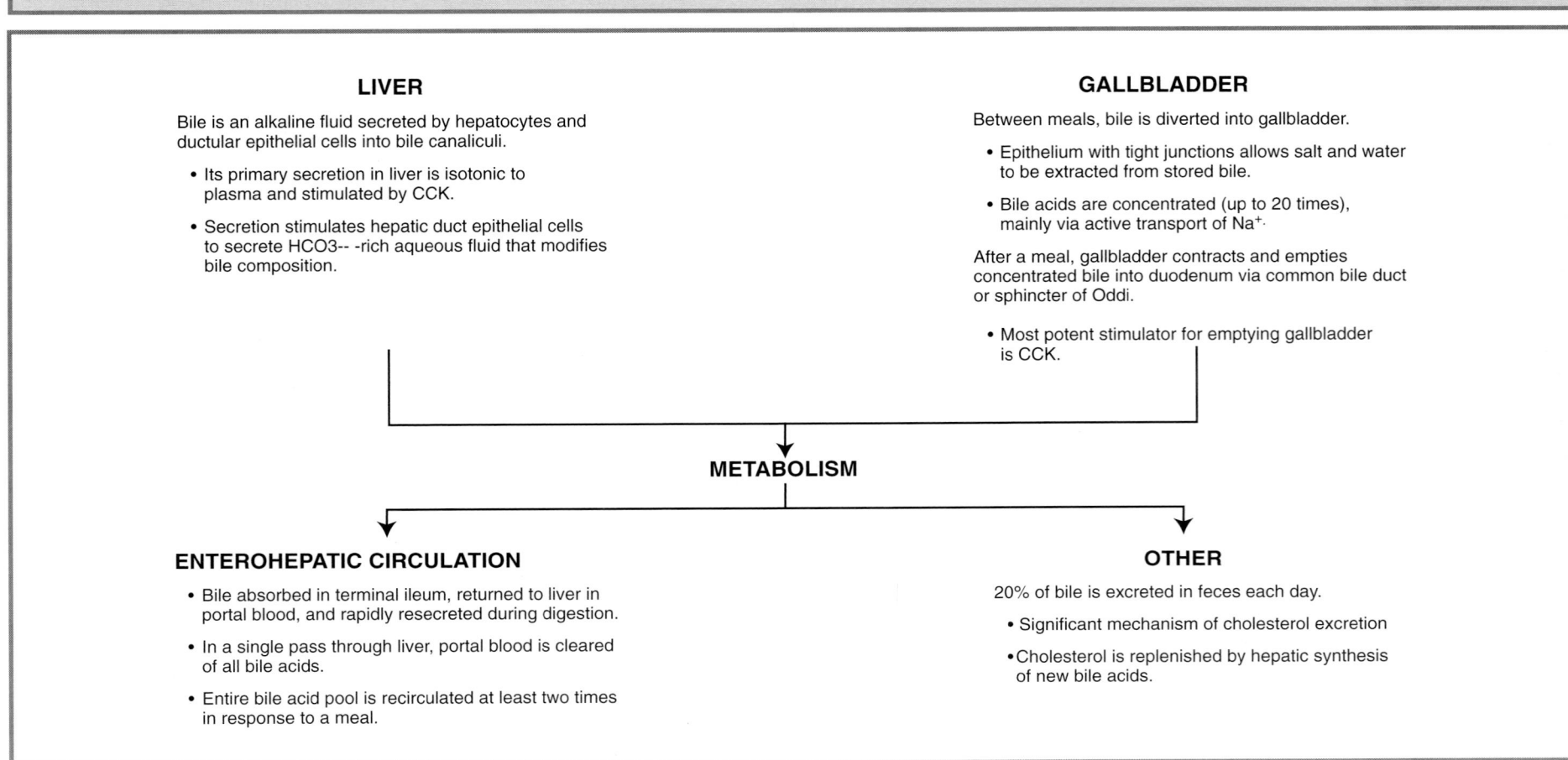

LIVER

Bile is an alkaline fluid secreted by hepatocytes and ductular epithelial cells into bile canaliculi.

- Its primary secretion in liver is isotonic to plasma and stimulated by CCK.

- Secretion stimulates hepatic duct epithelial cells to secrete HCO3-- -rich aqueous fluid that modifies bile composition.

GALLBLADDER

Between meals, bile is diverted into gallbladder.

- Epithelium with tight junctions allows salt and water to be extracted from stored bile.

- Bile acids are concentrated (up to 20 times), mainly via active transport of Na^+.

After a meal, gallbladder contracts and empties concentrated bile into duodenum via common bile duct or sphincter of Oddi.

- Most potent stimulator for emptying gallbladder is CCK.

METABOLISM

ENTEROHEPATIC CIRCULATION

- Bile absorbed in terminal ileum, returned to liver in portal blood, and rapidly resecreted during digestion.

- In a single pass through liver, portal blood is cleared of all bile acids.

- Entire bile acid pool is recirculated at least two times in response to a meal.

OTHER

20% of bile is excreted in feces each day.

- Significant mechanism of cholesterol excretion

- Cholesterol is replenished by hepatic synthesis of new bile acids.

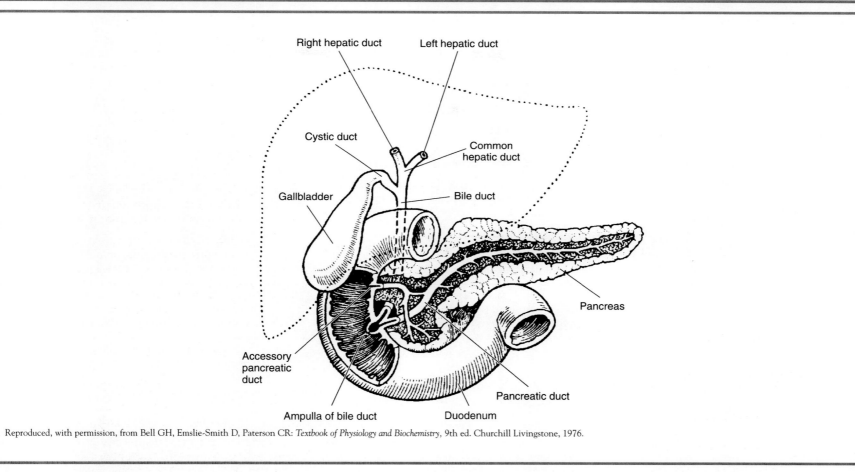

Right hepatic duct

Left hepatic duct

Cystic duct

Common hepatic duct

Gallbladder

Bile duct

Pancreas

Accessory pancreatic duct

Ampulla of bile duct

Duodenum

Pancreatic duct

Reproduced, with permission, from Bell GH, Emslie-Smith D, Paterson CR: *Textbook of Physiology and Biochemistry*, 9th ed. Churchill Livingstone, 1976.

FUNCTIONS OF STOMACH, EXOCRINE PANCREAS, AND GALLBLADDER IN DIGESTION

Phase	Stomach	Exocrine Pancreas	Gallbladder
Celiac	Sight, smell, and taste of food, chewing, and swallowing stimulate release of ACh from vagal fibers, which stimulates: • Parietal cells to secrete HCl. • G cells in antrum and duodenum to release gastrin. • Enterochromaffin-like cells in gastric mucosa to release histamine.	Vagal stimulation causes release of gastrin released from gastric antrum, which stimulates secretion of pancreatic juice.	• Vagal (parasympathetic, cholinergic) innervation and gastrin release mediate contraction and relaxation of sphincter of Oddi. • Stimulation of sympathetic nerves inhibits emptying of gallbladder.
Gastric	Stomach distention stimulates release of ACh, which stimulates parietal cells to secrete HCl and G cells to secrete gastrin.	Gastrin released in response to stomach distention, amino acids, and peptides, and neural reflexes stimulates secretion of pancreatic juice.	
Intestinal	• Protein digestion products in duodenum stimulate intestinal G cells with gastrin to stimulate parietal cells. • Intestinal endocrine cells stimulate parietal cells via entero-oxyntin.	• Greatest volume of pancreatic secretion. • Peptides, amino acids, fats and monoglycerides in duodenum stimulate secretion of pancreatic juice. • *CCK released from duodenum in response to digestion products is most important physiological mediator of enzyme component of pancreatic juice.* • CCK potentiates stimulatory effect of secretin on pancreatic ducts. • Secretin potentiates effect of CCK on acinar cells. • *Acid in duodenum causes release of secretin, which stimulates secretion of pancreatic juice rich in aqueous component and low in enzymes.*	• Highest rate of gallbladder emptying. • Emptying is stimulated by CCK, which causes gallbladder contraction and relaxation of sphincter of Oddi.

For the three phases of gastrointestinal acid secretion, think "Come and Get It": Celiac, Gastric, and Intestinal.

IV. Digestion and Absorption

DIGESTION AND ABSORPTION OF CARBOHYDRATES

Site	Mechanism	Products
Mouth and Salivary Glands	• Salivary amylase catalyzes hydrolysis of linear α-1,4 links (not branching α-1,6 links). • Salivary amylase not required for normal digestion and absorption of starch due to presence of pancreatic α-amylase, which is inactivated by low gastric pH.	Maltose, maltotriose, α-limit dextrins.
Pancreas	• α-Amylase activity in pancreas is greater than in saliva. • Within 10 minutes after entering duodenum, starch is entirely converted to oligosaccharides.	Maltose, maltotriose, α-limit dextrins.
Small Intestine	Oligosaccharides digested further via enzymes (eg, lactase, sucrase, isomaltase, and glucoamylase) in brush border membrane of duodenal and jejunal epithelium. • Enzyme activity highest at brush border of upper jejunum and declines gradually through rest of small intestine Duodenum and upper jejunum have highest capacity for absorbing sugars. • Na^+ in intestinal lumen enhances absorption of glucose and galactose and vice versa. • Fructose also transported but via different transporter.	• Lactose breaks down into glucose and galactose. • Sucrose breaks down into glucose and fructose. • α-Dextrinase cleaves α-1,6 branching points of starch, and glucoamylase cleaves terminal α-1,4 glycosidic bonds to break malto-oligosaccharides down to glucose units.
Colon	• Carbohydrate absorption normally does not occur. • If lactase is not present in small intestine, undigested lactose is metabolized by colonic bacteria that produce gas and release metabolic products that increase colonic motility, causing diarrhea.	

GLUCOSE TRANSPORT IN THE INTESTINE

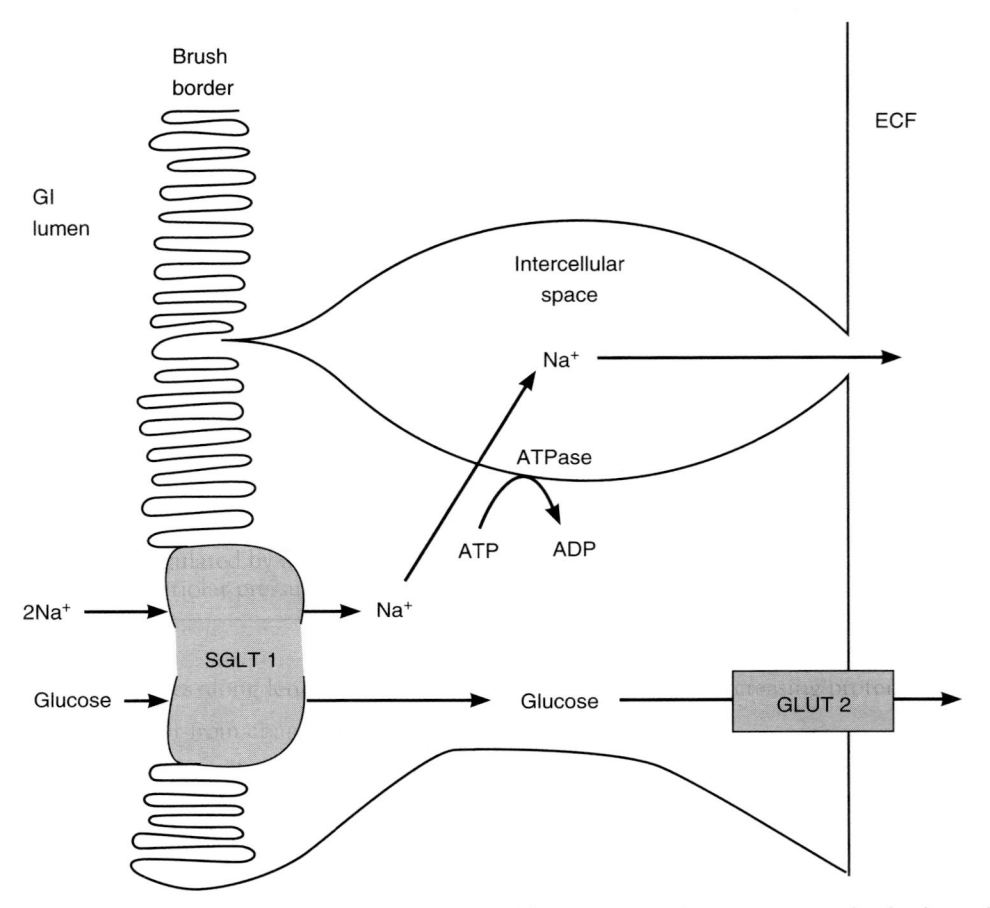

Glucose transport into intestinal cells is coupled to Na⁺ via SGLT 1 cotransporter. Glucose enters the interstitium by facilitated diffusion via GLUT 2, and then it diffuses into the blood. Na⁺ is actively transported out of the cell. ECF = extracellular fluid.

Reproduced, with permission, from Ganong WF: *Review of Medical Physiology*, 21st ed. McGraw-Hill, 2003:475.

DIGESTION AND ABSORPTION OF PROTEINS

Site	Mechanism	Products
Stomach	Chief cells secrete pepsinogens, which are converted in acid environment to active pepsins.	• Small peptides. • Single amino acids.
Small intestine	• 50% of ingested protein is digested and absorbed in duodenum. • Duodenum and upper jejunum contain peptidases that are integral membrane proteins. • Capacity is high enough that protein digestion in total absence of pepsins does not impair digestive process. • Essentially all ingested protein is digested and absorbed by time chyme has reached midjejunum.	
Pancreas	• Proteases (trypsin, chymotrypsin, carboxypeptidase) are active in duodenum. • Products of protein digestion are transported across brush border membrane into cytosol of intestinal epithelial cells, where they are hydrolyzed by peptidases, thus only single amino acids appear in portal blood.	

DIGESTION AND ABSORPTION OF LIPIDS

Site	Mechanism	Products
Mouth and Stomach	• Water insolubility of lipids separates them into oily phase and they are emptied from stomach later than other gastric contents. • Gastric lipase secreted by chief cells combines with lingual lipase produced by serous glands in tongue to produce preduodenal lipase. • Preduodenal lipase hydrolyzes triglycerides.	Glycerol and free fatty acids.
Small Intestine	• Absorption of lipid digestion products occurs in small intestine. • Emulsification: products of lipid digestion and fat soluble vitamins (A, D, E, K) combine with bile acids to form micelles.	Micelles.
	Micelles diffuse among microvilli and allow absorption of lipids along brush border into epithelial cells where they are processed by smooth endoplasmic reticulum into chylomicrons.	Chylomicrons.
	• Resulting chylomicrons are ejected from epithelial cells by exocytosis, and enter venous circulation via thoracic duct. • Terminal ileum absorbs bile acids.	Glycerol and free fatty acids.
Colon	• Ingested fat is completely absorbed. • Fat present in normal stool is from colonic bacteria and exfoliated intestinal epithelial cells.	None.
Pancreas	• Pancreatic lipase, cholesterol esterase, and phospholipase A_2 hydrolyze lipids. • Water-soluble pancreatic lipases access lipids at surfaces of fat droplets; *the surface available for digestion is increased by emulsification.* • Bile acids emulsify fats with aid of lecithins, thus aiding in digestion of fat droplets.	Glycerol and free fatty acids.
	Cystic fibrosis: • Autosomal recessive disorder. • Defective Cl⁻ channels make cells unable to secrete Cl⁻, Na⁺, and water into acinar lumen. • Resulting mucus obstructs pancreatic ducts and destroys pancreatic acinar cells. • Destruction of pancreatic cells causes deficiency of pancreatic enzymes, leading to poor lipid digestion, steatorrhea and malnutrition.	None.

WATER AND ELECTROLYTES IN DIGESTION AND ABSORPTION

Segment of Intestine	Electrolytes Absorbed	Electrolytes Secreted	Water Absorption
Duodenum and Jejunum	• Na^+ actively absorbed. • Cl^- passively absorbed. • K^+ passively concentrated by H_2O absorption; elevated $[K^+]$ drives net absorption of K^+. • HCO_3^- (via $CO_2 + H_2O$).	None.	• Highly permeable to water and ions. • "Loose tight junctions" allow large fluxes of water between lumen and blood (usually net flux from blood to lumen due to hypertonicity of chyme). • Intestinal permeability to water decreases as approach colon.
Ileum	• Na^+ actively absorbed. • Cl^- actively absorbed in exchange for HCO_3^-. • K^+ passively concentrated by H_2O absorption. • Elevated $[K^+]$ drives net absorption of K^+.	• HCO_3^- partly in exchange for Cl^-. • If $[HCO_3^-]$ in lumen > 45 mM, net absorption occurs.	• Lowest permeability to water of all intestinal segments. • *By time substances reach terminal ileum, 90–95% of H_2O in GI tract has been absorbed.*
Colon	• Na^+ actively absorbed ($[K^+]$ in lumen > 25 mM leads to net absorption). • Cl^- actively absorbed in exchange for HCO_3^-. • K^+ passively concentrated by H_2O absorption. • Elevated $[K^+]$ drives net absorption of K^+.	If $[K^+]$ in lumen < 25 mM, there is net secretion of HCO_3^-, partly in exchange for Cl^-.	Small net absorption of water (1–2 L/d).

GASTROINTESTINAL FLUID BALANCE

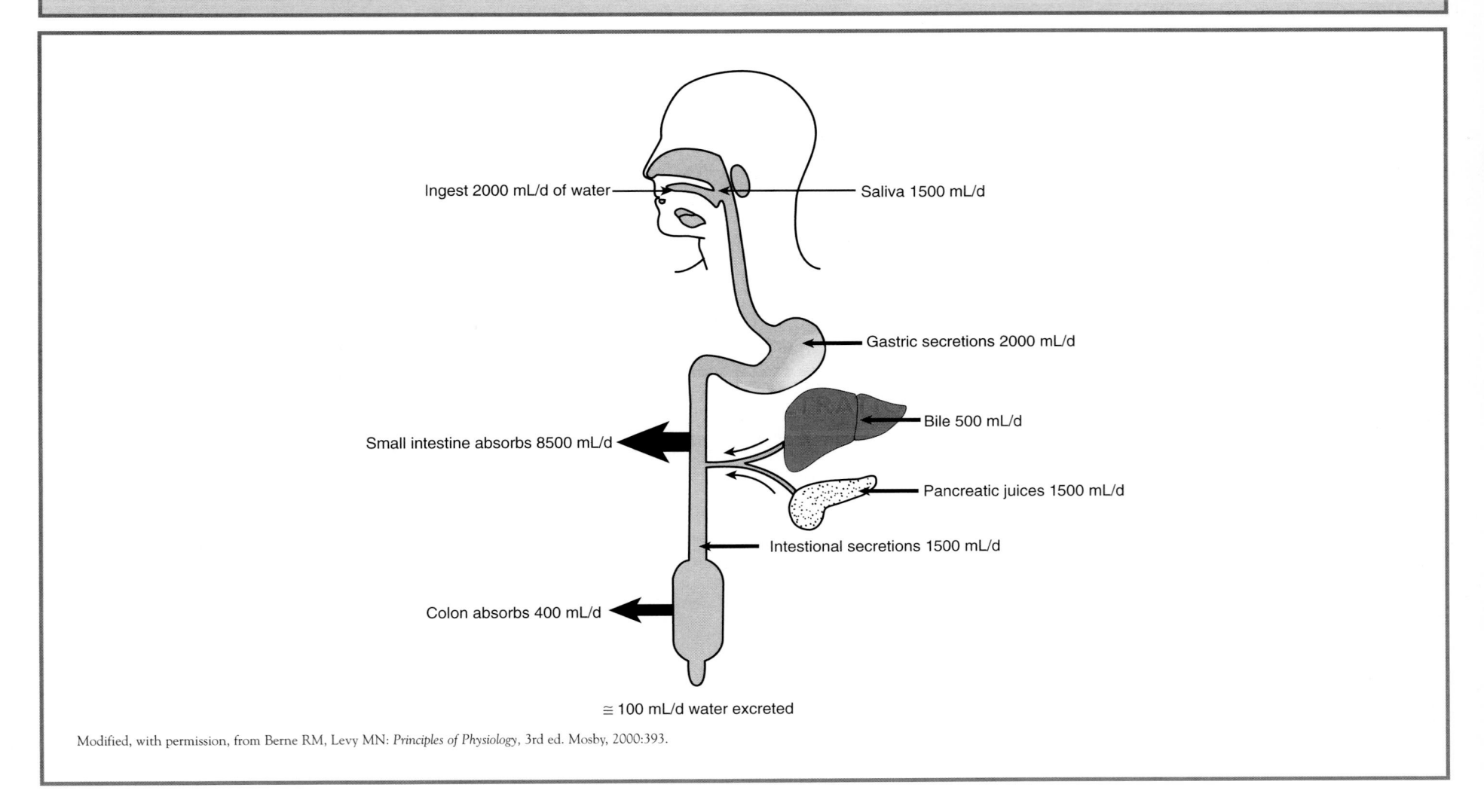

Ingest 2000 mL/d of water — Saliva 1500 mL/d

Gastric secretions 2000 mL/d

Bile 500 mL/d

Small intestine absorbs 8500 mL/d

Pancreatic juices 1500 mL/d

Intestional secretions 1500 mL/d

Colon absorbs 400 mL/d

≅ 100 mL/d water excreted

Modified, with permission, from Berne RM, Levy MN: *Principles of Physiology*, 3rd ed. Mosby, 2000:393.

IMPORTANT CONCEPTS IN INTESTINAL ABSORPTION OF WATER AND IONS

Stimulation of Water and Ion Absorption	Clinical Significance
Active absorption of Na^+ enhanced by sugars and neutral amino acids (and vice versa).	• Rehydration therapy promotes absorption of glucose, salt, and water. • Helps counteract secretory fluxes of salt and water in cholera and other secretory diarrheas.
Absorption of H_2O creates gradient favoring absorption of K^+, leading to high $[K^+]$ in lumen.	Diarrhea may lead to hypokalemia.
Net water absorption is powered by absorption of solutes from intestine (especially Na^+ and Cl^-) and occurs in small intestine in absence of significant osmotic pressure gradient.	Basis for osmotic laxatives (eg, magnesium sulfate): • Substances that cannot be absorbed in intestine will prevent an iso-osmotic equivalent of water from being absorbed. • Likewise, when nutrients are poorly absorbed (eg, lactose intolerance), osmotic effect of unabsorbed nutrient contributes to diarrhea.
• Stimulation of sympathetic nerves/elevated epinephrine levels increases absorption of Na^+, Cl^-, and H_2O. • Stimulation of parasympathetic nerves decreases ion and water absorption.	Stimulation of sympathetic nervous system during exercise or other stress increases availability of water and electrolytes to body.
Adrenal cortical hormones stimulate absorption of electrolytes and water: • Aldosterone increases K^+ secretion and Na^+ and H_2O absorption by ileum and colon (and by distal renal tubules). • Glucocorticoids increase K^+ secretion and Na^+ and H_2O absorption in colon.	Stimulation of renin-angiotensin-aldosterone system in setting of dehydration, hemorrhage, or hypotension.

DIGESTION AND ABSORPTION OF SELECTED SUBSTANCES

General Concepts	Mechanism of Absorption	Clinical Significance
Vitamin B$_{12}$		
• Vitamin B$_{12}$ is found in food bound to proteins. • *Normal absorption of B$_{12}$ requires intrinsic factor, a vitamin B$_{12}$-binding protein secreted by gastric parietal cells.*	• Low pH of stomach and digestion of proteins by pepsins release free B$_{12}$, which is then bound to R proteins in saliva and gastric juice. • Pancreatic proteases degrade R protein-B$_{12}$ complex, freeing vitamin B$_{12}$, which is taken up by intrinsic factor and becomes highly resistant to digestion. • Receptor proteins on brush border of ileal epithelium bind intrinsic factor–B$_{12}$ complex, leading to B$_{12}$ absorption. • Enteric bacteria synthesize B$_{12}$ and other B vitamins, but colonic epithelium lacks specific mechanism for their absorption.	• Impaired intestinal absorption of B$_{12}$ due to either dietary deficiency of B$_{12}$ or failure of parietal cells to produce intrinsic factor causes *pernicious anemia.* • Destruction of parietal cells is caused by autoimmune disorders or chronic bacterial infections. • Signs and symptoms of pernicious anemia include defective red blood cells; atrophy of gastric glands; defective gastric secretion of HCl, pepsins, and intrinsic factor; and chronically elevated gastrin. • Vitamin B$_{12}$ injections are used to treat pernicious anemia.
Iron		
• Duodenal epithelial cells are mainly responsible for absorption of nonheme iron. • Food inhibits iron absorption: iron tends to form insoluble salts with anions and insoluble complexes in food. • HCl secreted by stomach enhances iron absorption by making these complexes more soluble.	• Transport proteins in duodenal brush border bind ferrous iron (Fe^{2+}) (*not ferric iron, Fe^{3+}*). • Fe^{2+} is transported into duodenal epithelial cells bound to mobilferrin in cytosol, which helps it to diffuse through cytosol. • Fe^{2+} is then moved to transferrin on extracellular surface of basolateral membrane. • Fe^{2+}-transferrin complex is released to extracellular fluid and diffuses into blood.	• Iron absorption regulated according to body's needs. • Capacity of duodenum and jejunum to absorb iron increased in chronic iron deficiency, hemorrhage, growing children, pregnant women. • Vitamin C promotes iron absorption by forming soluble complexes with it and by reducing Fe^{3+} to the more soluble Fe^{2+}. • *Vitamin C should be taken with iron tablets.*

- Irreversible binding of iron to ferritin prevents excess iron absorption.

- This bound iron not available for transport into plasma and is excreted in feces.

- Synthesis of apoferritin is stimulated by iron, which protects against absorption of excessive amounts of iron.

Calcium

Absorption stimulated by vitamin D and parathyroid hormone.	Actively absorbed in all segments of intestine, especially duodenum and jejunum.	• Vitamin D deficiency causes rickets in which low Ca^{2+} absorption causes abnormal bone growth. • Bones are soft and flexible; patients may be "bowlegged."

CHAPTER 6
RENAL SYSTEM

IV. RENAL REGULATION

V. ACID-BASE RELATIONSHIPS

ABBREVIATIONS

ACE = angiotensin-converting enzyme

ACTH = adrenocorticotropic hormone

ADH = antidiuretic hormone

ANP = atrial natriuretic peptide

ATN = acute tubular necrosis

Cl_{CR} = creatinine clearance

ECF = extracellular fluid

FE_{Na} = fractional excretion of sodium

FF = filtration fraction

GFR = glomerular filtration rate

GI = gastrointestinal

ICF = intracellular fluid

JGA = juxtaglomerular apparatus

NAE = net acid excretion

P_i = inorganic phosphate

PTH = parathyroid hormone

RAAS = renin-angiotensin aldosterone system

RBC = red blood cell

RBF = renal blood flow

RFI = renal failure index

RPF = renal plasma flow

SIADH = syndrome of inappropriate secretion of antidiuretic hormone

SLE = systemic lupus erythematosus

WBC = white blood cell

TERMS TO LEARN

Term	Definition
Acidosis	State in which the acidity of body fluids and tissues is abnormally high and arterial pH is < 7.40.
Alkalosis	State in which the alkalinity of body fluids and tissues is abnormally high and arterial pH is > 7.40.
Antiporter	Protein transporter that exchanges one substance for another across cell membranes.
Autoregulation	Maintenance of RBF and GFR at a relatively constant level by kidneys, which adjust vascular resistance via afferent arterioles in response to changes in arterial pressure of 90–180 mm Hg.
Carbonic Anhydrase	Enzyme present in brush border of proximal tubule that catalyzes dehydration of H_2CO_3 in luminal fluid, facilitating resorption of HCO_3^-.
Countercurrent Flow	Describes the flow of fluid in nephron loops; two parallel limbs of tubular fluid flow in opposite directions.
Euvolemia	Normal volume; with respect to physiology, renal NaCl excretion equals dietary NaCl intake.
Glomerulotubular Balance	Mechanism in euvolemic state in which Na^+ resorption changes in parallel with GFR and filtered load of Na^+. This results in resorption of a constant fraction of filtered Na^+ and water from proximal tubule despite variations in GFR and ensures that spontaneous changes in GFR do not alter Na^+ balance.
Hemolytic Uremic Syndrome	Disorder in which sudden, rapid destruction of RBCs obstructs small renal arteries, leading to acute renal failure; occurs as a result of eclampsia, drug reaction, gastroenteritis, or septicemia.
Metabolic Acid-Base Disorder	Disturbance of acid-base balance that results from a change in $[HCO_3^-]$ of ECF; kidneys are primarily responsible for regulating $[HCO_3^-]$.
Micturition	Process of emptying the urinary bladder.
NAE (Net Acid Excretion)	Renal resorption of filtered load of HCO_3^- and renal excretion; an amount of acid equal to the amount of nonvolatile acid produced each day.
Nonvolatile Acid	Acid not derived directly from hydration of CO_2 (eg, lactic acid).
Osmotic Diuresis	Increased excretion of water and solutes (including Na^+) in urine due to decreased water resorption in proximal tubule. Compare with water diuresis.
Respiratory Acid-Base Disorder	Disturbance of acid-base balance that results from a change in P_{CO_2}; lungs are primarily responsible for regulating P_{CO_2}.

Symporter	Protein transporter that requires binding of more than one substance; bound substances are transported across cell membranes together.
Ultrafiltration	Filtration under pressure; first step in urine formation is ultrafiltration of plasma by glomerulus.
Volatile Acid	Acid that has potential to generate H^+ after hydration with H_2O (eg, CO_2).
Water Diuresis	Increased excretion of water in urine; amount of water resorbed in proximal tubule is normal. Compare with osmotic diuresis.

I. Introduction

RENAL FUNCTION

Function	Description	Examples
Regulatory	Regulates volume and composition of body fluids.	• *Major function of kidneys is resorption of NaCl and water.* • Acid-base balance (coordinated action of lungs, liver, and kidneys). • Body fluid osmolality (important to maintain normal cell volume in tissues). • Electrolyte balance (regulates Na^+, K^+, Cl^-, HCO_3^-, H^+, Ca^{2+} and P_i).
Excretory	• Excretes water and solutes. • Rids body of excess water and waste.	Excretes such end products of metabolism as urea (from amino acids), uric acid (from nucleic acids), and creatinine (from muscle creatine).
Endocrine	Produces and secretes hormones.	Renin: activates RAAS that helps regulate blood pressure and Na^+ and K^+ balance. Erythropoietin (85% made in kidneys, 15% in liver): • Stimulates RBC formation by bone marrow. • Decreased production causes anemia seen in chronic renal failure. • Stimulated by hypoxia, hemorrhage, adenosine, and catecholamines. • Inhibited by theophylline. Calcitriol (active metabolite of vitamin D_3): needed for normal resorption of Ca^{2+} by GI tract and for Ca^{2+} deposition in bone.

MOVEMENT OF TUBULAR FLUID

Process	Description	Steps in Urine Formation
Filtration	Passage of water and solutes through glomerular capillary membranes into renal tubule with aid of hydrostatic pressure.	1. Ultrafiltration of plasma by glomerulus.
Resorption	Movement of water and solutes from epithelial cell mucosa of tubular lumen to peritubular capillaries for redistribution in systemic circulation.	2. Resorption of water and solutes from ultrafiltrate.
Secretion	Movement of solutes from peritubular capillaries into tubular fluid for later excretion.	3. Secretion of solutes into tubular fluid.
Excretion	Removal of waste products of metabolism from body via urine (or feces in GI system).	4. Excretion: Average of 180 L of (essentially) protein-free fluid is filtered by glomerulus each day, but less than 1% of filtered substances are excreted in urine.

ANATOMY OF THE KIDNEY, URETERS, AND BLADDER

Structure	Description
Renal Cortex	• Outer region of kidney, lighter in color than medulla on gross inspection. • Contains nephrons. • Covers renal pyramids and extends between them to level of renal sinus as "renal columns of Bertin"; renal vessels travel in renal columns.
Renal Medulla	• Inner region of kidney, darker in color than cortex on gross inspection. • Contains renal pyramids.
Renal Pyramids	• Conical structures. • Bases are at corticomedullary border. • Apex of each is renal papilla that is cupped within a minor calyx.

Urine pathway: renal papilla → minor calyx → two or three major calyces → renal pelvis → ureter → bladder.

Continued

ANATOMY OF THE KIDNEY, URETERS, AND BLADDER (Continued)

Structure	Description
Renal Calyces	Calyces, pelves, and ureters are lined with transitional epithelium surrounded by spiral and longitudinal smooth muscle fibers.
Renal Pelvis	• Upper, expanded region of ureter that carries urine from major calyces to ureter. • Most commonly, near the level of the renal sinus, the renal vein is directly posterior to the ureter, and the renal artery is directly posterior to the renal vein.
Ureters	• Muscular tubes approximately 30 cm long. • Enter bladder posteriorly near bladder base above bladder neck. • Serve as conduits for urine. • Cross iliac vessels to enter pelvis near bifurcation of internal and external iliac arteries. • Course underneath gonadal vessels ("water under the bridge"). • Enter the bladder posteriorly.
Bladder	• Urachus anchors bladder apex to anterior abdominal wall. • Lined with transitional epithelium that lies superior to fibroelastic connective tissue and interlacing bundles of smooth muscle. • Includes fundus or body, detrusor muscle, and bladder neck. • At trigone, ureters converge.
Internal Sphincter	• Proximal sphincter made of smooth muscle. • Functions in involuntary urine control.
External Sphincter	• Distal sphincter made of striated muscle. • Functions in voluntary urine control.

STRUCTURE AND FUNCTION OF THE NEPHRON

Structure	Description	Function
Glomerulus	Network of capillaries supplied by afferent arteriole and drained by efferent arteriole.	Primary filtration of blood into renal tubule.
Podocytes	• Epithelial cells with foot-like processes that cover basement membrane of glomerular capillaries. • Separated by gaps called filtration slits bridged by thin diaphragm with pores.	Retard filtration of some proteins and macromolecules that pass through endothelium and basement membrane.
Filtration Barrier	• Made of capillary endothelium, basement membrane, and podocytes. • *Endothelium is fenestrated* and freely permeable to water, small solutes (eg, Na^+, urea, glucose), and proteins.	• Negatively charged glycoproteins on barrier surface retard filtration of molecules on basis of size and charge. • Cationic molecules are filtered more readily than anionic, as are molecules with radius of 2.0–4.2 nm. • Immunologic damage and inflammation of glomerulus may reduce negative charge on filtration barrier, causing increased filtration of proteins and *proteinuria*.
Mesangium	Includes contractile, phagocytic mesangial cells and mesangial matrix.	• Provides structural support for glomerular capillaries. • Secretes prostaglandins and cytokines. • Mesangial cells influence GFR by regulating glomerular capillary blood flow or by altering capillary surface area.
Bowman Capsule	Blind-ended beginning of nephron that encloses glomerulus.	Primary filtration of blood into renal tubule.
Renal Tubule	Proximal tubule: includes convoluted segment and straight segment (pars recta). Loop of Henle: includes thin descending limb, thin segment of ascending limb (present in juxtamedullary nephrons but not superficial nephrons), and thick segment of ascending limb. Distal tubule: includes convoluted segment and connecting tubule.	• Formation of urine via resorption and secretion of substances in ultrafiltrate. • Conduction of ultrafiltrate to renal pelvis.

Continued

STRUCTURE AND FUNCTION OF THE NEPHRON (Continued)

Structure	Description	Function
Collecting Duct	Includes cortical (outer) segment and medullary (inner) segment.	Carries urine to renal pelvis and ureter.
Vasa Recta	Capillary networks that form parallel sets of hairpin loops within medulla.	• Return blood to renal cortex and bring O_2 and nutrients to nephron segments. • *Function as countercurrent exchangers*: highly permeable to water and solutes, they remove excess water and solute from medullary interstitium and return resorbed water and solutes to circulation.
JGA	• Includes macula densa, extraglomerular mesangial (lacis) cells, and *renin-making juxtaglomerular cells of afferent arteriole*. • Macula densa: short segment near end of thick ascending limb that passes between afferent and efferent arterioles.	• JGA is component of glomerulotubular feedback involved in autoregulation of RBF and GFR. • Baroreceptor causes decreased renin secretion when arteriolar pressure at juxtaglomerular cells increases. • Macula densa acts as chemoreceptor: *sensation of low NaCl* → *release of renin*.
Renal Nerve Supply	• Sympathetic nerves originate in celiac plexus. • *There is no parasympathetic innervation*.	• Adrenergic fibers release norepinephrine and dopamine. • *Renin secretion and Na^+ resorption in renal tubule is stimulated by increased sympathetic activity*.

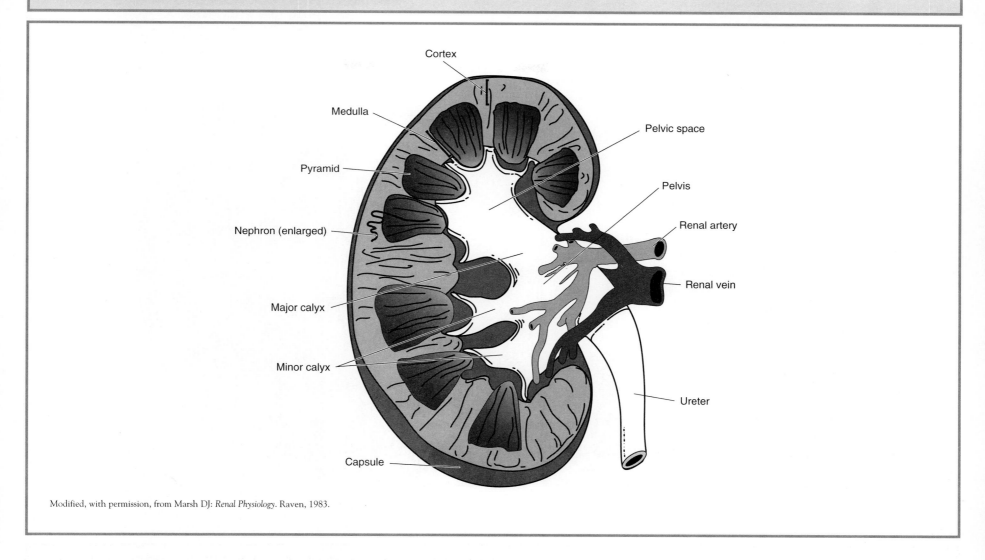

Modified, with permission, from Marsh DJ: *Renal Physiology*. Raven, 1983.

MICROSCOPIC STRUCTURE OF THE KIDNEY

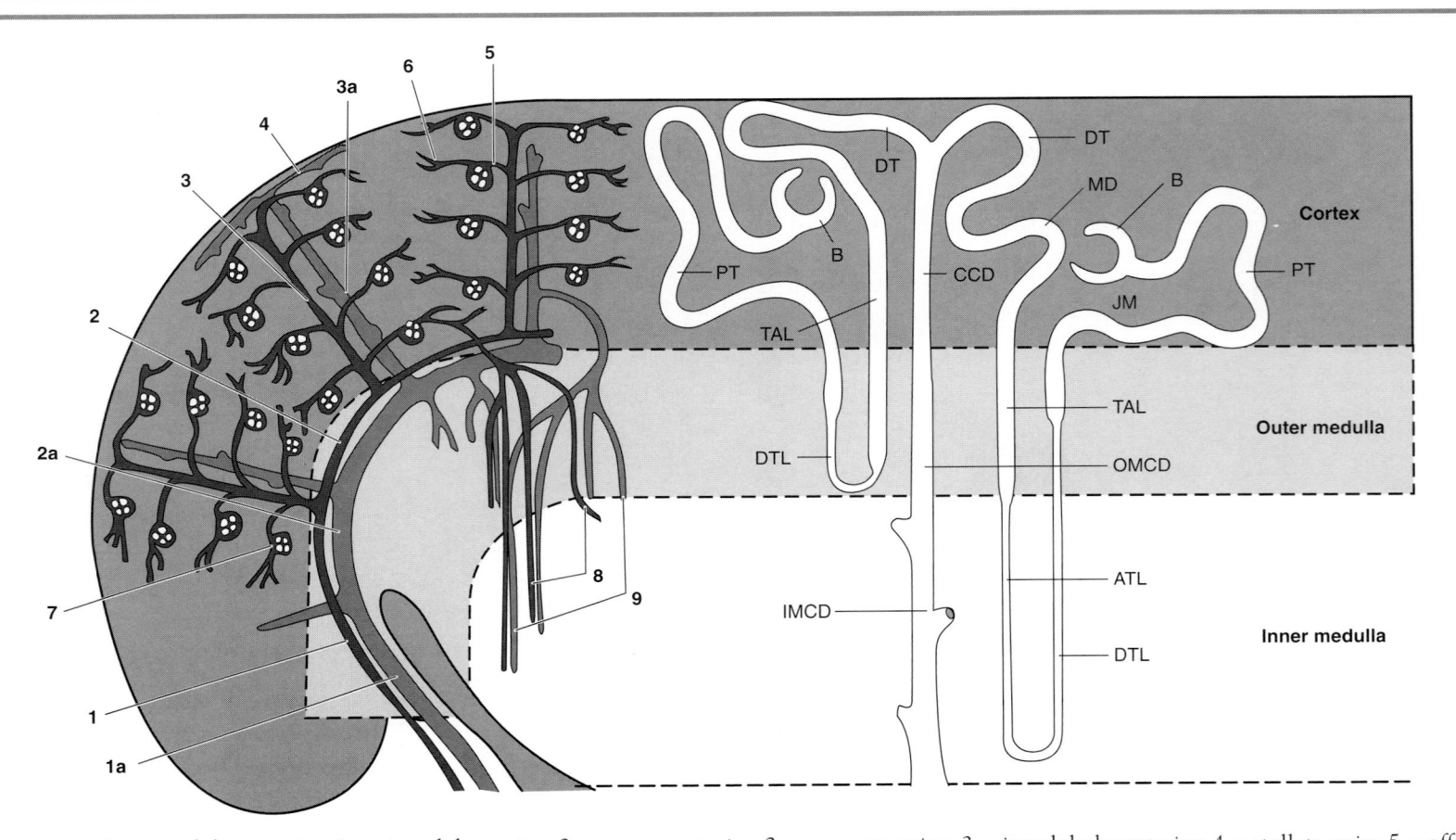

Vascular system: 1 = interlobar arteries; 1a = interlobar veins; 2 = arcuate arteries; 2a = arcuate veins; 3 = interlobular arteries; 4 = stellate vein; 5 = afferent arterioles; 6 = efferent arterioles; 7a, 7b, glomerular capillary networks; 8 = descending vasa recta; 9 = ascending vasa recta. Nephron: A superficial nephron is shown on the left, and a juxtamedullary nephron is shown on the right. PT = proximal tubule; DTL = descending thin limb; ATL = ascending thin limb; TAL = thick ascending limb. B, Bowman capsule; CCD = cortical collecting duct; DT = distal tubule; IMCD = inner medullary collecting duct; MD = macula densa; OMCD = outer medullary collecting duct; P = pelvis.

Modified, with permission, from Kriz W, Bankir LA: *Am J Physiol* 254:F1, 1988, and Koushanpour E, Kriz W: *Renal Physiology: Principles, Structure, and Function*, 2nd ed. Springer-Verlag, 1986.

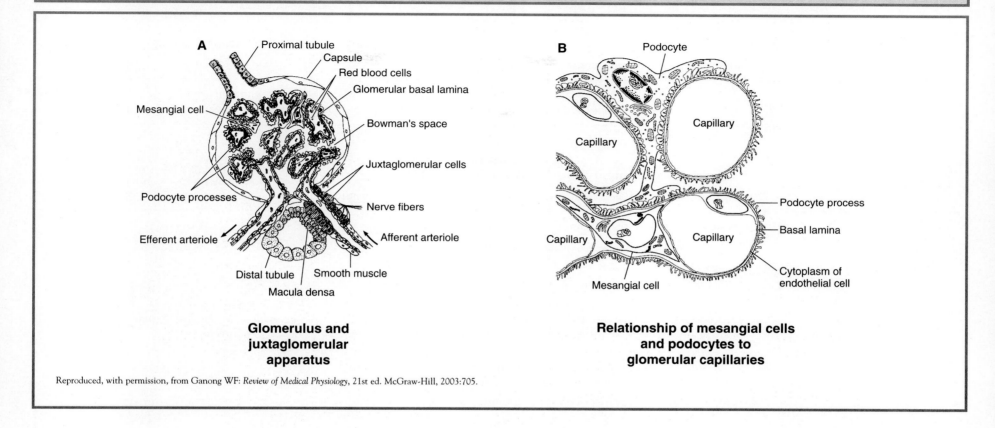

A

Proximal tubule

Capsule

Red blood cells

Glomerular basal lamina

Mesangial cell

Bowman's space

Juxtaglomerular cells

Podocyte processes

Nerve fibers

Efferent arteriole

Afferent arteriole

Distal tubule   Smooth muscle

Macula densa

**Glomerulus and
juxtaglomerular
apparatus**

B

Podocyte

Capillary

Capillary

Capillary

Podocyte process

Basal lamina

Capillary

Capillary

Cytoplasm of
endothelial cell

Mesangial cell

**Relationship of mesangial cells
and podocytes to
glomerular capillaries**

Reproduced, with permission, from Ganong WF: *Review of Medical Physiology*, 21st ed. McGraw-Hill, 2003:705.

SUMMARY OF RENAL TUBULAR FUNCTION

Structure	Function	Important Characteristics	Hormonal Regulation
Renal Corpuscle (glomerulus + Bowman capsule)	*Ultrafiltration* of plasma based on size and molecular charge of substances, and *Starling forces*.	• Capillary endothelium is freely permeable to water and small solutes (glucose, urea, sodium). • Capillary basement membrane is barrier to large plasma proteins. • Filtration slits of podocytes filter macromolecules. • Mesangium provides structural support, helps regulate blood flow, and secretes prostaglandins.	
Proximal Convoluted Tubule	Reabsorption of about 70% of filtered water and solutes, including: Na^+, Cl^-, K^+, HCO_3^-, Ca^{2+}, glucose, and amino acids.	• Na^+-K^+-ATPase in basolateral membrane actively pumps Na^+ from cell to blood in exchange for K^+ and other solutes. • *Reabsorption of all solutes and water is coupled to Na^+ reabsorption*. • *Water reabsorption follows solute transport*. • Tubular fluid is *isosmotic* with respect to plasma.	• PTH decreases NaCl, H_2O, Ca^{2+}, and phosphate reabsorption. • Angiotensin II increases NaCl and H_2O reabsorption.
Loop of Henle, Descending Thin Limb	Reabsorption of water concentrates tubular fluid as the bend of the loop is approached.	• Tubular fluid is *hyperosmotic* with respect to plasma. • Only segment of loop highly permeable to water in absence of ADH. • Impermeable to solutes.	
Loop of Henle, "The Bend"	Site of maximal concentration of tubular fluid (1200 mOsm/kg H_2O).	Tubular fluid is *hyperosmotic* with respect to plasma.	
Loop of Henle, Ascending Thin Limb	• Reabsorbs NaCl. • Secretes urea.	• Present only in juxtamedullary nephrons with long loops. • Impermeable to water but permeable to solutes.	

Loop of Henle, Thick Ascending Limb	Reabsorbs 20% of filtered solutes, including: Na^+, Cl^-, K^+, HCO_3^-, Ca^{2+}, and Mg^{2+}.	• *Impermeable to water.* • *Principal site of dilution of tubular fluid.* • Na^+-K^+-ATPase in basolateral membrane exchanges Na^+ for other solutes. • *Resorption of every solute is linked to Na^+-K^+-ATPase.* • Tubular *fluid is hypo-osmotic* with respect to plasma.	• Aldosterone, calcitonin, glucagon, ADH and PTH increase NaCl reabsorption. • PTH also increases Ca^{2+} reabsorption.
Distal Convoluted Tubule	• Reabsorbs about 10% of filtered solutes, including: Na^+, Cl^-, K^+, HCO_3^-, Ca^{2+}, and Mg^{2+}. • Secretes K^+ and H^+. • Distal segment reabsorbs 15% of filtered water.	*Initial segment* • Impermeable to water. • Tubular fluid is *hypo-osmotic* with respect to plasma. Distal segment • Reabsorbs water. • Tubular fluid may be hypo-osmotic or isosmotic with respect to plasma. • Contains *macula densa*, part of the JGA involved in renin-angiotensin-aldosterone system.	• ADH increases permeability to water, increases NaCl reabsorption, and increases K^+ secretion. • Aldosterone increases NaCl reabsorption and K^+ secretion. • PTH increases Ca^{2+} reabsorption. • Calcitonin increases NaCl reabsorption. • Prostaglandins and bradykinins decrease NaCl reabsorption.
Collecting Duct	• Reabsorbs Na^+, Cl^-, K^+, HCO_3^-, Ca^{2+}, and Mg^{2+}. • Secretes K^+.	• With distal convoluted tubule, contains *principal cells* that reabsorb Na^+ and water and secrete K^+ (mediated by Na^+-K^+-ATPase), and *intercalated cells* that secrete H^+ and reabsorb HCO_3^- (mediated by H^+-ATPase; $CO_2 + H_2O$ + carbonic anhydrase = HCO_3^-). • Inner medulla is permeable to urea. • Tubular fluid may be hypo-osmotic or isosmotic with respect to plasma.	• ADH increases permeability to water *and urea* in the inner medulla of the collecting duct. • Hormonal regulation otherwise same as in distal convoluted tubule.

RENAL BLOOD FLOW AND AUTOREGULATION

Description	Regulation Mechanisms	Functions
Renal Blood Flow		
• *Renal blood flow is 25% of cardiac output.* • Pathway: renal artery → interlobar artery → arcuate artery → interlobular artery → afferent arteriole → glomerular capillaries → efferent arteriole → peritubular capillaries and vasa recta (venous vessels parallel arterial vessels). • *Renal arteries are end arteries with no collateral circulation; destruction of a renal artery causes destruction of renal segment it supplies.*	• Norepinephrine, prostaglandins in renal medulla, and angiotensin II cause renal vasoconstriction. • Angiotensin II has greater effect on efferent arteriole than afferent arteriole. • Dopamine (which also causes natriuresis) and prostaglandins in renal cortex cause renal vasodilation.	• Delivers O_2, nutrients, and hormones to nephron. • Returns CO_2 and resorbed fluid and solutes to general circulation. • Helps concentrate and dilute urine. • Modifies rate of solute and water resorption by proximal tubule. • Indirectly determines GFR.
Autoregulation		
• *Process by which kidneys keep RBF and GFR constant.* • *Vascular resistance is adjusted via afferent arterioles (major resistance vessels) in response to changes in arterial pressure.* • *Effective only for arterial pressure changes of 90–180 mm Hg.* • Allows uncoupling of renal function from arterial pressure and ensures that fluid and solute excretion remain constant.	• Rise in arterial pressure stretches afferent arteriole, which contracts, increasing afferent arteriole resistance. • This action offsets increase in arterial pressure, allowing RBF and GFR to remain constant (constant $\Delta P/R$ allows constant RBF). • *Tubuloglomerular feedback:* macula densa senses tubular flow and generates signal that affects afferent arteriolar resistance.	Example: decreased GFR and tubular flow sensed by macula densa → JGA sends signal → renal vasodilation of primarily afferent arteriole → RBF and GFR increase (increased GFR has opposite effect).

STEPS IN MICTURITION

Step	Process
1	Collection of urine in renal calyces triggers pacemaker activity that generates action potentials and initiates peristaltic wave that spreads along smooth muscle syncytium of pelves and ureters, forcing urine toward bladder.
2	Bladder fills until critical pressure is reached that stimulates stretch receptors in bladder wall that trigger micturition reflex.
3	Sensory signals from bladder fundus enter spinal cord via pelvic nerves and return to bladder via parasympathetic fibers in those same nerves.
4	*Sacral parasympathetic (muscarinic) stimulation causes contraction of detrusor muscle.*
5	*Contraction of bladder neck causes opening of bladder neck.*
6	Cortical inhibition of pudendal nerve leads to voluntary relaxation of external sphincter, resulting in urine flow through external meatus and bladder emptying; *voluntary relaxation of external sphincter is required and may be initiating event in micturition.*

REGULATION OF MICTURITION

Type of Control	Description
Sympathetic	• Sympathetic stimulation results in urine storage (hypogastric nerves stimulate smooth muscle α-adrenergic receptors, causing urethral closure). • Interruption of hypogastric sympathetic nerves and pudendal nerves to lower urinary tract does not alter micturition reflex.
Parasympathetic	• Parasympathetic stimulation results in micturition. • Destruction of parasympathetic nerves causes complete bladder dysfunction.
Involuntary	• Internal sphincter is not under conscious control. • Inherent tone of internal sphincter prevents bladder emptying until certain stimuli initiate urination.
Voluntary	• External sphincter is under voluntary control. • Contraction of external sphincter prevents urination (more important for bladder control in men than in women).
Afferent	Visceral afferent pathways carry input from bladder receptors that detect fullness, pain, and temperature.

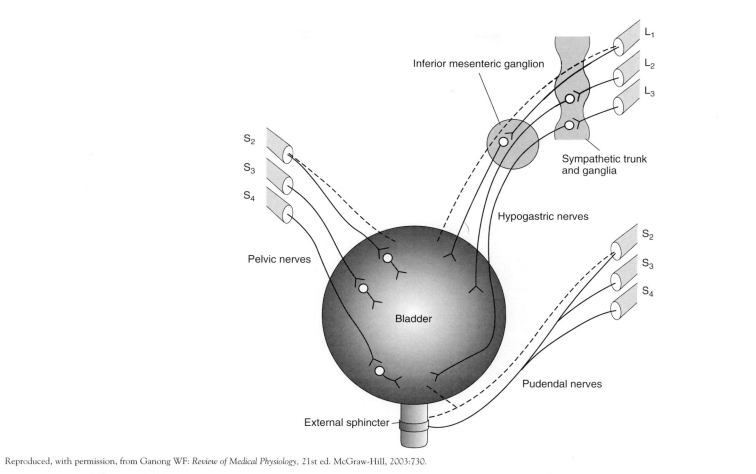

Reproduced, with permission, from Ganong WF: *Review of Medical Physiology*, 21st ed. McGraw-Hill, 2003:730.

EFFECTS OF ABNORMAL RENAL FUNCTION

Effects	Symptoms	Clinical Significance
Acidosis	Fatigue, headache, diarrhea, nausea, vomiting, loss of appetite, increased rate of breathing, dry skin, renal stones.	Associated with renal tubular acidosis.
Na$^+$ Retention	Edema.	• Associated with heart failure, hyperaldosteronism, nephritis, and nephrotic syndrome. • Nephrotic syndrome: increased capillary permeability leads to proteinuria, edema, hypoalbuminemia, and hyperlipidemia.
Loss of Concentrating Ability	Polyuria.	Loss of concentrating ability is first renal function lost in renal disease.
Loss of Diluting Ability	Oliguria, possibly leading to anuria.	Loss of diluting ability is last renal function lost in renal disease.
Accumulation of Breakdown Products of Protein Metabolism in Blood	Uremia: lethargy, anorexia, altered mental status, nausea/ vomiting, muscle spasm.	• If severe, may result in seizure or coma. • May require emergent hemodialysis.
Changes in Urine	Proteinuria, hematuria, pyuria, blood cell casts.	Changes in urine may be first sign of early renal disease.

RENAL DISEASES

Disease	Physiologic Disorder	Symptoms	Important Points
Chronic Renal Failure	• Inability to excrete phosphate. • Decreased plasma [Ca^{2+}] due to binding with phosphate. • Increased PTH secretion. • Decreased production of erythropoietin.	Osteitis fibrosa cystica (resorbed bone replaced by fibrous tissue), hyperparathyroidism, anemia.	• Associated hyperparathyroidism causes deposition of Ca^{2+} and P_i in soft tissue (eg, lung, heart, vessels). • This deposition can be prevented with low-phosphate diet or binding agents.
Nephrotic Syndrome	• Increased permeability of glomerular capillaries to proteins. • May be caused by immune complexes in mesangial cells.	Hyponatremia, edema, hypoalbuminemia, proteinuria.	• *Proteinuria may be indication of renal disease.* • Immune complexes may cause infiltration of inflammatory cells, resulting in scarring and destruction of glomeruli.
Fanconi Syndrome	• Impaired renal resorption of amino acids, glucose, and low-molecular-weight proteins at proximal tubule. • Decreased ATP and decreased function of Na^+-K^+-ATPase lead to generalized decrease in secondary active transport.	Osteomalacia, acidosis, hypokalemia, glycosuria, phosphaturia, amino aciduria.	Because other nephron segments cannot resorb these amino acids, glucose, or low-molecular-weight proteins, they are excreted in urine.
Liddle Syndrome	• Genetic abnormality causes mutation of Na^+ channels. • Increased number of Na^+ channels causes inappropriately elevated Na^+ absorption and increased ECF volume.	Hypertension, hypokalemia.	Rare genetic disorder.
Pseudohypoaldosteronism, Type I	Decreased number of functional Na^+ channels in collecting duct leads to decreased Na^+ resorption and decreased ECF volume.	Hypotension, hyponatremia, polyuria.	Dehydration with hyperosmotic serum.
Nephrogenic Diabetes Insipidus	Patients cannot maximally concentrate urine due to impaired renal response to ADH.	Polyuria, polydipsia; plasma {Na^+} near normal.	• *Polydipsia is required to maintain body fluid osmolality.* • Seen in 35% of patients taking lithium. • Treated with thiazide diuretics.

Continued

RENAL DISEASES (Continued)

Disease	Physiologic Disorder	Symptoms	Important Points
			• Central or neurogenic diabetes insipidus is due to failure of ADH secretion. • Central diabetes insipidus is treated with ADH replacement.
SIADH	• Elevated ADH (based on body fluid osmolality or blood pressure). • Decreased renal water excretion.	Low body fluid osmolality with urine concentrated more than would be expected.	Associated with infections, drugs, lung disease, or neoplasms of brain or lung.
Renal Artery Stenosis	RAAS is stimulated because kidney incorrectly perceives ECF volume contraction.	Hypertension, renal insufficiency.	• Associated with atherosclerosis. • Lowered blood pressure leads to significantly reduced RBF in affected kidney, which leads to decreased GFR and possible future renal failure. • Antihypertensives may be ineffective.

RENAL TUBULAR ACIDOSIS

Types	Physiologic Disorder	Symptoms	Clinical Significance
I (distal)	• Defect in H^+ secretion, OR • Impaired permeability to H^+ in distal renal tubule or collecting duct, OR • Inadequate production of NH_4^+.	• Symptoms depend on type. • May include confusion, fatigue, weakness, increased rate of breathing, renal stones, muscle pain.	• Seen in medullary sponge kidney, renal obstruction, result of treatment with drugs like amphotericin B, renal failure. • Associated with hypokalemia, hypercalcemia, osteomalacia, and renal stones. • Treat by alkalinizing urine.
II (proximal)	• Defect in H^+ secretion in proximal renal tubule causes decreased resorption of filtered load of HCO_3^- and increased HCO_3^- excretion. • Result is decreased plasma $[HCO_3^-]$.		• Hereditary or acquired. • Seen in Fanconi syndrome, cystinosis, result of treatment with inhibitors of carbonic anhydrase. • Associated with hypokalemia, hypercalcemia and osteomalacia, but *not renal stones*. • Treat by alkalinizing urine.
III	Combination of types I and II.		Very rare
IV (hyperkalemic)	Associated with mild renal insufficiency and hypoaldosteronism.		• Seen in diabetes, lupus, sickle cell anemia, obstructive nephropathy, Addison disease. • Seen with use of K^+-sparing diuretics. • Hyperkalemia increases risk of cardiac arrhythmia. • Treat with volume expansion.

II. Glomerular Filtration

STARLING FORCES ACROSS THE GLOMERULAR CAPILLARIES

GFR is sum of Starling forces that exist across capillaries: $GFR = K_f [(P_{GC} - P_{BS}) - \sigma(\pi_{GC} - \pi_{BS})]$

Components	Characteristics
Constant (K_f)	• Product of intrinsic permeability of glomerular capillary and glomerular surface area available for filtration. • K_f decreased when number of filtering glomeruli are decreased, resulting in less surface area (eg: renal disease, drugs, and hormones may constrict glomerular arterioles, leading to decreased K_f). • Agents that dilate glomerular arterioles increase K_f. • K_f is 100 × greater in glomerular capillaries than in systemic capillaries, accounting for its greater rate of filtration.
Hydrostatic Pressure in Glomerular Capillary (P_{GC})	• *Only force that favors filtration* (promotes movement of fluid from glomerular capillary into Bowman space). • P_{GC} normally decreases along length of glomerular capillary due to increasing resistance to flow. • Normally, GFR is regulated by alterations in P_{GC} that are mediated by changes in afferent or efferent arteriolar resistance and changes in renal arteriolar pressure.
Oncotic Pressure in Glomerular Capillary (π_{GC})	• Opposes filtration. • π_{GC} normally increases along length of glomerular capillary because of increasing protein concentration. • Changes in π_{GC} result from changes in protein synthesis outside kidneys. • For example, renal disease leads to proteinuria, which leads to decreased plasma [protein] and thus decreased π_{GC}.
Hydrostatic Pressure in Bowman Space (P_{BS})	Opposes filtration (eg, acute renal obstruction).
Oncotic Pressure in Bowman Space (π_{BS})	• Opposes filtration. • Value normally near zero.

Component	Characteristics
Reflection Coefficient for Proteins Across Glomerular Capillary (σ)	• If glomerular capillary impermeable to protein, σ = 1. • If glomerular capillary freely permeable to protein, σ = 0.

STARLING FORCES BETWEEN THE INTERCELLULAR SPACE AND PERITUBULAR CAPILLARIES

Component	Characteristics
$Q = K_f [(Pic - Pc) + \sigma(\pi c - \pi ic)]$	
Q = flow.	• *Sum of Starling forces normally favors movement of solute and water from interstitium of proximal tubule into peritubular capillaries.* • Starling forces affect proximal tubule but not loop of Henle, distal tubule, or collecting duct, which are less permeable to water.
Hydrostatic pressure in lateral intercellular space (Pic).	Favors movement of solute and water from interstitium into peritubular capillaries.
Oncotic pressure in peritubular capillary (πc).	Favors movement of solute and water from interstitium into peritubular capillaries.
	πc decreases in response to decreased GFR and FF when RPF is constant. • This increases backflow of NaCl and water from lateral intercellular space into tubular fluid, causing decreased net resorption of solute and water across proximal tubule. • Increased FF has opposite effect.
Hydrostatic pressure in peritubular capillaries (Pc).	Opposes movement of solute and water from interstitium into peritubular capillaries.
	Efferent arteriolar dilation increases Pc, while constriction decreases it. • Increased Pc inhibits solute and water resorption by increasing back leak of NaCl and water across tight junction; decreased Pc has opposite effect.
Oncotic pressure in lateral intercellular space (πic).	Opposes movement of solute and water from interstitium into peritubular capillaries.

SOLUTE AND WATER TRANSPORT ACROSS PROXIMAL TUBULE

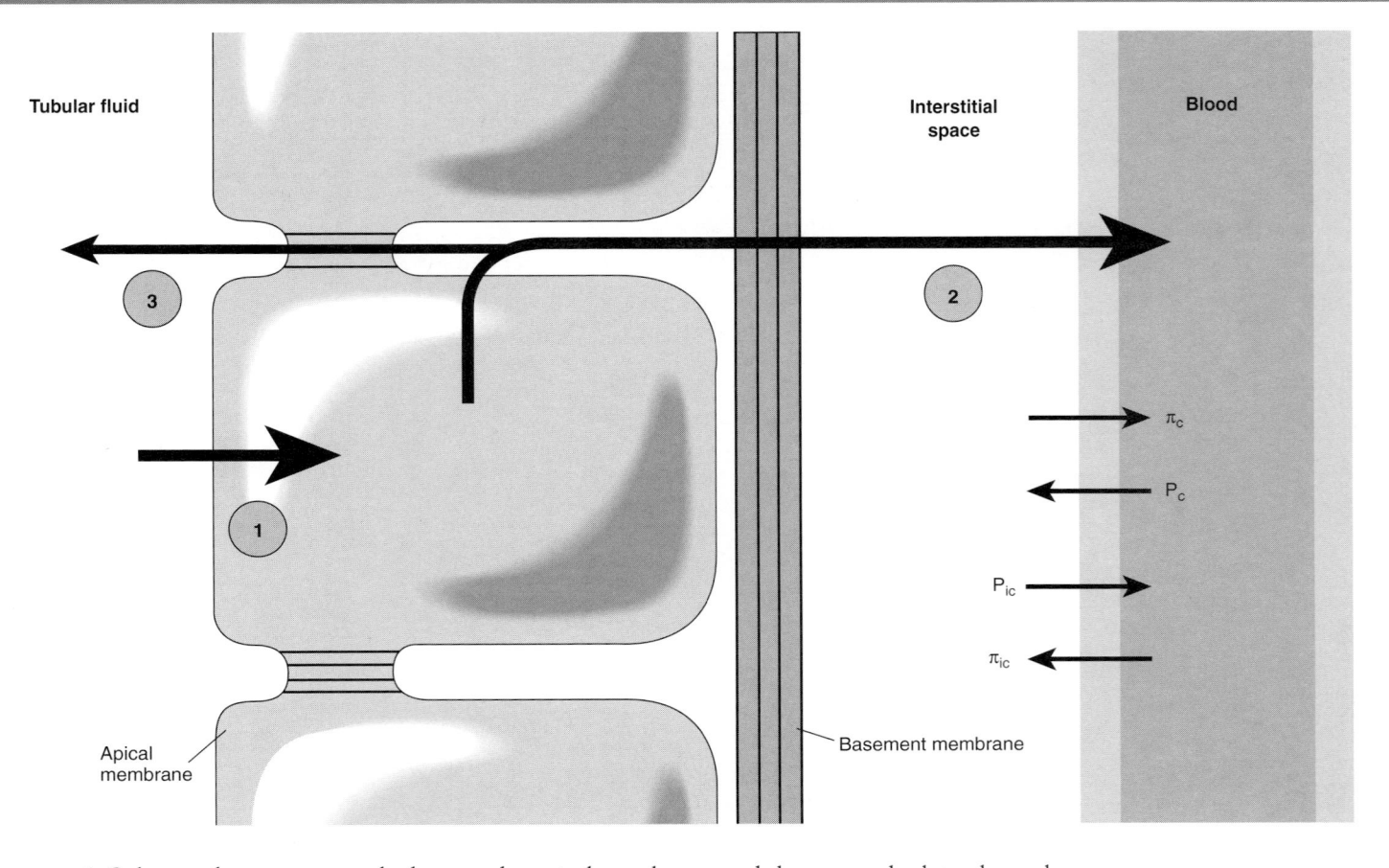

1 Solute and water are resorbed across the apical membrane, and then cross the lateral membrane.
2 Some solute and water flows from the interstitial space into the capillary.
3 Some solute and water reenters the tubular fluid.
  • Starling forces across the capillary wall determine the amount of fluid following pathway 2 versus pathway 3.

Modified, with permission, from Berne RM, Levy MN: *Principles of Physiology*, 3rd ed. Mosby, 2000:431

IMPORTANT FORMULAS AND VALUES IN GLOMERULAR FILTRATION

Term	Description	Formula	Normal Value
GFR	• Volume of glomerular filtrate formed per minute by kidneys. • Index of renal function. • *Decrease in GFR may be only clinical sign of kidney disease.* • 50% loss of functioning nephrons reduces GFR by only 25% (remaining nephrons compensate). • GFR must decline substantially before increase in plasma creatinine can be detected (eg, decrease in GFR from 120 to 100 mL/min (20% decrease) results in increase in creatinine from 1 to 1.2 mg/dL).	$GFR = (U_{CR} \times \dot{V})/P_{CR}$ • P_{CR} = plasma [creatinine] • U_{CR} = urine [creatinine] • $\dot{V}$ = urine flow per unit time	125 mL/min
Plasma Creatinine	• Used in clinical settings to assess renal function. • Inversely related to GFR.		0.5–1.5 mg/dL
Cl_{CR}	• Amount of creatinine excreted in urine per minute. • Used to determine GFR. • Substances that serve as markers for measurement of GFR must be freely filtered and not resorbed, secreted, metabolized, or produced by kidney, and cannot alter GFR (eg, urea or inulin).	• $Cl_{CR} = (U_{CR} \times \dot{V})/P_{CR}$ • Cl_{CR} = lean kg × (140 – age)/72 × CR for males; multiply result by 0.85 for females.	Average: 125 mL/min • Males: 90–140 mL/min • Females: 80–125 mL/min
FE_{Na}	• Determines amount of sodium excreted by kidneys. • Helps define extent of renal sodium conservation and etiology of renal disease. • Invalidated by diuretics unless dose is delayed 6–8 hours. • Can be low despite ATN.	$FE_{Na} = (U_{Na} \times P_{CR})/(P_{Na} \times U_{CR}) \times 100$	• Prerenal azotemia < 1%. • ATN > 1%. • Postrenal azotemia > 4%.
RFI	• Measures renal sodium conservation and concentrating ability. • Used in patients with oliguria for early differentiation between prerenal azotemia and ATN.	$RFI = (U_{Na} \times P_{CR})/U_{CR}$	RFI: • Prerenal azotemia < 1%. • ATN > 1%. • Postrenal azotemia > 1%.

Continued

IMPORTANT FORMULAS AND VALUES IN GLOMERULAR FILTRATION (Continued)

Term	Description	Formula	Normal Value
RFI			U_{Na} (mmol/L): • Prerenal azotemia > 20% • ATN > 40% • Postrenal azotemia > 40%.
FF	• That part of renal arterial plasma that passes through glomerulus and is filtered. • 80–85% passes through glomerular capillaries and eventually reaches systemic circulation via renal vein. • 10% of renal arterial plasma does not pass through glomerulus.	FF = GFR/RPF	0.15–0.20

SUBSTANCES THAT REGULATE GLOMERULAR FILTRATION

Type of Regulator	Substance	Site/Mechanism of Action
Vasoconstrictors (decrease GFR and RBF)	Angiotensin II.	Low ECF volume stimulates angiotensin II action in afferent and efferent arterioles.
	Endothelin.	Afferent and efferent arterioles.
	Sympathetic nerves (norepinephrine and epinephrine).	Low ECF volume stimulates SNS action in afferent arterioles.
Vasodilators (increase GFR and RBF)	Bradykinin.	Stimulates release of nitric oxide and prostaglandins.
	Dopamine.	Increases RBF and inhibits renin secretion.
	Nitric oxide.	• Dilation of afferent and efferent arterioles. • Decreased total peripheral resistance.
	Prostaglandins.	• During pathologic states (eg, hemorrhage), prostaglandins are produced within kidneys where they increase RBF by dampening vasoconstrictor effects, preventing renal ischemia. • There is no effect on GFR.

Other Substances	ACE.	Increases angiotensin II and decreases bradykinin, leading to decreased systemic blood pressure and vascular resistance, which results in decreased GFR and RBF.
	ANP.	Increased ECF volume dilates afferent arteriole and constricts efferent arteriole, leading to increased GFR with little change in RBF.
	ATP.	Constricts afferent arteriole, leading to decreased GFR and RBF.
	Glucocorticoids.	Increase GFR and RBF.
	Histamine.	Decreases resistance of afferent and efferent arterioles, leading to increased RBF with no effect on GFR.

HORMONAL REGULATION OF GLOMERULAR FILTRATION DURING ACUTE HEMORRHAGE

Step	Process
1	Hemorrhage → decreased arterial blood pressure → triggers baroreceptor reflex → stimulation of renal sympathetic nerves.
2	Release of norepinephrine → afferent and efferent arteriolar vasoconstriction → decreased GFR and RBF.
3	Release of epinephrine and angiotensin II → further vasoconstriction → decreased RBF.
4	Increased vascular resistance in kidneys and elsewhere → increase in total peripheral resistance.
5	Resulting tendency for blood pressure to increase (blood pressure is cardiac output multiplied by total peripheral resistance) offsets tendency of blood pressure to decrease in response to hemorrhage.
6	Result is preservation of arterial pressure at expense of maintaining normal GFR and RBF.

III. Body Fluid Volume and Osmolality

CHARACTERISTICS OF BODY WATER

Factor	Conditions Present	Effects
Water Movement	Plasma membranes are highly permeable to water.	• Allows water to move freely between body fluid compartments. • Except for transient changes, *ICF and ECF compartments are in osmotic equilibrium*. • Addition of NaCl to ECF without H_2O increases $[Na^+]$ and osmolality in ECF $\rightarrow$ increased ICF osmolality.
	Fluid shifts between ICF and ECF are primarily due to movement of water, not ions.	*Volume of body water determines body fluid osmolality.*
	The major determinant of plasma osmolality is Na^+.	• Disorders of water balance alter plasma $[Na^+]$. • *When abnormal plasma $[Na^+]$ is noted, problem most often relates to water balance, not Na^+ balance.* • Changes in Na^+ balance alter ECF volume, not its osmolality (ie, not its $[Na^+]$).
Renal Regulation of Water Balance	Normal intravascular volume.	• Urine osmolality: 50–1200 mOsm/kg water. • Urine volume: 0.5–18 L/d.
	Low intravascular volume (due to low water intake or high water loss).	Production of small volume, hyperosmotic (concentrated) urine conserves water.
	High intravascular volume.	Production of large volume, hypo-osmotic (diluted) urine removes excess water.

INTRAVENOUS FLUIDS

Solution Type	Mechanism of Action	Example
Isotonic	Does not induce an osmotic pressure gradient across plasma membrane of cells, so *entire volume of infused solution remains in ECF.*	0.9% NaCl.
	Oncotic pressure generated by albumin molecules retains fluid in vascular compartment, expanding its volume.	5% Albumin.
Hypotonic	• Increases both ICF and ECF volumes. • Used when vascular fluid is hyperosmotic.	0.45% NaCl or D_5W.
Hypertonic	• Expands ECF volume but decreases ICF volume by shifting water out of cells. • Used when vascular fluid is hypo-osmotic.	3% or 5% NaCl.

EUVOLEMIA

Key Concepts	Mechanisms of Regulation
Maintenance of euvolemia depends on delivery of constant fraction of filtered load of Na^+ to collecting duct.	• Autoregulation of GFR (and thus filtered load of Na^+). • Glomerulotubular balance: Na^+ resorption changes in parallel with GFR, so amount of Na^+ and water excreted remains relatively constant. • Loop of Henle (especially thick ascending loop) and distal tubule increase resorptive rates in response to increased delivery of Na^+.
	Aldosterone is primary regulator of Na^+ resorption by collecting duct and thus of Na^+ excretion. • Elevated aldosterone causes increased Na^+ resorption (decreased excretion) by principal cells of collecting duct. • Decreased aldosterone has opposite effect.
Urine NaCl excretion = NaCl intake.	ECF volume changes in parallel with Na^+. • With positive Na^+ balance (intake > excretion), ECF volume expands. • With negative Na^+ balance (intake < excretion), ECF volume contracts. • When Na^+ is in equilibrium, euvolemia exists.

EXTRACELLULAR FLUID VOLUME: CONTRACTION VERSUS EXPANSION

Sequence of Events	Volume Contraction	Volume Expansion
Volume Sensors Signal Kidneys	• Increase input from renal sympathetic nerves. • Decrease ANP from atrial myocytes. • Increase ADH from posterior pituitary. • Increase renin, stimulating angiotensin II, which increases release of aldosterone from adrenal cortex.	• Decrease input from renal sympathetic nerves. • Increase ANP from atrial myocytes. • Decrease ADH from posterior pituitary. • Decrease renin, inhibiting angiotensin II, which decreases release of aldosterone from adrenal cortex.
Kidneys Respond	• Decrease GFR, leading to decreased filtered load of Na^+. • Increase Na^+ resorption in proximal tubule and collecting duct.	• Increase GFR, leading to increased filtered load of Na^+. • Decrease Na^+ resorption in proximal tubule and collecting duct.
Result	• Decreased renal excretion of NaCl and H_2O. • Euvolemia is restored, and body fluid osmolality remains constant.	• Increased renal excretion of NaCl and H_2O. • Euvolemia is restored, and body fluid osmolality remains constant.

MAINTENANCE OF EXTRACELLULAR FLUID VOLUME BY BARORECEPTORS

Baroreceptors maintain ECF volume by regulating renal NaCl excretion.

Type of Baroreceptor	Location	Stimuli	Response	Example
Low Pressure	Cardiac atria, pulmonary vasculature.	Changes in vascular volume or distention of cardiac atria and pulmonary vasculature.	Baroreceptors signal brainstem via vagus nerve, which modulates sympathetic outflow and ADH secretion.	• Decreased filling of cardiac atria and pulmonary vessels increases sympathetic nerve activity and stimulates ADH. • Distention of these structures decreases sympathetic nerve activity.
			Changes in blood volume and pressure of 5–10% are necessary to evoke response.	Atrial myocytes release ANP when atria are distended, which helps reduce blood pressure and increase renal excretion of NaCl and H_2O.
High Pressure	Carotid sinus, aortic arch, afferent arterioles.	Changes in arterial blood pressure.	Baroreceptors in aortic arch and carotid sinus signal brainstem via vagus and glossopharyngeal nerves, which modulate sympathetic outflow and ADH secretion.	• Decreased blood pressure increases sympathetic nerve activity and ADH secretion. • Increased pressure decreases sympathetic nerve activity.
			Changes in blood volume and pressure of 5–10% are necessary to evoke a response.	• Afferent arterioles respond directly to pressure changes. • If perfusion pressure there is decreased, myocytes release renin. • *Renin is suppressed when perfusion pressure is increased* (renin determines levels of angiotensin II and aldosterone, both of which are important in regulating renal NaCl excretion).

RENAL RESPONSE IN CONGESTIVE HEART FAILURE AND HEPATIC CIRRHOSIS

Disease	Symptoms	Mechanism of Renal Response	ECF Volume	NaCl Excretion
Congestive Heart Failure	• Pulmonary and generalized edema. • Blood pressure and cardiac output may be reduced.	• Baroreceptors detect a reduced ECF volume. • Kidneys respond as they would to ECF volume contraction by retaining NaCl and water. • This response seems paradoxical in face of increased ECF volume, but *edema is not due to fluid in vascular system; it is in interstitial fluid compartment.* • There is decreased volume and pressure in portions of vascular system where baroreceptors are found.	Increased.	Decreased.
Advanced Hepatic Cirrhosis	Ascites (part of ECF).	• Baroreceptors detect a reduced ECF volume. • Kidneys respond as they would to ECF volume contraction by retaining NaCl and water, which results in accumulation of ascites. • Renal response seems paradoxical in face of increased ECF volume, but *this blood is pooled in splanchnic circulation.* • Damaged liver impedes drainage of blood from splanchnic circulation via portal vein, increasing portal system venous pressure and enhancing fluid transudation into peritoneal cavity. • This causes decreased volume and pressure in portions of vascular system where baroreceptors are found.	Increased.	Decreased.

URINE FORMATION IN DIURETIC AND ANTIDIURETIC STATES

Feature	Diuretic State	Antidiuretic State
Urine Tonicity	Low.	High.
Urine Volume	High.	Low.
Serum Osmolality	Low.	High.
Serum ADH Levels	Low.	High.
Key Process Within Nephron	In ascending thin limb (which is impermeable to water but permeable to solutes), the following occurs: • NaCl is passively resorbed and urea passively diffuses into tubular fluid. • Tubular fluid becomes diluted but volume remains same.	Countercurrent multiplication: NaCl resorbed in ascending thin and thick limbs accumulates in medullary interstitium, increasing its osmolality and creating driving force for water resorption by collecting duct. Loop of Henle, descending limb: because descending limb is highly permeable to water, increased osmolality of medullary interstitium causes water to be absorbed, increasing the concentration of tubular fluid. Collecting duct: in presence of ADH, permeability to water is increased, allowing water to diffuse out of tubule lumen, and increasing urine osmolality.
Result	• Urine can be formed with an osmolality as low as 50 mOsm/kg H_2O with low [NaCl] and low [urea]. • Volume up to 18 L/d (10% of GFR).	• Urine with osmolality as high as 1200 mOsm/kg H_2O with high [urea] and other nonresorbed solutes. • Volume as low as 0.5 L/d.

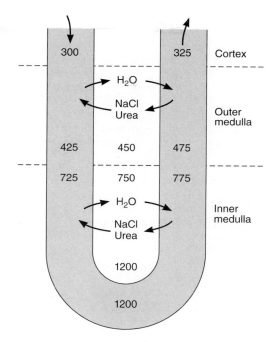

Water diffuses out of the descending limb and into the ascending limb. NaCl and urea diffuse out of the ascending limb and into the descending limb.

Reproduced, with permission, from Ganong WF: *Review of Medical Physiology,* 21st ed. McGraw-Hill, 2003:721.

NaCl AND H₂O RESORPTION IN THE PROXIMAL TUBULE

Segment of Proximal Tubule	Mechanism	Effects
First Half	• Na⁺ resorbed mainly with HCO₃⁻ and organic molecules (glucose, amino acids, Pᵢ, lactate). • Organic molecules that enter cell with Na⁺ across apical membrane leave across basolateral membrane via passive transport.	• Resorption of NaHCO₃ and organic molecules (organic molecules are almost completely removed from tubular fluid here). • H⁺ secretion. • *Resorption of nearly all organic solutes, ions, and water is coupled to Na⁺ resorption, so changes in Na⁺ resorption influence the resorption of water and other solutes by proximal tubule.* • Solvent drag—some solutes (K⁺, Ca²⁺) are resorbed with fluid.
	Na⁺ that enters across apical membrane leaves cell and enters blood via Na⁺-K⁺-ATPase.	Transtubular osmotic gradient is established that provides driving force for passive resorption of water by osmosis.
Second Half	• Na⁺ resorbed mainly with Cl⁻, via both transcellular and paracellular pathways. • Na⁺ leaves cell and enters blood via Na⁺-K⁺-ATPase.	• *Resorption of NaCl and other solutes establishes transtubular osmotic gradient that drives passive resorption of water by osmosis.* • Resorption of more Cl⁻ than water causes increase in [Cl⁻] along length of proximal tubule. • H⁺ secretion .
	• Cl⁻ leaves cell and enters blood via K⁺-Cl⁻ symporter in basolateral membrane. • Cl⁻ gradient set up in first half of proximal tubule leads to diffusion of Cl⁻ from tubular lumen into lateral intercellular space, and creates luminal fluid that is positively charged relative to blood.	Positive transepithelial voltage causes passive diffusion of Na+ out of tubular fluid into blood.

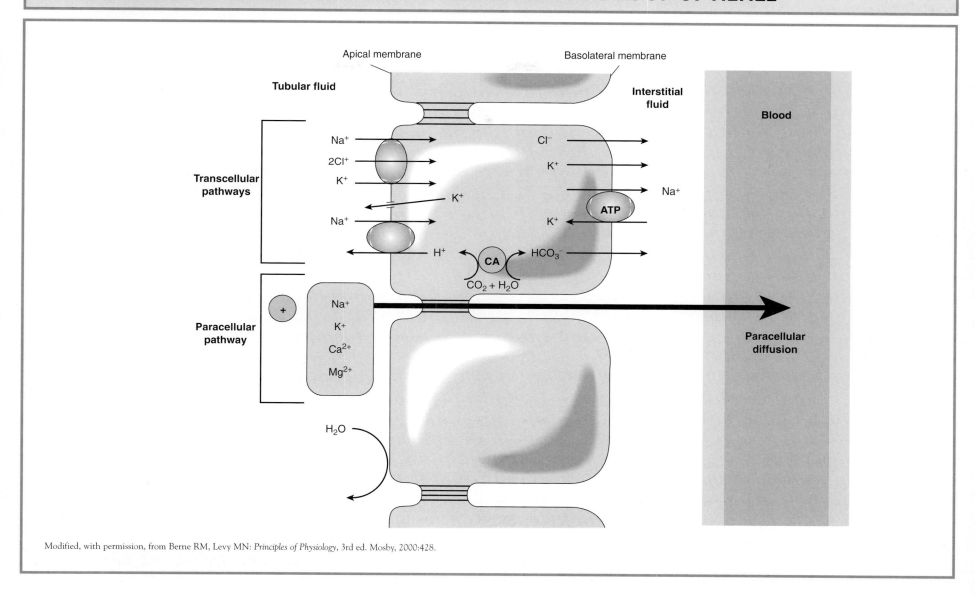

Modified, with permission, from Berne RM, Levy MN: *Principles of Physiology*, 3rd ed. Mosby, 2000:428.

EFFECTS OF DIURETICS ON THE KIDNEY

Type of Diuretic	Example(s)	Mechanism of Action/Result
Carbonic Anhydrase Inhibitors	Acetazolamide (Diamox).	• Decreases H^+ secretion in proximal tubule of loop of Henle. • Increase in Na^+ and K^+ excretion.
Loop	Furosemide (Lasix), bumetanide (Bumex).	• Inhibits $1Na^+$-$1K^+$-$2Cl^-$ cotransporter in medullary portion of thick ascending limb of loop of Henle by reducing positive voltage that drives paracellular resorption of these ions. • Inhibits water resorption by decreasing osmolality of medullary interstitial fluid. • Increase in urinary NaCl, K^+, Ca^{2+}, and H_2O excretion.
Potassium-sparing	Amiloride (Midamor), spironolactone (Aldactone), triamterene (Dyrenium).	• Inhibits Na^+ channels in distal tubule and collecting ducts which reduces net luminal charge, leading to decreased driving force for Cl^- resorption and inhibition of K^+ secretion. • Increase in urinary NaCl excretion and increased K^+ resorption.
Thiazide	Hydrochlorothiazide.	• Inhibits $1Na^+$-$1K^+$-$2Cl^-$ cotransporter in proximal portion of distal tubule. • Stimulates Ca^{2+} resorption. • Increase in urinary K^+ excretion, and decreased Ca^{2+} excretion.
Xanthines	Caffeine, theophylline.	Decrease in tubular reabsorption of Na^+.

ACTIONS OF DIURETICS ON THE NEPHRON

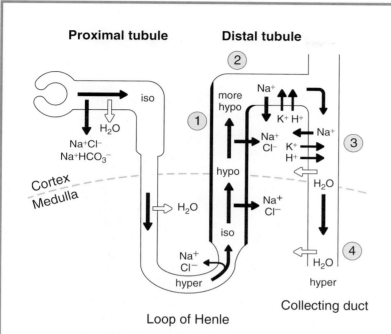

Proximal tubule

Distal tubule

iso

H_2O

Na^+Cl^-
$Na^+HCO_3^-$

Cortex
Medulla

more
hypo

Na^+

K^+ H^+

Na^+
Cl^- K^+ H^+ Na^+

hypo

H_2O

H_2O

Na^+
Cl^-

iso

Na^+
Cl^-

hyper

Na^+
Cl^-

hyper

Collecting duct

Loop of Henle

① Loop diuretics act on the thick ascending limb of Henle.

② Thiazide diuretics act on the first part of the distal convoluted tubule.

③ Aldosterone antagonists, amiloride, and triamterene primarily act on the collecting duct.

④ Antagonists to V_2-vasopressin receptors act on the collecting duct.

Reproduced, with permission, from Ganong WF: Review of Medical Physiology, 20th ed. McGraw-Hill, 2001:700.

COMPETITION FOR SECRETION AMONG ORGANIC ANIONS AND CATIONS IN THE KIDNEY

Substances Secreted by Proximal Tubule		Examples	Clinical Significance
Organic Cations		Cimetidine reduces urinary excretion of procainamide by competing with it for organic cation secretory pathway.	• Administration of organic anions together or organic cations together can increase plasma concentration of both drugs to levels much higher than those seen when drugs are given alone.
Endogenous cations:	Drugs:		• This process may cause drug toxicity.
• Creatinine.	• Amiloride.		
• Dopamine.	• Atropine.		
• Epinephrine.	• Cimetidine.		
• Norepinephrine.	• Isoproterenol.		
	• Morphine.		
	• Procainamide.		
	• Quinine.		
Organic Anions		Infusion of *para*-aminohippuric acid reduces urinary excretion of penicillin by competing with it for organic cation secretory pathway.	• Reduction of penicillin excretion due to administration of *para*-aminohippuric acid extends biological half-life of penicillin.
Endogenous anions:	Drugs:		• Hippurates were given with penicillin during World War II, when penicillin was in short supply.
• Bile salts.	• Acetazolamide.		
• Hippurates.	• Bumetanide.		
• Oxalate.	• Chlorothiazide.		
• Prostaglandins.	• Furosemide.		
• Urate.	• Hydrochlorothiazide.		
	• Penicillin.		
	• Probenecid.		
	• Salicylate.		

REGULATION OF POTASSIUM SECRETION

Regulating Factor	Effect	Mechanisms
Plasma [K^+]	Hyperkalemia stimulates K^+ secretion.	• Stimulates Na^+-K^+-ATPase. • Increases permeability of apical membrane to K^+. • Stimulates aldosterone secretion. • Increases flow rate of tubular fluid.
	Hypokalemia inhibits K^+ secretion.	Mechanisms opposite to those listed immediately above.
Aldosterone	Stimulates K^+ secretion.	• Aldosterone is stimulated by hyperkalemia and angiotensin II and is inhibited by hypokalemia and ANP. • Aldosterone acts synergistically with plasma [K^+] to stimulate K^+ secretion. • It increases Na^+-K^+-ATPase and permeability of apical membrane to K^+.
ADH	Stimulates K^+ secretion.	• Increases electrochemical driving force for K^+ exit across apical membrane (increases K^+ secretion). • Decreases tubular flow by stimulating water resorption (decreases K^+ secretion). • Inhibitory effect of decreased flow of tubular fluid offsets stimulatory effect on electrochemical driving force for K^+ exit. • As a result, urinary K^+ excretion is kept constant despite wide fluctuations in water excretion.
Metabolic Acid-Base Balance	• Acute acidosis decreases K^+ secretion. • Acute alkalosis increases K^+ secretion.	• Acute acidosis inhibits Na^+-K^+-ATPase, reducing cell [K^+] and electrochemical driving force for K^+ exit across apical membrane; it also decreases permeability of apical membrane to K^+. • Acute alkalosis has opposite effects.
	Chronic metabolic acidosis may either inhibit or stimulate K^+ excretion, depending on duration of disturbance.	• When metabolic acidosis lasts for days, renal K^+ excretion is stimulated. • Na^+-K^+-ATPase is inhibited, causing decreased resorption of water and NaCl in proximal tubule and increased tubular fluid flow via distal tubule and collecting duct. • ECF is also decreased, which stimulates aldosterone.

Continued

REGULATION OF POTASSIUM SECRETION (Continued)

Regulating Factor	Effect	Mechanisms
		• Long-term acidosis increases plasma [K^+], which stimulates aldosterone, leading to increased tubular fluid flow.
		• All these events offset effects of acidosis on cell [K^+] and apical membrane permeability, causing increased K^+ secretion.
Tubular Fluid Flow	Increased tubular fluid flow (eg, ECF volume expansion, diuretic treatment) stimulates K^+ secretion.	• K^+ secretion increases [K^+] in tubular fluid.
		• This increase reduces electrochemical driving force for K^+ across apical membrane and thereby reduces rate of K^+ secretion (like negative feedback loop).
		• Increased tubular fluid flow minimizes rise in tubular fluid [K^+] as secreted K^+ is excreted.
		• Diuretics increase tubular fluid flow and increase renal K^+ secretion and excretion.
		• Increased tubular flow also increases amount of Na^+ entering distal tubule and collecting duct, causing increased Na^+ resorption that stimulates K^+ uptake across basolateral membrane by increasing Na^+-K^+-ATPase.
	Decreased tubular fluid flow (eg, ECF volume contraction, diarrhea, vomiting, hemorrhage) decreases K^+ secretion.	Mechanisms opposite to those listed immediately above.

EFFECT OF CERTAIN PHYSIOLOGIC STATES ON POTASSIUM HOMEOSTASIS

Physiologic State	Effect	Mechanism
Metabolic Acid-Base Disorders	• Metabolic acidosis increases plasma $[K^+]$. • Metabolic alkalosis decreases plasma $[K^+]$.	• Low pH promotes movement of H^+ into cells and reciprocal movement of K^+ out of cells. • High pH has opposite effect.
Plasma Osmolality	• High ECF osmolality increases plasma K^+. • Low ECF osmolality decreases plasma K^+.	• Increased plasma osmolality causes water to leave cells until ICF and ECF osmolality are equal. • Water loss shrinks cells, causing increase in intracellular $[K^+]$ that drives K^+ from cells, increasing plasma $[K^+]$.
Cell Lysis	Hyperkalemia.	• Destroyed cells release K^+ and other solutes into ECF. • Examples: severe trauma, rhabdomyolysis, tumor lysis syndrome, digestion of RBCs in gastric ulcer disease.
Exercise	Hyperkalemia.	• More K^+ is released from skeletal muscle cells during exercise than during rest. • Severity of hyperkalemia depends on degree of exercise. • Exercise-induced hyperkalemia is usually asymptomatic and normalizes after rest. • Exercise can cause life-threatening hyperkalemia in individuals with impaired ability to excrete K^+ (eg, renal failure); those with endocrine disorders that affect insulin, epinephrine, or aldosterone; and those who take β-blockers.
Postprandial	Hyperkalemia.	• Minutes after GI tract K^+ absorption, plasma $[K^+]$ rises and stimulates secretion of insulin, epinephrine, and aldosterone. • Insulin, epinephrine, and aldosterone increase K^+ uptake in bone, liver, RBCs, and skeletal muscle by stimulating Na^+-K^+-ATPase. • Rapid uptake into cells prevents potentially life-threatening hyperkalemia. • *Insulin is the most important hormone that shifts K^+ into cells after a meal.* • In individuals with diabetes mellitus, infusion of insulin (and glucose to prevent hypoglycemia) corrects hyperkalemia.

FACTORS THAT INFLUENCE POTASSIUM MOVEMENT IN THE NEPHRON

Type of Movement	Location	Mechanism	Influencing Factors
K$^+$ Resorption	Proximal tubule, loop of Henle, distal tubule, and collecting duct.	• Active K$^+$ resorption in proximal tubule via Na$^+$-K$^+$-ATPase. • Mechanism in distal tubule and collecting duct not well understood.	Dietary K$^+$: • Amount K$^+$ resorbed is a constant fraction of amount filtered. • For example, low dietary K$^+$ stimulates K$^+$ resorption in distal tubule and collecting duct.
K$^+$ Secretion	Distal tubule and collecting duct.	K$^+$ actively transported across basolateral membrane via Na$^+$-K$^+$-ATPase, then diffuses across apical membrane into tubular fluid.	Dietary K$^+$: • When K$^+$ excreted > K$^+$ filtered, K$^+$ secretion increases. Acid-base status: • Acidosis decreases K$^+$ secretion. • Alkalosis increases K$^+$ secretion. Hormones: • ADH and aldosterone increase K$^+$ secretion. Hyperkalemia increases K$^+$ secretion.
K$^+$ Excretion	Distal tubule and collecting duct.	Rate of renal K$^+$ excretion is determined by K$^+$ secretion in distal tubule and collecting duct.	Dietary K$^+$: • In average diet, renal K$^+$ excretion is 15% of amount filtered. • Low dietary K$^+$ may cause K$^+$ excretion to fall to 1% of that filtered. Acid-base status: • Chronic acidosis and alkalosis increase K$^+$ excretion. • Acute acidosis decreases K$^+$ excretion. Hormones: • Aldosterone and glucocorticoids increase K$^+$ excretion. Hyperkalemia increases K$^+$ excretion.

RENAL PROCESSING OF CALCIUM AND PHOSPHATE

Substance	Important Points	Factors that Increase Resorption	Factors that Increase Excretion
Calcium	• 99% is resorbed by nephron: 70% in proximal tubule, 20% in loop of Henle (mainly thick ascending limb). • Resorption of Ca^{2+} and Na^+ parallel each other. • 10% of filtered load is excreted.	• Volume contraction. • Alkalosis. • Hormones: PTH, calcitriol.	• Volume expansion. • Acidosis. • Hormones: calcitonin.
Phosphate	• Normally resorbed at maximum rate, determined by diet: 80% in proximal tubule, 10% in distal tubule. • High-phosphate diets decrease maximal resorptive rate, and low-phosphate diets increase (independent of PTH levels).	• Volume contraction. • Alkalosis. • Hormones: PTH, calcitriol.	• Volume expansion. • Acidosis. • Hormones: calcitonin, glucocorticoids. • Because P_i is resorbed maximally, any increase in amount filtered causes a rise in urinary P_i excretion.

IV. Renal Regulation

THE THREE COMPONENTS OF THE RENIN-ANGIOTENSIN-ALDOSTERONE SYSTEM

Feature	Renin	Angiotensin II	Aldosterone
Description	Renal hormone (proteolytic enzyme) produced by juxtaglomerular cells in afferent arterioles.	• Protein produced on surface of vascular endothelial cells in lungs and kidneys. • Angiotensin I is converted to angiotensin II by ACE. • Secretagogue for aldosterone.	Renal hormone produced in glomerulosa cells of adrenal cortex.
Function	Converts angiotensinogen (made in liver) to angiotensin I.	• Produces arteriolar vasoconstriction, which increases systemic blood pressure. • Increases NaCl resorption by proximal tubules. • Stimulates contraction of mesangial cells, resulting in decreased GFR. • Stimulates ADH secretion and thirst.	• Stimulates NaCl resorption in distal tubule, collecting duct, and, in thick ascending loop, resulting in decreased NaCl excretion and increased water resorption. • Stimulates K^+ secretion by distal tubule and collecting duct.
Regulation	See "Regulation of Renin Secretion", p. 348.	• Factors that inhibit renin indirectly inhibit angiotensin II. • ACE-inhibitors (eg, captopril) inhibit angiotensin II.	• Pituitary ACTH stimulates adrenal cortex to secrete aldosterone. • Elevated plasma $[K^+]$ stimulates adrenal cortex to secrete aldosterone. • Elevated renin (via angiotensin II) stimulates aldosterone. • ANP inhibits aldosterone.

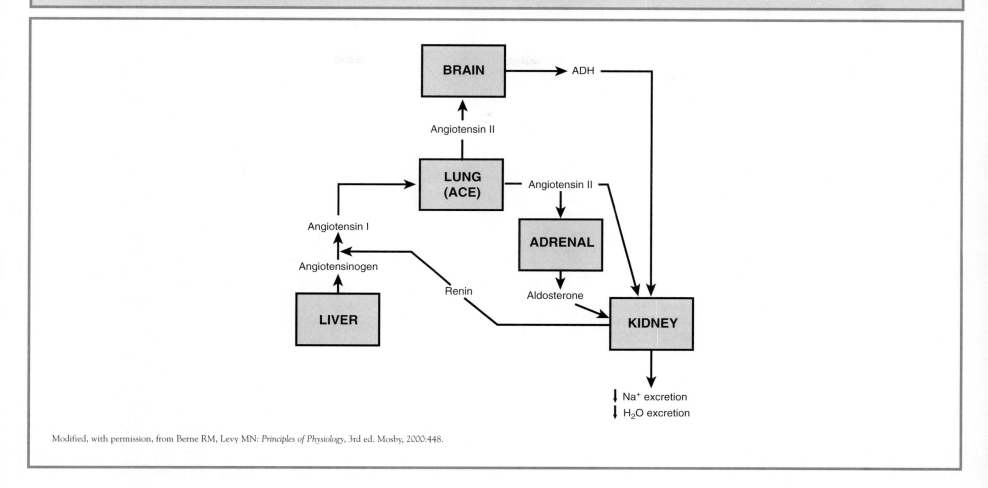

Modified, with permission, from Berne RM, Levy MN: *Principles of Physiology*, 3rd ed. Mosby, 2000:448.

REGULATION OF RENIN SECRETION

Factors	Mechanism
Sympathetic Nervous System	1. ECF volume contraction and negative Na^+ balance stimulate sympathetic nervous system.
	2. Sympathetic nervous system stimulation leads to:
	• Stimulation of juxtaglomerular cell renin secretion via β_1-adrenergic receptors.
	• Constriction of afferent and efferent arterioles (greater effect on afferent arterioles) via α-adrenergic receptors.
	• *Stimulation of NaCl resorption*, especially in proximal tubule.
Prostaglandin Activity	• Prostaglandins directly stimulate juxtaglomerular cells to secrete renin.
	• Note: inhibition of prostaglandins with indomethacin and propanolol inhibit renin secretion.
Perfusion Pressure	Afferent arteriole functions as high-pressure baroreceptor.
	• When afferent arteriole senses decreased perfusion pressure, renin secretion is stimulated.
	• Increased perfusion pressure inhibits renin.
Delivery of NaCl to Macula Densa	• Tubuloglomerular feedback: decreased NaCl delivery increases GFR, leading to increased renin (increased NaCl delivery inhibits renin).
	• This mechanism helps maintain systemic arterial pressure under conditions of reduced vascular volume.
	• Pathway: volume contraction → decreased perfusion to body tissues (including kidneys) → decreased GFR → decreased filtered load of NaCl → decreased delivery of NaCl to macula densa → renin stimulation → angiotensin II → vasoconstriction → increased blood pressure that helps maintain tissue perfusion.
Angiotensin II and Aldosterone	• Inhibit renin secretion via negative feedback on juxtaglomerular cells.
	• Note: elevated aldosterone can be associated with elevated renin in pathologic conditions such as secondary hyperaldosteronism, cirrhosis, and nephrosis.
ADH	Not completely understood.

RENAL ARTERY STENOSIS AND THE DEVELOPMENT OF RENAL HYPERTENSION

Step	Event
1	Renal artery constriction (eg, due to atherosclerotic plaque) reduces perfusion pressure to that kidney.
2	Afferent arteriole senses reduced perfusion pressure, leading to increased renin secretion.
3	Elevated renin increases production of angiotensin II.
4	Angiotensin II causes arteriolar vasoconstriction throughout vascular system, leading to increased systemic blood pressure.
5	Afferent arterioles of contralateral, nonstenosed kidney sense increased systemic blood pressure, leading to suppression of renin secretion from that kidney.
6	Elevated angiotensin II also works via negative feedback loop to inhibit renin secretion by contralateral, nonstenosed kidney.

ATRIAL NATRIURETIC PEPTIDE

Site of Origin	Stimuli	Functions	Mechanisms
• Produced and stored primarily in atrial myocytes. • Also produced in brain.	Released with atrial stretch in response to: • Positive Na⁺ balance. • ECF volume expansion. • Increased blood pressure.	• *Antagonizes RAAS.* • *Increases renal NaCl and water excretion and relaxes vascular smooth muscle, resulting in decreased systemic vascular resistance and blood pressure and extravasation of fluid.*	• Inhibits posterior pituitary ADH secretion and ADH-stimulated water resorption across collecting duct. • Inhibits renin secretion by afferent arterioles by its action on juxtaglomerular cells. • Inhibits aldosterone secretion by acting on adrenal cortex and via its inhibition of renin. • Counteracts pressor effects of catecholamines and angiotensin II. • Inhibits NaCl resorption by medullary collecting duct, directly and via its inhibition of aldosterone. • Dilates afferent arterioles by relaxing mesangial cells, which increases GFR and filtered load of Na⁺. • Constricts efferent arterioles, which increases GFR and filtered load of Na⁺. • Relaxes vascular smooth muscle of arterioles and venules.

REGULATION OF ANTIDIURETIC HORMONE

Description	Function	Stimulatory Factors	Inhibitory Factors
• Hormone that is produced in neuroendocrine cells of supraoptic and paraventricular nuclei of hypothalamus and stored in neurohypophysis (posterior pituitary). • Only major hormone that directly regulates renal H_2O excretion. • Homeostasis when osmolality is 280–295 mOsm/kg H_2O. • 5–10% decrease in blood volume or arterial pressure is required before ADH is stimulated.	• Increases permeability of collecting duct to water, leading to net absorption of water from tubule lumen into blood. • Increased osmolality of medullary interstitial fluid also increases permeability of medullary collecting duct to urea (which adds to effect of ADH). • Stimulates K^+ secretion. • High levels of ADH result in antidiuresis with small volumes of concentrated urine. • Low levels of ADH result in water diuresis with large volumes of dilute urine.	• Many factors that stimulate production of ADH also stimulate the thirst center (located in the anterolateral hypothalamus). • Volume contraction (decreased ECF volume). • Increased plasma oncotic pressure. • Angiotensin II. • Nausea and vomiting. • Pain, stress, exercise.	• Volume expansion (increased ECF volume). • Decreased plasma oncotic pressure. • ANP. • Alcohol.

SUMMARY OF THE REGULATION OF RENAL NaCl AND H²O RESORPTION

Factor	Major Stimulus	Action in Nephron
ADH	Increased plasma osmolality, decreased ECF volume.	Increases water resorption in distal tubule and collecting duct.
Aldosterone	Increased angiotensin II, increased [K+].	• Increases NaCl resorption in thick ascending limb. • Increases NaCl and water resorption in distal tubule and collecting duct.
Angiotensin II	Increased renin.	Increases NaCl and water resorption in proximal tubule.
ANP	Increased ECF volume, increased blood pressure.	• Increases GFR. • Decreases renin, aldosterone, and ADH. • Decreases water and NaCl resorption in collecting duct.
Urodilatin	Increased ECF volume, increased blood pressure.	Decreases water and NaCl resorption in collecting duct.
Dopamine	Increased ECF volume.	Decreases water and NaCl resorption in proximal tubule.
Sympathetic Nervous System	Decreased ECF volume.	• Decreases GFR. • Increases renin secretion. • Increases NaCl resorption in thick ascending limb. • Increases NaCl and water resorption in proximal tubule, distal tubule, and collecting duct.

V. Acid-Base Relationships

GENERAL CONCEPTS IN ACID-BASE PHYSIOLOGY

Concept	Description
Normal pH	• ECF is maintained within narrow range of pH (7.35–7.45). • Life cannot exist outside pH 6.8 to 7.8.
Normal Arterial Blood Gas	pH = 7.4, P_{CO_2} = 40 mm Hg, ECF $[HCO_3^-]$ = 24 mEq/L.
Primary Reaction	$CO_2 + H_2O \leftrightarrow H_2CO_3 \leftrightarrow H^+ + HCO_3^-$ • First part of reaction is hydration and dehydration of CO_2. • *This rate-limiting step is catalyzed by carbonic anhydrase.*
Henderson-Hasselbach Equation	pH = pK + log ($[A^-]/[HA]$). • A^- = any anion. • HA = dissociated acid. • Shows that pH of ECF varies when either HCO_3^- or P_{CO_2} is altered. • pH = 6.1 + log ($[HCO_3^-]/0.03\ P_{CO_2}$).
Regulation	• *Kidneys are primarily responsible for regulating $[HCO_3^-]$.* • *Lungs are primarily responsible for regulating P_{CO_2}.*
Compensatory Responses	• Minimize pH changes but do not correct underlying processes that produce acid-base disorders. • Such underlying causes of disorders must be corrected to restore blood pH to normal. • See "Compensatory Responses of ECF to Changes in pH", p. 354.

COMPENSATORY RESPONSES OF EXTRACELLULAR FLUID TO CHANGES IN pH

Compensatory Response	Description	Mechanism
Extracellular Buffering	• HCO_3^- buffer system is principal ECF buffer. • Additional ECF buffers are phosphate and plasma proteins.	• Addition of nonvolatile acid or loss of base neutralizes acid load and consumes HCO_3^-, resulting in decreased $[HCO_3^-]$ in ECF. • Addition of nonvolatile base or loss of acid leads to consumption of H^+, resulting in HCO_3^- production (from dissociation of H_2CO_3) and increased $[HCO_3^-]$ in ECF.
	ECF buffering by bone.	• Acidosis promotes binding of Ca^{2+}-containing salts to H^+ in exchange for Ca^{2+}. • This leads to Ca^{2+} release and demineralization of bone.
Intracellular Buffering	ICF buffering.	• Buffering of nonvolatile acid promotes movement of H^+ into cells. • Buffering of nonvolatile alkali promotes movement of H^+ out of cells. • H^+ is titrated inside cell by HCO_3^-, phosphate, and proteins.
Alterations in Ventilatory Rate	• Ventilatory rate adjusts blood P_{CO_2} and pH and vice versa. • Response may be initiated within minutes but may require hours to achieve maximal effect.	• Metabolic acidosis increases $[H^+]$, decreases pH, and increases ventilatory rate (metabolic alkalosis has opposite effects). • Increased ventilation decreases P_{CO_2}, which increases pH and creates respiratory alkalosis (decreased ventilation has opposite effects). • Maximal hyperventilation can reduce P_{CO_2} to 10 mm Hg. • Hypoventilation cannot raise $P_{CO_2} > 60$ mm Hg. • Respiratory acidosis (increased P_{CO_2}) causes CO_2 to move into cell where it is hydrated to form H_2CO_3, resulting in H^+ production (respiratory alkalosis has opposite effects).
Adjustments in Renal NAE	• Kidneys adjust excretion of net acid and HCO_3^- to alter pH and P_{CO_2}. • Response may take days to complete.	• Metabolic acidosis (increased $[H^+]$ or P_{CO_2}) stimulates H^+ secretion and entire filtered load of HCO_3^- is resorbed. • Renal production and excretion of NH_4^+ is also stimulated. • Result is increased NAE, production of new HCO_3^-, and increased plasma $[HCO_3^-]$ (metabolic alkalosis (decreased $[H^+]$ or P_{CO_2}) has opposite effects).

VOLATILE AND NONVOLATILE ACID PRODUCTION

Body State	Dietary Source	Product(s) of Metabolism	Result
Normal	Carbohydrates and fats.	CO_2 and H_2O.	CO_2 is eliminated from body by lungs and has no impact on acid-base balance.
	Amino acids.	Net nonvolatile acids: • Cysteine and methionine $\rightarrow$ sulfuric acid. • Lysine, arginine, and histidine $\rightarrow$ hydrochloric acid.	• Nonvolatile acids do not circulate throughout body but are immediately buffered. • Acids and alkalis from diet and cellular metabolism, and HCO_3^- lost in feces add a net of about 1 mEq/kg of nonvolatile acid to body weight each day.
		Bicarbonate aspartate and glutamate $\rightarrow HCO_3^-$.	HCO_3^- in ECF is important buffer: • $H_2SO_4 + 2NaHCO_3 \leftrightarrow Na_2SO_4 + 2CO_2 + 2H_2O$ • $HCl + NaHCO_3 \leftrightarrow NaCl + CO_2 + H_2O$ • $CO_2 + H_2O \rightarrow HCO_3^- + H^+$
			• Buffering process yields Na^+ salts of strong acid anions and removes HCO_3^- from ECF. • Kidneys excrete Na^+ salts and replenish HCO_3^- lost by neutralization of nonvolatile acids.
	Organic anions (eg, citrate).	HCO_3^-.	See HCO_3^- above.
Low Insulin Levels	Carbohydrates and fats.	Organic ketoacids (eg, β-hydroxybutyric acid).	• Ketoacids serve as source of energy during starvation. • Individuals with diabetes mellitus are at risk for diabetic ketoacidosis.
Hypoxic State	Carbohydrates and fats.	Organic acids (eg, lactic acid) due to anaerobic metabolism.	• Organic acids accumulate and body fluid pH decreases (acidosis). • Occurs in normal patients during vigorous exercise. • Poor tissue perfusion (eg, during reduced cardiac output) can also lead to anaerobic metabolism and thus to acidosis.
			Treatment: • Insulin in case of diabetes mellitus. • Improved oxygen delivery to tissues, which promotes metabolism of these organic acids to CO_2 and H_2O and helps correct acid-base disorder.

NET ACID EXCRETION

Description	Mechanism	Formula

- Renal resorption of filtered load of HCO_3^- and renal excretion of acid equals amount of nonvolatile acid produced each day.

- *To maintain acid-base balance, net acid excretion must equal nonvolatile acid production.*

Normally, very little HCO_3^- is excreted, and net acid excretion reflects titratable acid and NH_4^+ excretion.

- Titratable acid = 1/3 of net acid excretion.

- NH_4^+ = 2/3 of net acid excretion.

Resorption of filtered HCO_3^- and excretion of acid occurs via H^+ secretion by nephron:

- Kidneys excrete salts of free acids and excrete H^+ with titratable acids such as phosphate (they cannot excrete free acids).

- Kidneys synthesize and excrete NH_4^+ and return HCO_3^- to systemic circulation (replenishing HCO_3^- lost during neutralization of nonvolatile acid).

- Minimal urine pH attainable by kidneys is 4–4.5.

- Renal acid excretion normally creates acidic urine.

$NAE = [(U_{NH4+} \times \dot{V}) + (U_{TA} \times \dot{V})] - (U_{HCO3}^- \times \dot{V})$

- $(U_{NH4+} \times \dot{V})$ = rate of excretion of NH_4^+ (mEq/d).

- $(U_{TA} \times \dot{V})$ = rate of excretion of titratable acid (mEq/d).

- $(U_{HCO3}^- \times \dot{V})$ = amount of HCO_3^- lost in urine (equivalent to adding H^+ to body).

FORMATION OF NEW HCO$_3^-$ FROM NH$_4^+$ IN THE NEPHRON

Structure	Primary Process	Result	Mechanism(s)
		To maintain acid-base balance, kidneys replace HCO$_3^-$ lost during buffering of nonvolatile acids via HCO$_3^-$ resorption and the synthesis and excretion of NH$_4^+$.	
Proximal Tubule	NH$_4^+$ metabolized from glutamine.	*If NH$_4^+$ is excreted, new HCO$_3^-$ is formed.*	HCO$_3^-$ exits across basolateral membrane and is resorbed into blood as new HCO$_3^-$.
		NH$_4^+$ excretion can be used as a "marker" of glutamine metabolism in proximal tubule.	• Systemic acidosis stimulates cell enzymes in proximal tubule responsible for glutamine metabolism → increased NH$_4^+$ → increased "new" HCO$_3^-$ (alkalosis has opposite effect). • Hypokalemia stimulates NH$_4^+$ production, and hyperkalemia inhibits it. • NH$_4^+$ exits cell across apical membrane and is secreted into tubular fluid via Na$^+$-H$^+$ antiporter, with NH$_4^+$ substituting for H$^+$. • NH$_3$ can also diffuse out of cell into tubular fluid, where it is protonated to NH$_4^+$.
		If NH$_4^+$ is not excreted but is resorbed into systemic circulation, it is converted into urea by liver.	• Urea formation generates H$^+$, which is then buffered by HCO$_3^-$. • Urea production from NH$_4^+$ consumes HCO$_3^-$ and negates formation of HCO$_3^-$ through renal synthesis and excretion of NH$_4^+$.
Thick Ascending Limb	NH$_4^+$ resorption.	NH$_4^+$ resorption.	• 1Na$^+$-1K$^+$-2Cl$^-$-symporter with NH$_4^+$ substituting for K$^+$. • Positive transepithelial gradient in lumen also drives paracellular resorption of NH$_4^+$.
Collecting Duct	H$^+$ secretion.	• H$^+$ secretion in collecting duct results in excretion of NH$_4^+$ being resorbed by thick ascending limb. • Inhibition of H$^+$ secretion in collecting duct results in return to circulation of NH$_4^+$ being resorbed by thick ascending limb and its conversion to urea by liver.	Active H$^+$ secretion parallels passive diffusion of NH$_3$. (Collecting duct does not have specific transport mechanism for NH$_4^+$ secretion and is not significantly permeable to it; however, it is permeable to NH$_3$.)

Continued

FORMATION OF NEW HCO$_3^-$ FROM NH$_4^+$ IN THE NEPHRON (Continued)

Structure	Primary Process	Result	Mechanism(s)
Medullary Interstitium	Nonionic diffusion and diffusion trapping leads to NH$_4^+$ excretion.	NH$_4^+$ resorbed by thick ascending limb accumulates in medullary interstitium, exits in chemical equilibrium with NH$_3$, and then reenters tubular fluid of collecting duct.	Nonionic diffusion: • NH$_3$ diffusing from medullary interstitium into lumen of collecting duct lumen. • NH$_3$ is protonated to NH$_4^+$ by acidic tubular fluid (collecting duct is less permeable to NH$_4^+$ than to NH$_3$). Diffusion trapping: • NH$_4^+$ is trapped in tubule lumen and is excreted in urine.

RESORPTION OF FILTERED HCO$_3^-$ IN THE NEPHRON

Location	Mechanism(s)
Proximal Tubule (80%)	• H$^+$ secreted across apical membrane via Na$^+$-H$^+$ antiporter and H$^+$-ATPase. • Inside cell, H$^+$ and HCO$_3^-$ production is catalyzed by carbonic anhydrase. • H$^+$ is secreted into tubular fluid. • HCO$_3^-$ exits across basolateral membrane and returns to blood via 1Na$^+$-3HCO$_3^-$ symporter and Cl$^-$-HCO$_3^-$ antiporter,
Thick Ascending Limb (15%)	Mechanisms identical to those in proximal tubule, except carbonic anhydrase is not present in brush border of thick ascending limb.
Distal Tubule and Collecting Duct (5%)	• In intercalated cells, H$^+$ and HCO$_3^-$ production is catalyzed by carbonic anhydrase. • H$^+$ is secreted via apical membrane ATPase and H$^+$-K$^+$ ATPase. • *H$^+$ secretion predominates under normal conditions.* • HCO$_3^-$ exits across basolateral membrane via Cl$^-$-HCO$_3^-$ antiporter and enters blood. • Second population of intercalated cells in collecting duct have H$^+$-ATPase in basolateral membrane and Cl$^-$-HCO$_3^-$ antiporter in apical membrane, causing HCO$_3^-$ to be secreted into tubular fluid instead of H$^+$. • Activity here is increased during metabolic alkalosis when kidneys must excrete excess HCO$_3^-$.

FACTORS THAT INCREASE H⁺ SECRETION[1]

Factor	Mechanism
Acidosis (decreased plasma [HCO_3^-] or increased P_{CO_2})	• Acidosis decreases pH of nephron cells, creating cell-to-tubular fluid H⁺ gradient that stimulates H⁺ secretion. • Acidosis also increases Na^+-H^+ antiporter in apical membrane and Na^+-$3HCO_3^-$ symporter in basolateral membrane of proximal tubule. • Intercalated cells of collecting duct increase H^+-ATPase in apical membrane.
ECF Volume Contraction/ Negative Na^+ Balance	Activation of RAAS increases Na^+ resorption: • Angiotensin II stimulates Na^+-H^+ antiporter in apical membrane of proximal tubule and thick ascending limb, which stimulates H⁺ secretion. • Aldosterone stimulates intercalated cells to secrete H⁺ in addition to stimulating Na^+ resorption.
Increased Filtered Load of HCO_3^-	• H⁺ secretion in proximal tubule and thick ascending limb is linked to Na^+ resorption via Na^+-H^+ antiporter. • Therefore, factors that alter Na^+ resorption secondarily affect H⁺ secretion. • Example: when GFR is increased, filtered load of Na^+ is increased (glomerulotubular balance) and more fluid (including HCO_3^-) is resorbed.
Hypokalemia	Acidifies cells.
PTH	PTH inhibits Na^+-H^+ antiporter in apical membrane of proximal tubule, which decreases proximal tubular resorption of HCO_3^-.

[1]Contrasting factors (alkalosis, volume expansion, decreased filtered HCO_3^-, hyperkalemia) have opposite effects

ACID SECRETION BY PROXIMAL TUBULE CELLS IN THE KIDNEY

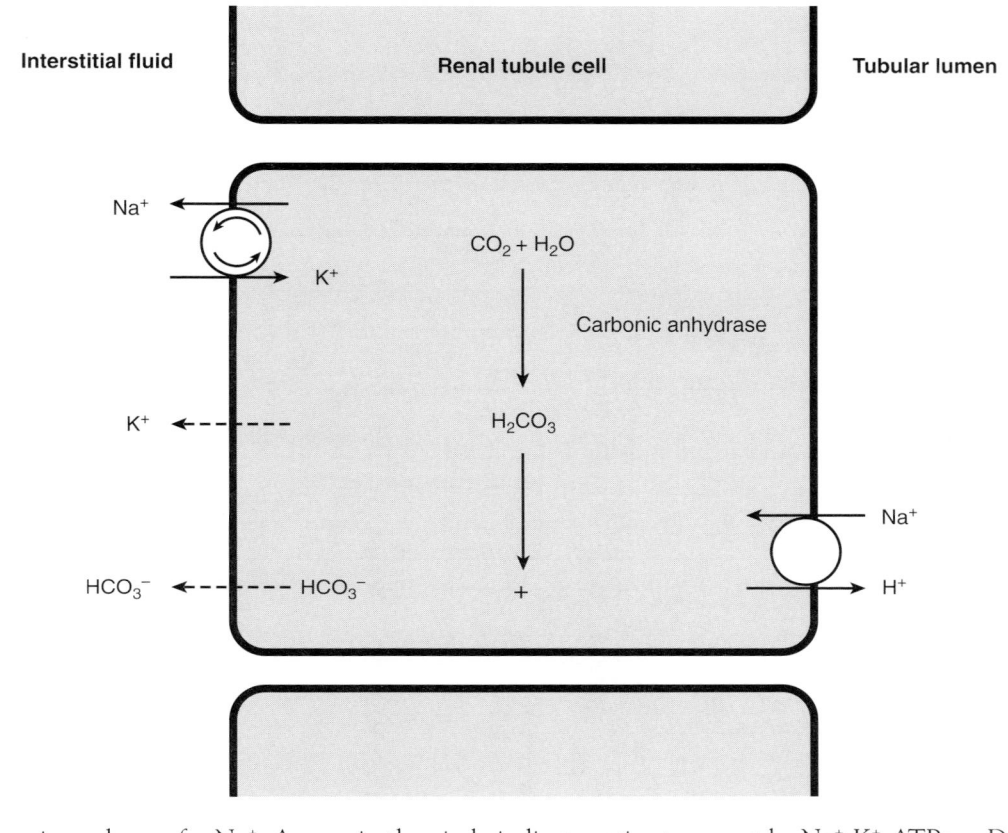

H+ is transported into tubular lumen in exchange for Na+. Arrows in the circle indicate active transport by Na+-K+-ATPase. Dashed arrows indicate diffusion.

EVALUATION OF THE ANION GAP

Anion Gap Value	Description	Associated Conditions
Normal	• Difference between concentrations of the major plasma cation (Na^+) and major plasma anions (Cl^- and HCO_3^-). • Anion gap = $[Na^+] - ([Cl^-] + [HCO_3^-])$. • 8–16 mEq/L. • Tool used to analyze cause of metabolic acidosis.	• Diarrhea. • Renal tubular acidosis.
Increased	• Decrease in $[HCO_3^-]$ is not matched by an increase in $[Cl^-]$ but rather by an increase in unmeasured anions. • Anion of nonvolatile acid is not Cl^- (eg, lactate, β-hydroxybutyrate). • Seen with increase in organic anions or decreased plasma $[K^+]$, $[Ca^{2+}]$, or $[Mg^{2+}]$.	☞ Remember SLUMPED: • Salicylates (acetylsalicylic acid). • Lactic acidosis. • Uremia (renal failure). • Methanol (and alcohol). • Paraldehyde. • Ethylene glycol. • Diabetic ketoacidosis. Other causes include: carbon monoxide, cyanide, toluene, isoniazid, and iron.
Decreased	• May occur with dissociation of protons from plasma proteins. • May occur from an increase in unmeasured cations (Ca^{2+}, Mg^{2+}, γ-globulins, and lithium).	• Acidemia. • Hypoalbuminemia. • Hemodilution. • Assay artifacts (eg, Cl^- in bromide therapy).

TECHNIQUE FOR USING ARTERIAL BLOOD GAS MEASUREMENTS TO IDENTIFY ACID-BASE DISORDERS

Step	Question to Ask	Aspect of ABG to Examine	Answer
1	Is there an underlying acidosis or alkalosis?	pH.	• pH indicates origin of initial disorder. • *There is not an over compensation for the primary abnormality.*
2	Is the disorder primarily metabolic or respiratory?	$[HCO_3^-]$ and P_{CO_2}.	• If primary metabolic disorder, $[HCO_3^-]$ is either significantly decreased (acidosis) or elevated (alkalosis). • If primary respiratory disorder, P_{CO_2} is either significantly elevated (acidosis) or depressed (alkalosis).
3	Is there a compensatory response?	$[HCO_3^-]$ and P_{CO_2}.	Compensatory response for a primary metabolic disorder involves changes in ventilation (and thus changes in P_{CO_2}): • Appropriately compensated metabolic acidosis leads to a decrease in P_{CO_2}. • Appropriately compensated metabolic alkalosis leads to an increase in P_{CO_2}. Compensatory response for a primary respiratory disorder involves changes in renal acid excretion (and thus changes in $[HCO_3^-]$): • Appropriately compensated respiratory acidosis leads to an increase in $[HCO_3^-]$. • Appropriately compensated respiratory alkalosis leads to a decrease in $[HCO_3^-]$

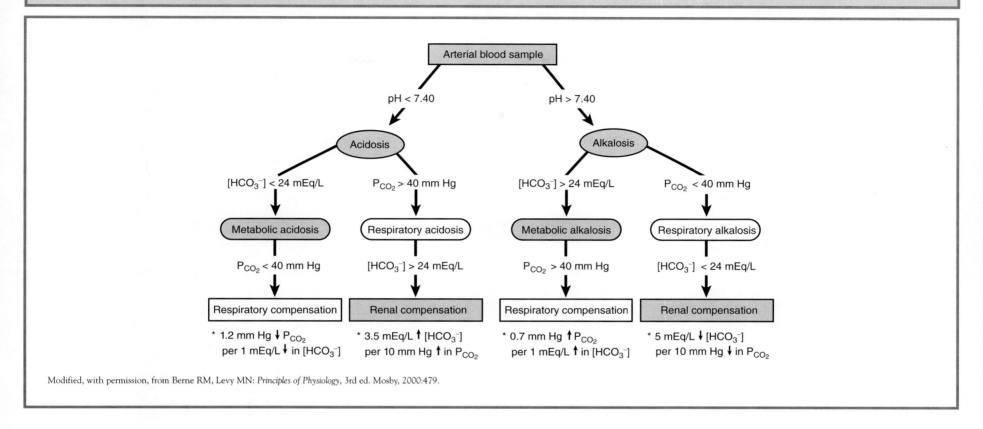

Modified, with permission, from Berne RM, Levy MN: *Principles of Physiology*, 3rd ed. Mosby, 2000:479.

SUMMARY OF ACID-BASE DISORDERS

Disorder	Plasma pH	Primary Abnormality	Compensatory Mechanism	Associated Conditions
Metabolic Acidosis	Decreased.	Decreased plasma $[HCO_3^-]$.	• ECF and ICF buffers. • *Hyperventilation* decreases P_{CO_2}. • Decreased renal HCO_3^- excretion increases plasma $[HCO_3^-]$.	• Diabetic ketoacidosis (addition of nonvolatile acid). • Diarrhea (loss of nonvolatile base). • Renal tubular acidosis and renal failure (kidneys fail to excrete enough net acid to replenish HCO_3^- used to neutralize nonvolatile acids).
Metabolic Alkalosis	Increased.	Increased plasma $[HCO_3^-]$.	• ECF and ICF buffers. • *Hypoventilation* increases P_{CO_2}. • Increased renal HCO_3^- excretion decreases plasma $[HCO_3^-]$ and creates *paradoxically acidic urine*.	• Ingestion of antacids (addition of nonvolatile base). • Hemorrhage (volume contraction). • Vomiting or nasogastric suction (loss of HCl, a nonvolatile acid).
Respiratory Acidosis	Decreased.	Increased P_{CO_2}.	• ICF buffers. • Decreased renal HCO_3^- excretion increases plasma $[HCO_3^-]$.	• Drugs or trauma that depress respiratory centers (inadequate ventilation). • Pulmonary edema (impaired gas diffusion).
Respiratory Alkalosis	Increased.	Decreased P_{CO_2}.	• ICF buffers. • Increased renal HCO_3^- excretion decreases plasma $[HCO_3^-]$.	• Elevated emotional state (anxiety, pain, or fear) associated with hyperventilation. • Drugs or central nervous system disorders that stimulate respiratory centers (cause hyperventilation).
Mixed Acid-Base Disorder	Normal.	Decreased P_{CO_2} and decreased plasma $[HCO_3^-]$.		• Ingestion of large amounts of acetylsalicylic acid (stimulates respiratory centers and causes hyperventilation). • Note: salicylic acid simultaneously produces metabolic acidosis and respiratory alkalosis.

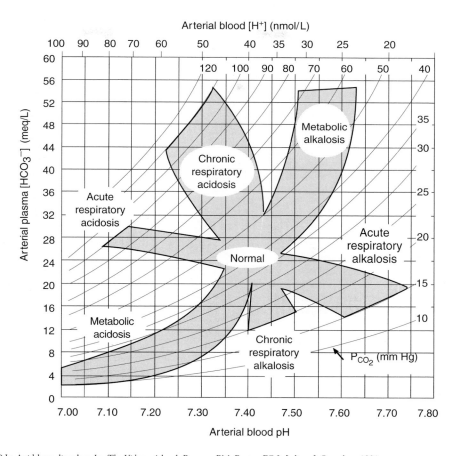

Reproduced, with permission from Cogan MG, Rector FC Jr: Acid-base disorders. In: *The Kidney*, 4th ed. Brenner BM, Rector FC Jr [editors]. Saunders, 1991.

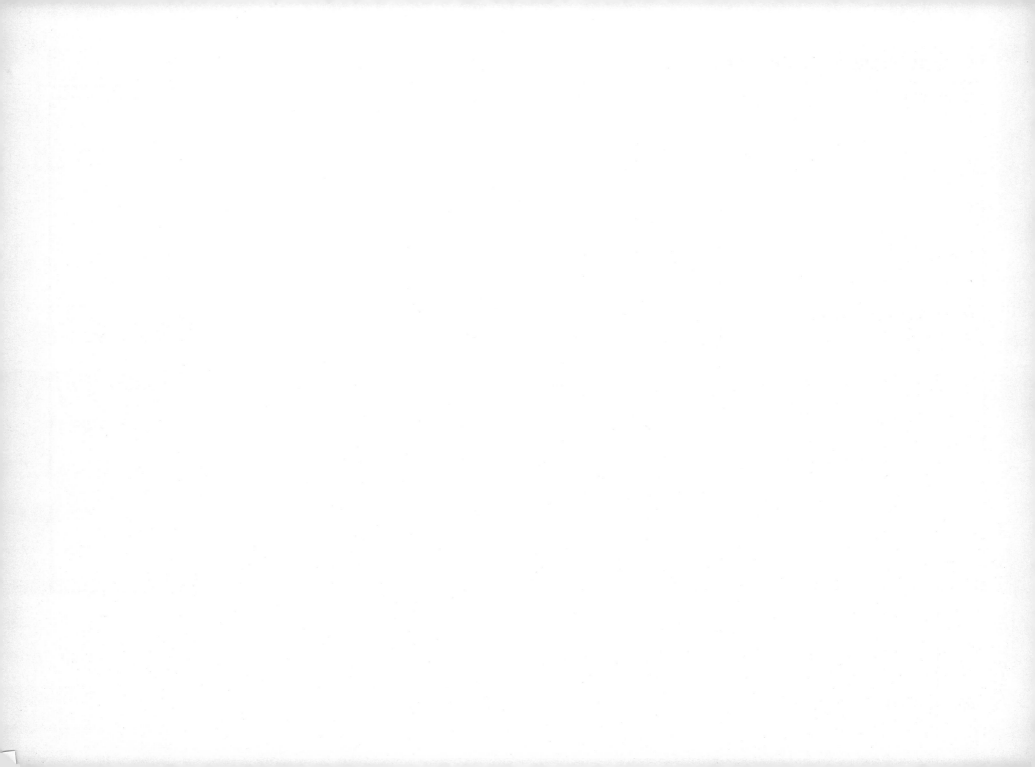

CHAPTER 7

METABOLISM

ABBREVIATIONS

ADP = adenosine diphosphate

ATP = adenosine triphosphate

CoA = coenzyme A

COX = cyclooxygenase

DM = diabetes mellitus

DNA = deoxyribonucleic acid

FFA = free fatty acid

HDL = high-density lipoprotein

G6P = glucose 6-phosphate

G6PD = glucose-6-phosphate dehydrogenase

GI = gastrointestinal

HDL = high-density lipoprotein

HMG-CoA = 3-hydroxy-3-methylglutaryl coenzyme A

IDL = intermediate-density lipoprotein

LDL = low-density lipoprotein

NADP = nicotinamide adenine dinucleotide phosphate

NADH = reduced nicotinamide adenine dinucleotide

NSAID = nonsteroidal anti-inflammatory drug

RNA = ribonucleic acid

TCA = tricarboxylic acid

VLDL = very low density lipoprotein

Anabolism	Formation of energy-storing substances such as proteins, fats, and carbohydrates from simpler molecules.
Apoproteins	Protein constituents of lipoproteins (apoproteins B, C, and E) that are synthesized in liver and intestine, interact with specific cell receptors, and serve catalytic functions.
Basal Metabolic Rate	Minimal energy expenditure at rest, linearly related to lean body mass and body surface area; equals 2000 kcal/d in average adult male.
Catabolism	Utilization of energy; oxidation of carbohydrates, proteins, and fats, producing mainly CO_2 and H_2O.
Cyclooxygenase	Enzyme that converts arachidonic acid to prostaglandins, prostaclcyins, and thromboxanes; two types are COX-1 and COX-2.
Eicosanoids	Substances derived from arachidonic acid (a 20-carbon [eicosa-] polyunsaturated fatty acid) and linoleic and linolenic acids, including prostaglandins, prostacyclin, thromboxanes, lipoxins, and leukotrienes.
Essential Fatty Acids	Those fatty acids that cannot be synthesized by humans and must be obtained in the diet—linolenic, linoleic, and arachidonic acid. Vegetable oils are sources of linolenic and linoleic acids, and arachidonic acid results from the synthesis of linoleic acid.
Gluconeogenesis	Synthesis of glucose from noncarbohydrate sources such as amino acids; occurs mainly in liver and kidneys. Gluconeogenesis meets the body's need for glucose when carbohydrates are not available in sufficient amounts (eg, during stress or starvation).
Glycogen	Storage form of glucose, with major supplies in liver and skeletal muscle.
Glycogenesis	Synthesis of glycogen, which is derived from glucose, galactose, and fructose, or formed de novo from pyruvate, lactate, glycerol, and amino acids (except leucine); occurs in liver and kidney.
Glycogenolysis	Breakdown of glycogen.
Glycolysis	Conversion of glucose to pyruvate or lactate; *phosphofructokinase 1 is the rate-limiting enzyme*.
Lipoproteins	Complex particles made of triglycerides, cholesterol, phospholipids, and apolipoproteins that increase solubility of lipids, allowing water-insoluble phospholipids, triglycerides, and cholesterol to travel in plasma. Examples include chylomicrons, HDL, LDL, and VLDL.
Oxidation	Combination of a substance with O_2, loss of hydrogen, or loss of electrons; *reduction is the reverse process*. Oxidation is catalyzed by specific enzymes (cofactors or coenzymes), as in dehydrogenation: $R\text{-}OH \rightarrow R = O$.

Continued

β-Oxidation	Process in which fatty acyl CoAs are oxidized in mitochondria, yielding two carbons at a time as acetyl CoA until the entire fatty acid molecule is broken down; the resulting acetyl CoA enters the citric acid cycle.
Oxidative Phosphorylation	Production of ATP associated with oxidation by the flavoprotein-cytochrome system; metabolism of fats, glucose, and amino acids produces protons that are translocated across the inner mitochondrial membrane. Diffusion of these substances down the concentration gradient drives ATP synthesis; *90% of O$_2$ consumption in the basal state is mitochondrial, and 80% of that is coupled to ATP synthesis.*
Triglyceride	Three fatty acids bound to glycerol; *the major component of both dietary and storage fat.* Naturally occurring fatty acids contain an even number of carbon atoms; no fatty acids with more than 16 carbon atoms are made. Saturated signifies no double bonds, and unsaturated signifies dehydrogenated, or various numbers, of double bonds.

I. Energy Metabolism

OXIDATIVE PHOSPHORYLATION

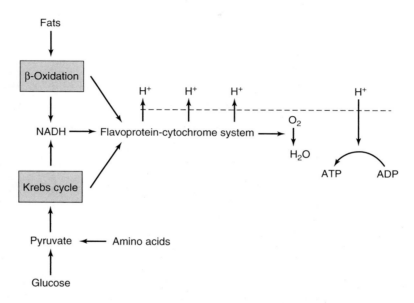

Oxidative phosphorylation, the coupling of oxidation with the formation of ATP, involves the transfer of protons across the inner mitochondrial membrane (indicated by the dashed line), down a concentration gradient.

H^+ = proton.

Reproduced, with permission, from Ganong WF: *Review of Medical Physiology*, 21st ed. McGraw-Hill, 2003:288.

ENERGY BALANCE

Status	Description	Clinical Significance
Neutral	Equilibrium; energy (caloric) input = energy output.	State in healthy adults.
Positive	Anabolic; energy (caloric) intake > energy loss due to heat and work.	State in growing children. • Energy is stored. • Weight is gained.
Negative	Catabolic; energy (caloric) intake < energy output.	State in elderly individuals. • Endogenous energy stores are used, and weight is lost. • Muscle wasting may occur.

ENERGY STORAGE

Substance	Kcal Per Gram	Fate of Excess[1]
Carbohydrate (glycogen)	4	75% is stored.
Protein	4	100% is converted to either fats or carbohydrates.
Fat (triglycerides)	9	97% is stored.

[1]Not used for energy.

II. Carbohydrate and Glucose Metabolism

ENERGY TRANSFER BETWEEN ORGANS

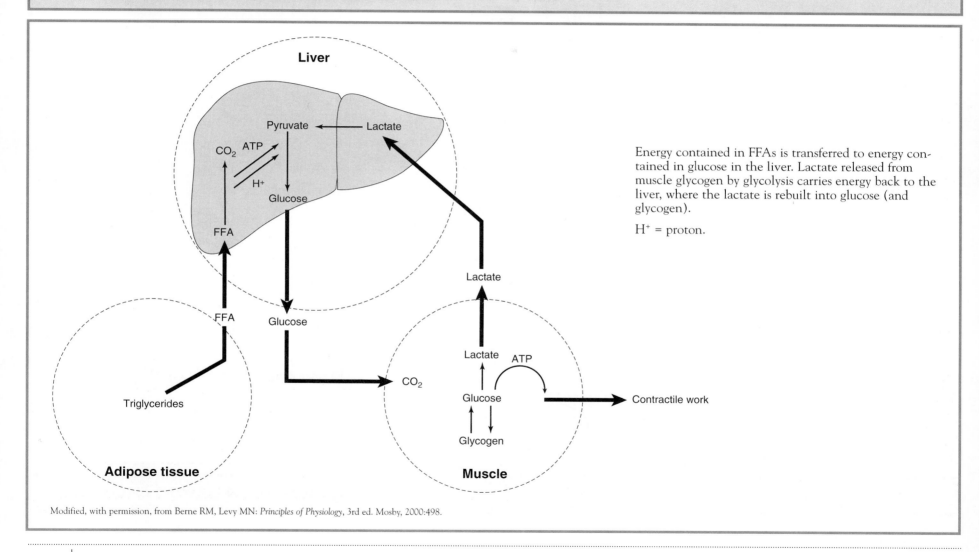

Energy contained in FFAs is transferred to energy contained in glucose in the liver. Lactate released from muscle glycogen by glycolysis carries energy back to the liver, where the lactate is rebuilt into glucose (and glycogen).

H^+ = proton.

Modified, with permission, from Berne RM, Levy MN: *Principles of Physiology*, 3rd ed. Mosby, 2000:498.

CARBOHYDRATE METABOLISM

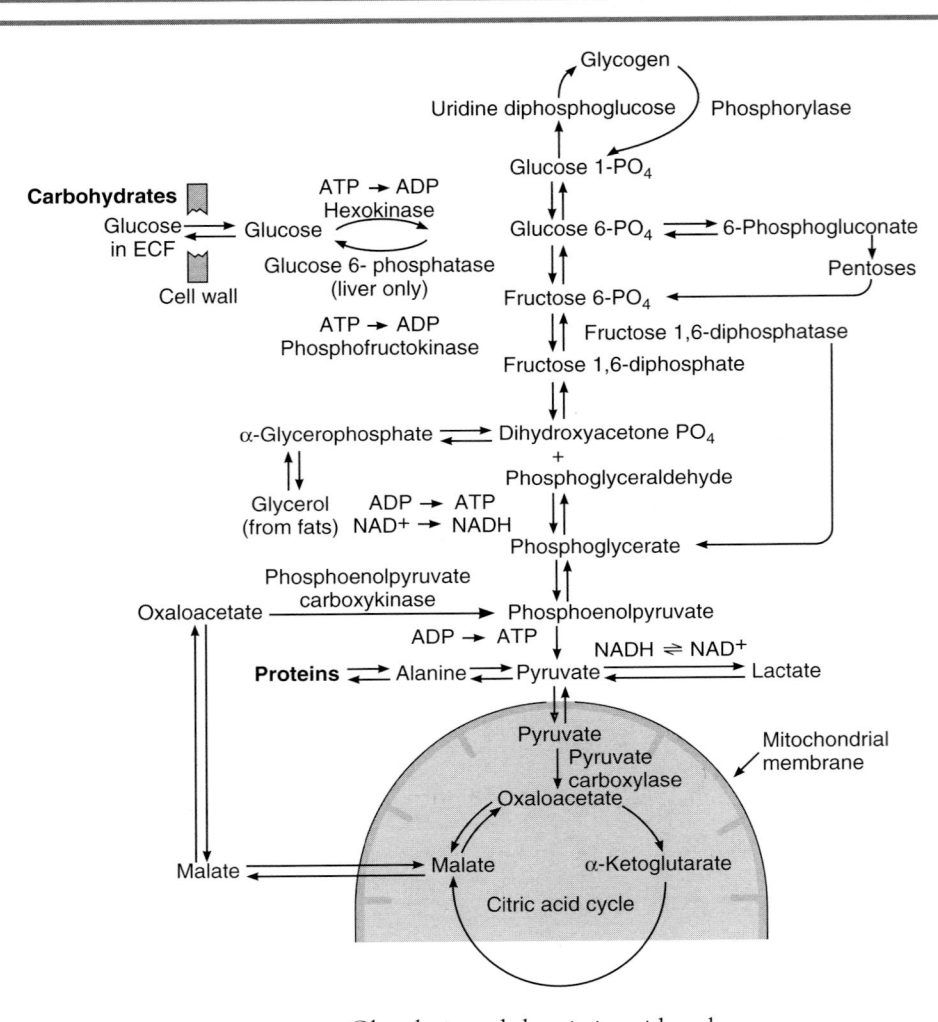

Glycolysis and the citric acid cycle.

Reproduced, with permission, from Ganong WF: *Review of Medical Physiology*, 21st ed. McGraw-Hill, 2003:290.

PATHWAYS OF CARBOHYDRATE/GLUCOSE METABOLISM

Pathway	Description	Reactions	Important Points
Aerobic Glycolysis (hexose monophosphate shunt or pentose phosphate pathway)	• Glucose catabolism via oxidation and decarboxylation to pentoses. • First stage of cellular respiration. • Net production of two ATP.	Glucose → pentoses → pyruvate.	• First reaction step catalyzed by glucose 6-phosphate dehydrogenase (G6PD). • Deficiency of G6PD is caused by X-linked recessive disorder that causes hemolytic anemia (Asian men, Mediterranean men, men of African descent).
Anaerobic Glycolysis (Embden-Meyerhof Pathway)	• Glucose catabolism via cleavage through fructose to trioses. • Major source of energy for rapidly contracting skeletal muscle. • Net production of three ATP (glucose enters glycolysis from glycogen).	Glucose → trioses → pyruvate → lactate.	• Provides energy for short periods of time when O_2 consumption exceeds demand (eg, during bursts of intense muscular activity). • Ischemia may produce very high concentrations of lactate, causing metabolic acidosis and muscle cramping.
Citric Acid Cycle (Krebs cycle or TCA cycle)	• Common pathway for complete aerobic oxidation of carbohydrates, fats, and some amino acids to CO_2 and H_2O. • Including aerobic glycolysis, net production of 38 ATP.	• Pyruvate → acetyl CoA + oxaloacetate → citrate, and so on. • Each turn of cycle provides four NADH, one $FADH_2$, one GTP, and three CO_2.	• Glucose can be converted to fat through acetyl CoA, but fats are not converted to glucose via this pathway (conversion of pyruvate to acetyl CoA is irreversible). • *Fats are not converted to carbohydrates in body* (except from glycerol).
Gluconeogenesis (glucogenesis)	Synthesis of glucose from *lactate*, amino acids, or oxaloacetate, via pyruvate.	*Cori cycle*: muscle glycolysis → lactate → liver → gluconeogenesis (and storage as glycogen).	*Gluconeogenesis is not simple reversal of glycolysis.*
Glycogenesis	Synthesis of *glycogen, the storage form of glucose*.	Glucose 1-phosphate → glycogen via glycogen synthase.	• Glycogen is derived from dietary sugars or is formed de novo from pyruvate, lactate, glycerol, and amino acids. • Glycogen formation occurs primarily in liver.

Continued

PATHWAYS OF CARBOHYDRATE/GLUCOSE METABOLISM (Continued)

Pathway	Description	Reactions	Important Points
Glycogenolysis	Breakdown of glycogen.	Glycogen → glucose 1-phosphate (via phosphorylase) → G6P.	• Continuous production of glucose by liver is critical in fasting state (80% glycogenolysis; 20% gluconeogenesis). • *Glucose-6-phosphatase in liver allows conversion of G6P to glucose*, which enters bloodstream. • Muscle and other tissues do not have glucose-6-phosphatase, so G6P there is catabolized via glycolysis. • Liver disease (alcoholic hepatitis, cirrhosis) causes inability to store glucose as glycogen; this results in hypoglycemia during fasting and inability to take up lactate, causing high plasma lactate levels and metabolic acidosis.

III. Protein Metabolism

PROTEIN BALANCE

A. **Protein balance is reflected by nitrogen balance.**

- Nitrogen balance:
  nitrogen in urine = nitrogen content of dietary protein.

- Daily dietary protein intake of 0.8g/kg is needed to maintain balance.

- Protein requirements increase in growing children, pregnant women, and people recovering from illness-induced weight loss.

Negative nitrogen balance
Nitrogen losses exceed intake (eg, starvation, forced immobilization, elevated hormone secretion from the adrenal cortex).

Positive nitrogen balance
Nitrogen intake exceeds excretion (eg, during growth or recovery from severe illness, after administration of anabolic steroids).

B. **Amino acid metabolism maintains protein balance**

Transamination
Conversion of one amino acid to corresponding keto acid, with simultaneous conversion of another keto acid to amino acid.
- Alanine + α-ketoglutarate $\rightleftharpoons$ pyurate + glutamate
- Serum transaminase levels rise when many active cells are damaged (eg, myocardial infarction results in an increase in plasma aspartate aminotransferase [AST]).

Amination
Addition of amino group (NH_4^+).

Deamination
Oxidative deamination of amino acids in the liver.
- Amino acid + NAD^+ $\rightarrow$ imino acid + H^+
- Imino acid + H_2O $\rightarrow$ keto acid + NH_4^+

CATEGORIZATION OF AMINO ACIDS

Category	Description	Examples
Essential	• Amino acids that cannot be synthesized by humans and must be obtained in diet. • Required as precursors for membrane phospholipids and glycolipids, and for synthesis of eicosanoids. • *Deficiency of even one essential amino acid disrupts normal protein synthesis.*	Histidine, isoleucine, leucine, lysine, methionine (and/or cysteine), phenylalanine (and/or tyrosine), threonine, tryptophan, valine.
Nonessential	• Amino acids that can be synthesized endogenously. • Their carbon skeletons can be built from glucose metabolites in citric acid cycle.	• All amino acids other than those listed above. • Alanine, aspartic acid, cystine, glycine, proline, serine, tyrosine, and so on.
Glucogenic	Amino acids that produce compounds that can readily be converted to glucose.	*All amino acids except leucine can contribute carbon atoms for glucose synthesis.*
Ketogenic	Amino acids that are converted to acetoacetate (ketone body).	Leucine, isoleucine, phenylalanine, tyrosine.

METABOLISM OF SPECIFIC PROTEINS

Protein	Description	Important Points
Creatine	Liver: methionine, glycine, and arginine → creatine.	• Creatinuria may occur normally in children and pregnant women. • It is also seen in myopathy, poorly controlled DM, starvation, and hyperthyroidism.
	Skeletal muscle: ATP + creatine → phosphorylcreatine + ADP. • *Phosphorylcreatine is important energy store for ATP synthesis.* • During exercise, reaction is reversed, maintaining ATP to supply energy for muscle contraction.	• *Creatine is not converted directly to creatinine.* • Creatine ↔ phosphorylcreatine → creatinine. • Phosphorylcreatine in skeletal muscle → creatinine in urine. • Rate of creatinine excretion is relatively constant.
Urea	• Deamination of amino acids in liver involves conversion of ammonia to urea. • Urea is excreted by kidneys.	• In severe liver disease, ammonia cannot be detoxified; blood urea nitrogen decreases, and blood NH_3 increases. • Congenital deficiency of ornithine carbamoyltransferase may also lead to NH_3 intoxication.
Purines and Pyrimidines	• Building blocks of DNA and RNA. • Released by breakdown of nucleotides and may be reused or catabolized. • Purines are converted to uric acid and excreted in urine. • Pyrimidines are catabolized to CO_2 and NH_3.	• Most nucleic acids are synthesized from amino acids in liver, and some are obtained from diet. • RNA is in dynamic equilibrium with amino acid pool. • Once formed, DNA is stable for life.
Uric Acid	• Formed from breakdown of purines and from direct synthesis from 5-phosphoribosyl pyrophosphate and glutamine. • Excreted in urine in humans.	• Elevated serum uric acid levels are associated with gout. • Elevated urine uric acid levels are associated with increased risk of renal stones (serum uric acid levels may or may not be increased).

UREA CYCLE

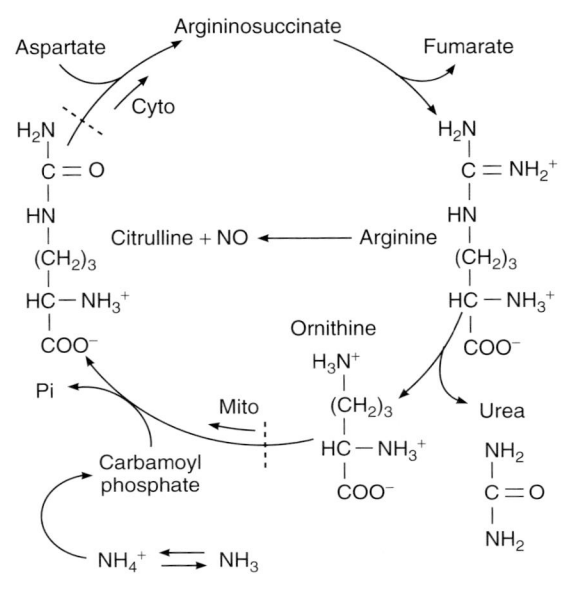

Most of the NH$_4^+$ formed by deamination of amino acids in the liver is converted to urea. Production of carbamoyl phosphate and its conversion to citrulline occurs in the mitochondria.

Cyto = cytoplasm; mito = mitochondrion; NO = nitric oxide.

ARACHIDONIC ACID DERIVATIVES

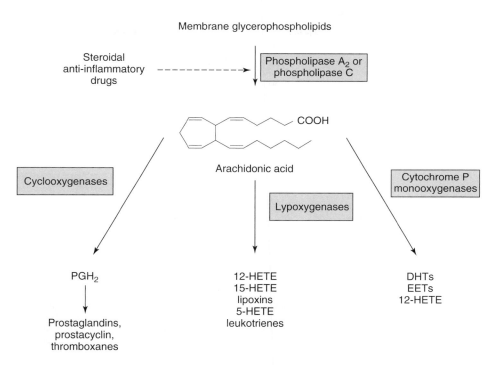

Membrane glycerophospholipids

Steroidal anti-inflammatory drugs

Phospholipase A$_2$ or phospholipase C

COOH

Arachidonic acid

Cyclooxygenases

Lypoxygenases

Cytochrome P monooxygenases

PGH$_2$

Prostaglandins, prostacyclin, thromboxanes

12-HETE
15-HETE
lipoxins
5-HETE
leukotrienes

DHTs
EETs
12-HETE

DHT = dihydroeicosatetraenoic acid; EET = epoxyeicosatrienoic acid; HETE = hydroyeicosatetraenoic acid; PGH$_2$ = prostaglandin H$_2$.

Reproduced, with permission, from Ganong WF: *Review of Medical Physiology*, 20th ed. McGraw-Hill, 2001:299.

SELECTED EICOSANOIDS

Type	Functions
Leukotrienes	• Mediate allergic responses and inflammation. • Constrict arterioles and bronchioles. • Increase vascular permeability. • Attract neutrophils and eosinophils to inflammatory sites.
Lipoxin	Dilates vessels and inhibits cytoxic effects of natural killer cells.
Prostacyclin	• Produced by vascular endothelial and smooth muscle cells away from site of vessel injury. • Maintains patency of rest of vessel by inhibiting platelet aggregation and working as vasodilator.
Prostaglandins	Important in inflammatory response, cardiovascular system, reproduction, parturition (cause uterine contraction), and pain.
Thromboxane A_2	• Promotes vasoconstriction, platelet aggregation, and clot formation at site of vessel injury. • Synthesized in platelets.

CYCLOOXYGENASE

Types	Description	Clinical Significance
COX-1	• Expressed constitutively. • Inhibition is undesirable because of its involvement in homeostasis.	• *NSAIDs inhibit all forms of COX, thus causing an anticoagulant effect that helps prevent strokes and myocardial infarction.* • NSAIDs used to treat pain, fever, and inflammation may also cause unwanted renal and GI side effects (elevated creatinine, gastritis) because they inhibit both COX-1 and COX-2. • Cortisol inhibits release of arachidonic acid from phospholipid stores via phospholipase A_2, inhibiting formation of all arachidonic acid derivatives.
COX-2	• Induced by growth factors, cytokines, and tumor promoters. • *Inhibition reduces inflammation, pain, and fever.*	• *Celecoxib (Celebrex) and rofecoxib (Vioxx) are COX-2–specific inhibitors.* • They treat pain, fever, and inflammation and result in minimal renal or GI side effects.

IV. Fat Metabolism

ENZYMES INVOLVED IN FATTY ACID METABOLISM

Enzyme	Location	Function	Factors That Affect Enzyme Levels
Lipoprotein Lipase	Surface of capillary endothelium.	• Clears chylomicrons from circulation by *catalyzing breakdown of triglycerides in chylomicrons to FFA and glycerol*, which then enter adipose cells and are reesterified (FFA may remain in circulation). • With cofactor heparin, it also removes triglycerides from circulating VLDLs.	**Increase:** feeding. **Decrease:** fasting and stress.
Hormone-Sensitive Lipase	Intracellular adipose tissue.	• Catalyzes breakdown of stored triglycerides into glycerol and fatty acids. • Fatty acids enter circulation.	**Increase:** fasting, stress; growth hormone, glucocorticoids, thyroid hormone. • Indirectly via catecholamines, glucagon, adrenocorticotropic hormone, thyroid-stimulating hormone, and luteinizing hormone. **Decrease:** feeding, *insulin*, prostaglandin E.

REGULATION OF HORMONE-SENSITIVE LIPASE BY CATECHOLAMINES

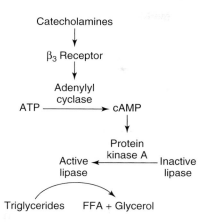

Catecholamines increase the activity of hormone-sensitive lipase with the aid of ATP.

Reproduced, with permission, from Ganong WF: *Review of Medical Physiology*, 21st ed. McGraw-Hill, 2003:309.

PATHWAYS OF FATTY ACID OXIDATION AND SYNTHESIS

Form of Fatty Acid	Pathway	Clinical Significance
Triglycerides	Fat contributes to carbohydrate stores via conversion of three-carbon glycerol moieties of triglycerides (via glycerol phosphate) to glucose.	• Glucose and fatty acids act as alternative or competing energy substrates. • *Increased carbohydrate use shifts fat metabolism from oxidation to storage* (ie, glycolysis increases, and gluconeogenesis and glycogenesis decrease). • Increased use of fat as fuel shifts carbohydrate metabolism from oxidation to storage.
FFAs	β-Oxidation: • Long-chain fatty acids bind carnitine and cross inner mitochondrial membrane. • *Two carbons are removed at a time as acetyl CoA* until entire fatty acid is broken down. • Acetyl CoA enters citric acid cycle.	• Increased insulin, cortisol, and endorphin levels and decreased levels of growth hormone favor fat deposition. • In the liver, β-oxidation yields ketones (acetoacetic acid and β-hydroxybutyrate).
Ketones (acetoacetate, acetone, β-hydroxybutyrate)	Free acetoacetate is formed in liver. • Converted into β-hydroxybutyrate and acetone. • Metabolized to CO_2 and H_2O via TCA cycle. Ketone bodies are also metabolized via other pathways.	• *Three conditions result in deficient intracellular glucose: starvation; diabetic ketoacidosis; and high-fat, low-carbohydrate diet.* • Decreased products of glucose metabolism cause depressed entry of acetyl CoA into TCA cycle. • High levels of acetyl CoA cause more acetoacetate to be formed in liver, resulting in accumulation of ketones in bloodstream (*ketosis*). • Acetone odor on breath of vomiting child is caused by ketosis of starvation. • *Metabolic acidosis that develops in diabetic ketosis can be severe and fatal.* • *Glucose abolishes ketosis (carbohydrates are antiketogenic).*

Two pathways for formation of acetoacetete

$$CH_3-\overset{\overset{\displaystyle O}{\|}}{C}-S-CoA + CH_3-\overset{\overset{\displaystyle O}{\|}}{C}-S-CoA \underset{\beta\text{-Ketothiolase}}{\rightleftharpoons} CH_3-\overset{\overset{\displaystyle O}{\|}}{C}-CH_2-\overset{\overset{\displaystyle O}{\|}}{C}-S-CoA + HS\text{-}CoA$$

2 Acetyl-CoA Acetoacetyl-CoA

$$CH_3-\overset{\overset{\displaystyle O}{\|}}{C}-CH_2-\overset{\overset{\displaystyle O}{\|}}{C}-S-CoA + H_2O \xrightarrow[\text{(liver only)}]{\text{Deacylase}} CH_3-\overset{\overset{\displaystyle O}{\|}}{C}-CH_2-\overset{\overset{\displaystyle O}{\|}}{C}-O^- + H^+ + HS\text{-}CoA$$

Acetoacetyl-CoA **Acetoacetate**

$$Acetyl\text{-}CoA + Acetoacetyl\text{-}CoA \longrightarrow CH_3-\overset{\overset{\displaystyle OH}{|}}{\underset{\underset{\displaystyle CH_2-COO^-}{|}}{C}}-CH_2-\overset{\overset{\displaystyle O}{\|}}{C}-S-CoA + H^+$$

HMG-CoA

$$HMG\text{-}CoA \longrightarrow \textbf{Acetoacetate} + H^+ + Acetyl\text{-}CoA$$

Formation of β-Hydroxybutyrate and acetone

Acetoacetate

$$CH_3-\overset{\overset{\displaystyle O}{\|}}{C}-CH_2-\overset{\overset{\displaystyle O}{\|}}{C}-O^- + H^+ \xrightarrow{\text{Tissues except liver}} CO_2 + ATP$$

$$\xrightarrow{-CO_2} CH_3-\overset{\overset{\displaystyle O}{\|}}{C}-CH_3$$

Acetone

+2H ⇅ −2H

$$CH_3-CHOH-CH_2-\overset{\overset{\displaystyle O}{\|}}{C}-O^- + H^+$$

β-Hydroxybutyrate

LIPOPROTEINS THAT TRANSPORT PLASMA LIPIDS

Lipoprotein	Description	Function	Clinical Significance
Chylomicrons	• Lipoproteins with lowest density and highest lipid content. • Formed from intestinal triglycerides.	Absorb cholesterol from intestine and release triglycerides to adipose tissue.	Type I hyperlipidemia/familial hyperchylomicronemia causes extremely high levels of chylomicrons despite normal dietary fat intake.
Chylomicron Remnants	Chylomicrons depleted of their triglycerides that remain in circulation.	Carry cholesterol to liver, where they bind to receptors and are absorbed.	
VLDL	• Largest lipoprotein. • Most liver cholesterol is incorporated into VLDL.	Transports triglycerides produced in liver to extrahepatic tissues, where they are broken down and either used for energy by muscle or stored in adipose tissue.	Type IV hyperlipidemia/familial hypertriglyceridemia. • Common disease. • Associated with elevated VLDL. • Ideal value = 25–50% of total cholesterol.
IDL	After triglycerides are removed from VLDL by lipoprotein lipase, VLDL remnant becomes IDL.	• Some IDL is taken up by liver. • Remainder lose more triglycerides and become LDL.	Type III hyperlipidemia/familial dysbetalipoproteinemia results in elevated levels of IDL and significant atherosclerotic disease by middle age.
LDL	• "Bad" cholesterol. • After triglycerides are removed from IDL by lipoprotein lipase, IDL remnant becomes LDL.	*Transports cholesterol to tissues.*	• *Elevated LDL is associated with increased incidence of atherosclerotic disease.* • Ideal value < 130 mg/dL (< 100 mg/dL if congenital adrenal hyperplasia is present).
HDL	• "Good" cholesterol. • Produced in liver and intestine.	• *Transports cholesterol to liver, where it is excreted in bile.* • Facilitates conversion of free cholesterol to esterified cholesterol and release of FFAs from chylomicrons.	• *HDL lowers plasma cholesterol; elevated HDL lowers incidence of atherosclerotic disease.* • Ideal value > 60 mg/dL.

LIPOPROTEIN SYNTHESIS

Chylomicrons rich in dietary triglycerides are converted to chylomicron remnants rich in cholesteryl esters by lipoprotein lipase.

VLDLs rich in triglycerides are secreted by the liver and converted to IDLs and then to LDLs rich in cholesteryl esters.

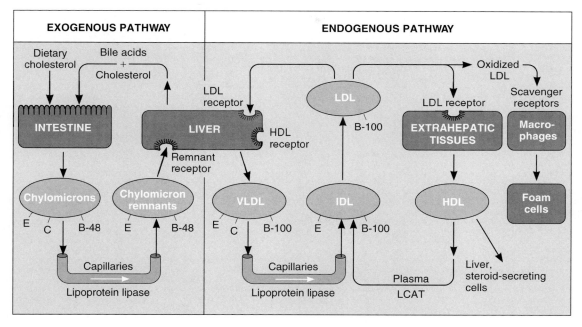

LCAT = lecithin-cholesterol acyltransferase.

Reproduced, with permission, from McPhee SJ, Lingappa VR, Ganong WF [editors]: *Pathophysiology of Disease*, 4th edition. McGraw-Hill, 2003.

SYNTHESIS AND DEGRADATION OF CHOLESTEROL

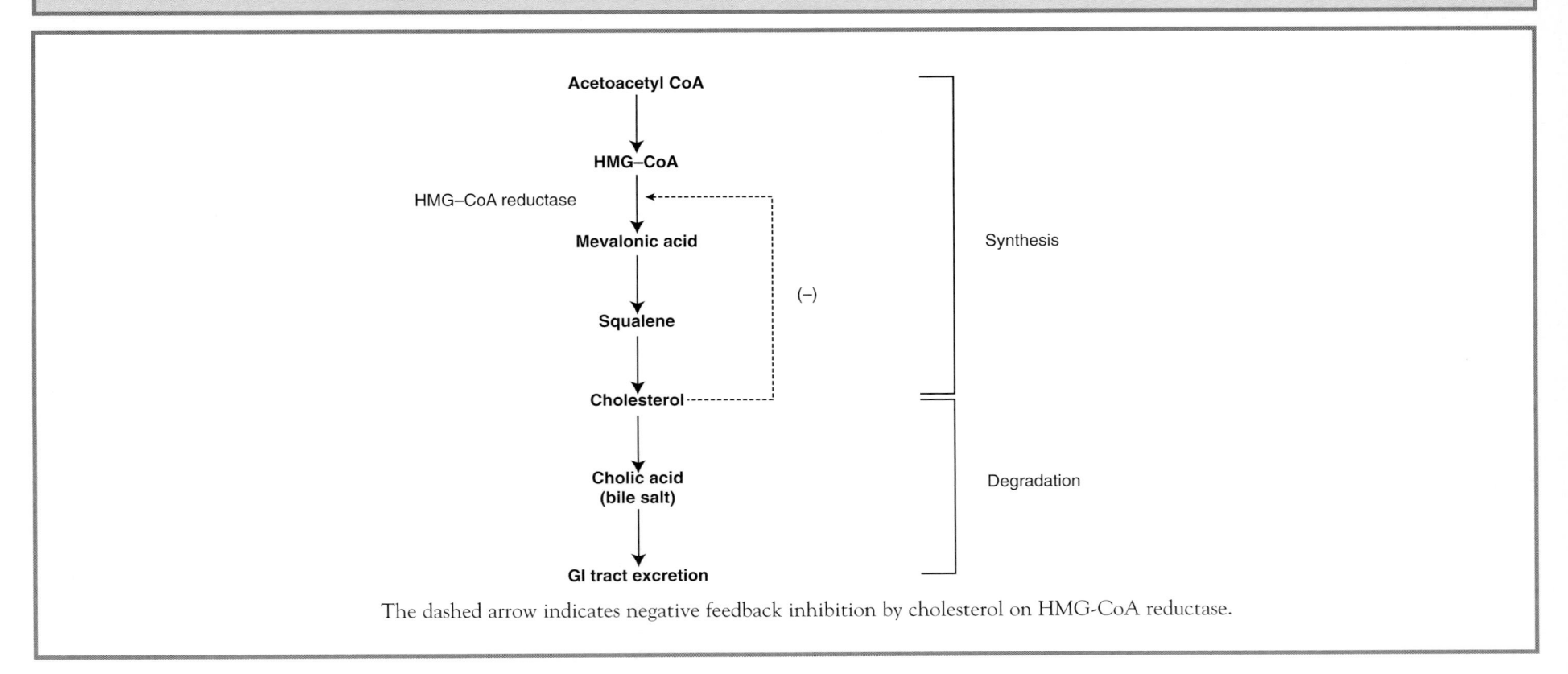

The dashed arrow indicates negative feedback inhibition by cholesterol on HMG-CoA reductase.

INHIBITION OF CHOLESTEROL SYNTHESIS

Inhibiting Factor	Mechanism	Clinical Significance
Feedback Inhibition		
Cholesterol	• *Cholesterol feedback inhibits at HMG-CoA reductase.* • It also stimulates esterification of any excess cholesterol and inhibits synthesis of new LDL receptors.	Widely used and highly effective drug class known as "statins" inhibit HMG-CoA reductase (eg, lovastatin).
Hormones	Thyroid hormones (T_3 and T_4) increase number of LDL receptors in liver.	• Hypercholesterolemia often seen with hypothyroidism. • Fewer LDL receptors in liver leads to more cholesterol in circulation.
	Estrogens increase plasma HDL and lower LDL by increasing its catabolism.	Women more commonly have higher HDL and lower risk of atherosclerotic disease than men.
	Glucagon phosphorylates and inactivates HMG-CoA reductase.	Glucagon is released in response to hypoglycemia.
	Low insulin inactivates HMG-CoA reductase.	Untreated DM is associated with high cholesterol levels.
Drugs		
Atorvastatin (Lipitor)	Directly inhibits HMG-CoA reductase.	• Rare side effects include hepatotoxicity and rhabdomyolysis. • *Periodic liver function studies should be obtained.*
Ezetimibe (Zetia)	Inhibits absorption of cholesterol at brush border of small intestine.	Rare side effects include diarrhea and abdominal pain.
Clofibrate	Increases fatty acid oxidation in muscle and liver, reducing lipoprotein secretion from liver.	Not often used because of its side effects, including cholelithiasis, myositis, nausea, and anticoagulation.
Niacin	Inhibits mobilization of FFAs from peripheral fat deposits, reducing VLDL synthesis in liver.	Not often used because of its side effects, including flushing, pruritus, and orthostatic hypotension.
Cholestyramine	Binds intestinal bile acids and is excreted in feces.	Common side effects include constipation, dyspepsia, and impaired absorption of fat-soluble vitamins.

V. Vitamins and Minerals

ESSENTIAL VITAMINS

Vitamin	Source(s)	Function(s)	Deficiency Symptoms/Disorders
A (fat soluble)	Fruit, yellow vegetables.	Component of visual pigment; fetal development.	*Night blindness*, dry skin.
B$_1$ (thiamin)	Liver, cereal grains.	Cofactor in decarboxylation.	*Beriberi*. • Wet beriberi (nerve degeneration, edema). • Dry beriberi (emaciation). • Common in polished rice–based diets. Neuritis.
B$_2$ (riboflavin)	Liver, milk.	Component of flavoproteins.	*Cheilosis* (swollen, cracked, bright-red lips), glossitis.
B$_3$ (niacin, nicotinic acid)	Liver, meat, yeast.	Component of NAD^+ and $NADP^+$.	*Pellagra*. • Scaly dermatitis, dementia, diarrhea, glossitis. • Common in corn-based diets.
B$_5$ (pantothenic acid)	Eggs, liver, yeast.	Component of CoA.	Alopecia (baldness), adrenal insufficiency, dermatitis, enteritis.
B$_6$ (pyridoxine)	Corn, liver, yeast, wheat.	Forms prosthetic group of decarboxylases and transaminases.	Convulsions, hyperirritability.
B$_9$ (folic acid)	Leafy green vegetables.	• Coenzymes in carbon transfer. • Involved in methylating reactions.	Anemia, *neural tube defects in infants of folate-deficient women*, sprue (disease of small intestine associated with anemia, diarrhea, glossitis, malabsorption, steatorrhea, weight loss).

B_{12} (cyanocobalamin)	Eggs, liver, meat, milk.	• Coenzyme in amino acid metabolism. • Stimulates erythropoiesis.	*Pernicious anemia* (megaloblastic anemia; nervous system affected if severe).
C (ascorbic acid)	Citrus fruits, leafy green vegetables.	• Scavenges free radicals. • Keeps prosthetic metal ions in reduced form.	*Scurvy.* • Swollen, bleeding gums and subcutaneous bleeding. • Results from diet devoid of fresh fruit and vegetables.
D (fat soluble)	Fish liver.	Increases intestinal absorption of calcium and phosphate.	*Rickets* (soft, malformed bones).
E (fat soluble)	Eggs, leafy green vegetables, meat, milk.	Antioxidant.	Ataxia, spinocerebellar dysfunction.
H (biotin)	Egg yolks, liver, tomatoes.	Catalyzes CO_2 fixation in various synthetic processes.	Dermatitis, enteritis.
K (fat soluble)	Leafy green vegetables.	*Promotes blood clotting.*	*Hemorrhage.*

CLINICAL FINDINGS ASSOCIATED WITH VITAMIN EXCESS

Vitamin	Associated Symptoms
A	Anorexia, bone pain, headache, hepatosplenomegaly, hyperostosis, irritability, patchy hair loss, scaly dermatitis.
B_6 (pyridoxine)	Peripheral neuropathy.
D	Weight loss, soft tissue calcification, renal failure.
K	Anemia, GI disturbance.

CLINICAL FINDINGS ASSOCIATED WITH ABNORMAL MINERAL INGESTION

Element	Deficiency Symptoms	Toxicity Symptoms/Disorders
Aluminum	Undetermined.	Dementia.
Chromium	Insulin resistance.	Arrhythmias.
Cobalt	Deficiency of vitamin B_{12}, leading to megaloblastic anemia.	Anorexia.
Copper	Anemia, changes in ossification.	Wilson disease (autosomal recessive disorder resulting in brain damage).
Fluorine	Dental caries.	Anorexia, weakness.
Iodine	Thyroid disorders.	Similar to deficiency (eg, goiter).
Iron	Anemia.	Hemochromatosis.
Zinc	Skin ulcers, immune depression, hypogonadal dwarfism.	GI discomfort, dizziness.

VI. Disorders of Metabolism

SELECTED METABOLIC DISORDERS

Disease	Pathogenesis	Clinical Significance
Carnitine deficiency	• Genetic defects in enzymes involved in transfer of fatty acids into mitochondria. • Results in deficient β-oxidation of fatty acids.	• Often fatal condition associated with cardiomyopathy and hypoketonemic hypoglycemia with coma. • Triggered by fasting, causing depletion of glucose stores and lack of fatty acid oxidation to provide energy. • Ketone bodies are not formed in normal amounts because of lack of adequate CoA in liver.
Dyslipidemia	Elevated plasma cholesterol levels caused by various mutations in apoprotein and lipid receptors. • In familial hypercholesterolemia, mutant LDL receptors prevent normal cellular uptake of cholesterol. • Hyperlipidemia results in accumulation of IDL and cholesterol remnants.	• *Increased risk of atherosclerotic disease*, with increased risk of such conditions as myocardial infarction, cerebral thrombosis, and ischemia of extremities. • Infiltration of cholesterol and appearance of foam cells in lesions of arterial walls. • Proliferative lesions that eventually calcify, distorting vessels and making them rigid.
Galactosemia	• Accumulation of ingested galactose in the circulation. • Caused by inborn error of metabolism, resulting in a congenital deficiency of galactose 1-phosphate uridyl transferase. • This transferase catalyzes reaction between galactose 1-phosphate and uridine diphosphate glucose.	• Disturbances of growth and development. • Treat with galactose-free diet.

Continued

SELECTED METABOLIC DISORDERS (Continued)

Disease	Pathogenesis	Clinical Significance
Gout	• Primary: enzyme abnormalities result in increased uric acid production or deficit in renal tubular transport of uric acid. • Secondary: elevated uric acid levels in body fluids as result of decreased excretion or increased production secondary to another disease process.	• Recurrent attacks of arthritis. • Urate deposits in the joints (*usually metatarsophalangeal joint of great toe*), kidneys, and elsewhere. • Elevated blood and urine uric acid levels. • Renal disease and thiazide diuretics result in decreased excretion and increased production of uric acid. • Leukemia and pneumonia cause increased breakdown of uric acid–rich white blood cells. • Colchicine or NSAIDs relieve arthritis. • Colchicine inhibits phagocytosis of uric acid crystals by leukocytes. • Probenecid inhibits uric acid reabsorption in kidneys. Allopurinol, which inhibits xanthine oxidase, decreases uric acid production and helps in prevention.
Kwashiorkor	Malnutrition caused by *diet sufficient in calories but deficient in protein*.	Low plasma albumin levels; edema; fragile, red-brown hair; depressed immune function; deficiency of lymphocytes; reduced wound healing; increased infections; fatty infiltration of liver; protuberant abdomen; dry, scaling skin; failure to thrive or grow.
Marasmus	Malnutrition caused by *diet deficient in both calories and protein*.	Infant or child looks "old." • No skin fat. • Pale.
McArdle disease (myophosphorylase deficiency glycogenosis)	• Deficiency of muscle phosphorylase causes accumulation of glycogen in skeletal muscle. • Accumulated glycogen cannot be broken down to provide energy for muscle contraction.	• Muscle pain and stiffness on exertion and reduced exercise tolerance. • Glucagon or epinephrine causing normal rise in plasma glucose indicates normal hepatic phosphorylase.

CHAPTER 8
ENDOCRINE SYSTEM

ABBREVIATIONS

ACTH = adrenocorticotropic hormone

ADH = antidiuretic hormone (vasopressin)

ANP = atrial natriuretic peptide

CCK = cholecystokinin

CRH = corticotropin-releasing hormone

DHEA = dehydroepiandrosterone

DIT = diiodotyrosine

DM = diabetes mellitus

ECF = extracellular fluid

FFA = free fatty acid

FSH = follicle-stimulating hormone

GH = growth hormone

GI = gastrointestinal

GnRH = gonadotropin-releasing hormone

HDL = high-density lipoprotein

LDL = low-density lipoprotein

LH = luteinizing hormone

MIT = monoiodotyrosine

MSH = melanocyte-stimulating hormone

P_i = inorganic phosphate

PRL = prolactin

PTH = parathyroid hormone

T_3 = triiodothyronine

T_4 = thyroxine

TRH = thyrotropin-releasing hormone

TSH = thyroid-stimulating hormone

TERMS TO LEARN

Chvostek Sign	Rapid contraction of ipsilateral facial muscles elicited by tapping over facial nerve at angle of jaw; sign of tetany in hypocalcemia.
Circadian	Exhibiting 24-hour periodicity; circadian rhythms are synchronized to day-night (light-dark) cycle. ACTH secretion, melatonin secretion, sleep-wake cycle, and the "biological clock" all follow circadian rhythms.
Endocrine	Relating to a process in which cells secrete a regulatory substance directly into the bloodstream, thereby affecting cells that may be some distance away.
Hormones	Chemical messengers produced by ductless glands and transported in the circulation to target cells, where they regulate metabolic processes. Amines, amino acids, polypeptides, proteins, and steroids may act as hormones.
Hypercalcemia of Malignancy	Common complication of breast, renal, ovarian, and skin cancers; occurs when disease metastasizes to bone, causing erosion (osteolytic hypercalcemia) and when PTH-related protein is produced (humoral hypercalcemia of malignancy).
Insulin Shock	Result of severe hypoglycemia caused by endogenous or exogenous hyperinsulinemia (eg, insulinoma or patient with DM who takes too much insulin, respectively). Blood glucose falls to 50–70 mg/dL and the central nervous system becomes excitable, leading to hallucinations, nervousness, trembling, and sweating; when blood glucose is 20–50 mg/dL, convulsions and loss of consciousness occur. Lower blood glucose levels result in coma; the *acetone breath and Kussmaul breathing present in hyperglycemic diabetic coma are not present in hypoglycemic coma.*
(IGFs) Insulin-Like Growth Factors	Somatomedins that promote growth; inhibit GH–releasing hormone and have nonsuppressible insulin-like activity that persists despite pancreatectomy or antibodies (but does not prevent DM). IGF-I is stimulated by GH after birth, has growth-stimulating activity, peaks at puberty, and declines in old age. IGF-II is independent of GH and plays a role in fetal growth.
Negative Feedback	Conditions or products resulting from prior hormone action that suppress further hormone release; *primary mechanism of hormone regulation.*
Neurocrine	Process by which a neuron releases regulatory substances into the bloodstream to affect distant cells; the signaling molecules are neurohormones (eg, vasopressin and oxytocin from hypothalamus).
Positive Feedback	Products of initial hormone action that stimulate further hormone secretion.
Somatomedins	Protein hormones secreted by liver in response to stimulation by GH that promote protein synthesis and growth as well as feedback inhibit GHRH. Lack of somatomedins causes retarded growth despite high GH levels (eg, IGF-I and -II) and somatomedin C.

Somatostatin (GH–Inhibiting Factor)	Hormone secreted from hypothalamus, pancreas, and GI tract that inhibits secretion of GH, insulin, glucagon, and pancreatic polypeptide; it is stimulated by glucose, amino acids, and CCK. Excess somatostatin (eg, pancreatic tumor) causes hyperglycemia and other manifestations of DM, dyspepsia, decreased gastric acid secretion, and inhibition of CCK (which causes decreased gallbladder contraction and formation of gallstones).
Tetany	Twitching of muscles, especially those of face, hands, and feet, caused by *hypocalcemia*; most often due to inadvertent parathyroidectomy during thyroid surgery. Calcium provides temporary relief, and PTH injections can correct the abnormality.
Thyroid-Binding Globulin	Protein that binds thyroid hormones; 99% of circulating thyroid hormones are bound to thyroid-binding globulin, transthyretin, and albumin. Thyroid-binding globulin is increased in acute hepatic disease, pregnancy, and in response to estrogen therapy and tranquilizers and decreased in cirrhosis, nephrotic syndrome, and in response to glucocorticoids and androgens. Only free or unbound thyroid hormones are physiologically active.
Trousseau Sign	Spasm of muscles of upper extremity that causes flexion of wrist and thumb with extension of fingers; sign of tetany in hypocalcemia.

I. Hypothalamus and Pituitary Gland

FUNCTIONAL AREAS OF THE HYPOTHALAMUS

Area	Location	Function
Suprachiasmatic Nuclei	One nucleus on each side of optic chiasm.	Control circadian rhythms.
Feeding Center	Medial forebrain.	• Stimulation evokes eating behavior. • Lesions cause severe, fatal anorexia. • Leptin and gastrointestinal hormones (CCK, glucagons, somatostatin) inhibit food intake.
Satiety Center	Ventromedial nucleus.	• Stimulation (by glucose) causes cessation of eating. • Lesions cause hyperphagia. • If food is abundant, hypothalamic obesity results.
Cold Center (heat production center)	Posterior hypothalamus.	Stimulation by cold results in shivering, cutaneous vasoconstriction, and piloerection.
Heat Center (heat loss center)	Anterior hypothalamus.	• Stimulation by heat results in cutaneous vasodilation and sweating. • Lesion causes hyperthermia.
Thirst Center	Anterior hypothalamus.	• Osmoreceptors help regulate thirst. • Water intake is increased by increased osmotic pressure of plasma, decreased ECF volume, and increased plasma osmolality (eg, hemorrhage causes increased drinking even with no change in plasma osmolality). • Effect of ECF volume on thirst is mediated partly by renin-angiotensin system (stimulated by hypovolemia).

HYPOTHALAMIC AND PITUITARY HORMONES

Location	Hormone	Primary Actions
Median Eminence of Hypothalamus	TRH.	Stimulates TSH.
	CRH.	Stimulates ACTH.
	GHRH.	Stimulates GH.
	Somatostatin.	Inhibits GH.
	GnRH.	Stimulates LH and FSH.
	PRL-inhibiting hormone (dopamine).	*Tonically inhibits PRL.*
	PRL-releasing factor.	TRH, TSH, estrogens, and various polypeptides stimulate PRL.
Anterior Pituitary	TSH (thyrotropin).	• Stimulates thyroid secretion and growth of thyroid gland. • TSH, LH, FSH, and human chorionic gonadotropin have same α-subunits and different β-subunits that confer hormonal specificity.
	ACTH (corticotropin).	• Stimulates zona fasciculata and zona reticularis to secrete hormones (cortisol and sex steroid precursors, respectively). • Works with MSH to stimulate secretion of brown pigment melanin.
	GH (somatotropin).	• Accelerates body growth and metabolism. • Opposes actions of insulin: increases hepatic glucose output, inhibits glucose uptake by muscle and adipose cells, leading to increase in plasma glucose (ie, diabetogenic). • Increases lipolysis, leading to increase in FFA levels and providing energy (ie, ketogenic). • Stimulates protein anabolism. • Stimulates secretion of IGF-I and somatostatin (negative feedback). • Regulation of electrolytes: increases gastrointestinal Ca^{2+} absorption, decreases Na^+ and K^+ excretion, increases plasma phosphorus.
	FSH.	Stimulates ovarian follicle growth and spermatogenesis.

Continued

HYPOTHALAMIC AND PITUITARY HORMONES (Continued)

Location	Hormone	Primary Actions
	LH.	Females: stimulates ovulation and luteinization of ovarian follicles. Males: stimulates testosterone secretion.
	PRL (mammotropin).	Females: • Stimulates breast development, secretion of milk, and maternal behavior, and is increased during pregnancy. • Stimulates dopamine (negative feedback loop). • Excess amounts inhibit GnRH. • Hyperprolactinemia (associated with chromophobe adenomas of anterior pituitary) may cause galactorrhea. • Elevated PRL levels occur in 20% of women with secondary amenorrhea. Males: associated with impotence, hypogonadism, and osteoporosis (due to estrogen deficiency).
Intermediate Lobe of Pituitary (rudimentary in humans)	MSH (melanotropin).	• Stimulates synthesis of brown pigment melanin in epidermal melanocytes. • Pigmentary changes seen in endocrine disorders are caused by interaction between ACTH and melanotropin-1 receptors (eg, hyperpigmentation in primary adrenal insufficiency and abnormal pallor in hypopituitarism). • Secondary adrenal insufficiency (decreased ACTH) associated with normal pigmentation. • Albinos have congenital inability to make melanin. • Piebaldism caused by congenital defects in melanin precursors.
Posterior Pituitary	ADH (vasopressin).	• Increases water reabsorption by kidney by increasing permeability of collecting duct, leading to concentrated urine with decreased volume and increased osmolality of body fluid. • Causes vasoconstriction.
	Oxytocin.	• Causes milk ejection and contraction of pregnant uterus. • Enhanced by estrogen. • Inhibited by progesterone. • May also act on nonpregnant uterus to facilitate sperm transport.

A FLAGTOP (8 major pituitary hormones)—Antidiuretic, Follicle stimulating, Luteinizing, Adrenocorticotropic, Gonadotropic, Thyroid Stimulating, Oxytocin, Prolactin

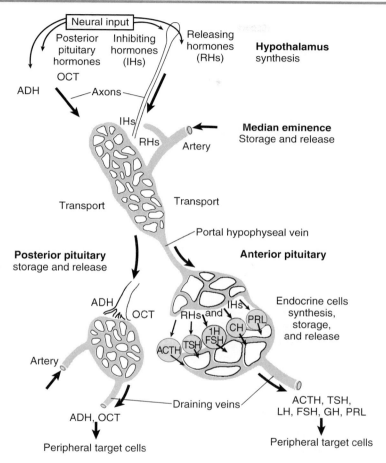

Axons from supraoptic and paraventricular nuclei connect to the posterior pituitary through the hypothalamohypophyseal tract.
Blood vessels from the median eminence of the ventral hypothalamus connect to the anterior pituitary through the portal hypophyseal vessels.

OCT = oxytocin.

HYPOTHALAMIC AND PITUITARY DISORDERS

Disorder	Description	Symptoms
Acromegaly	• Excessive secretion of GH caused by pituitary or hypothalamic tumors. • In children, acromegaly is called gigantism.	• Abnormal growth of hands, feet, and facial bones, abnormal glucose tolerance, lactation in absence of pregnancy, hyperprolactinemia, osteoarthritis. • Tumors may cause enlargement of sella turcica, leading to headache and visual disturbances caused by compression of optic nerves.
Diabetes Insipidus	Central diabetes insipidus is caused by hypothalamic or posterior pituitary disease leading to deficiency of ADH (vasopressin).	Polyuria and polydipsia.
	Nephrogenic diabetes insipidus is caused by failure of kidneys to respond to ADH because of genetic defects in its ADH receptor.	Polyuria and polydipsia.
Dwarfism	• Short stature caused by either deficiency of GRH, GH, IGF. or mutated GH receptors that are unresponsive. • Achondroplasia is most common form of dwarfism in humans. • Caused by autosomal dominant disorder believed to result from mutation of fibroblast growth factor receptor 3 gene.	Short limbs, normal head and trunk, normal intelligence.
Kallmann Syndrome	Hypogonadism caused by low levels of circulating gonadotropins (hypogonadotropic hypogonadism).	• Hypogonadism, partial or complete loss of sense of smell (hyposmia or anosmia). • Most commonly seen in men.
Nelson Syndrome	Removal of bilateral hyperplastic adrenals, leading to development of rapidly growing ACTH-secreting pituitary tumors.	• Skin hyperpigmentation and neurologic signs caused by pressure on structures in sellar region. • High ACTH (MSH and ACTH activity account for pigmentation). • Some of these tumors are malignant.

Sheehan Syndrome	Acute infarction of pituitary gland secondary to acute postpartum hemorrhage.	• Amenorrhea, fatigue, inability to breastfeed. • *Permanently damaged pituitary.*
Syndrome of Inappropriate Antidiuretic Hormone (SIADH)	• Excess secretion of ADH. • Associated with cerebral and pulmonary disease (eg, lung tumors). • Postoperative patients may develop elevated ADH associated with pain and hypovolemia.	• *Low plasma osmolality and dilutional hyponatremia.* • *High fluid intake can cause water intoxication in patients with hypersecretion of ADH.* • It is essential to treat underlying disease.

II. Thyroid Gland

THYROID GLAND HISTOLOGY

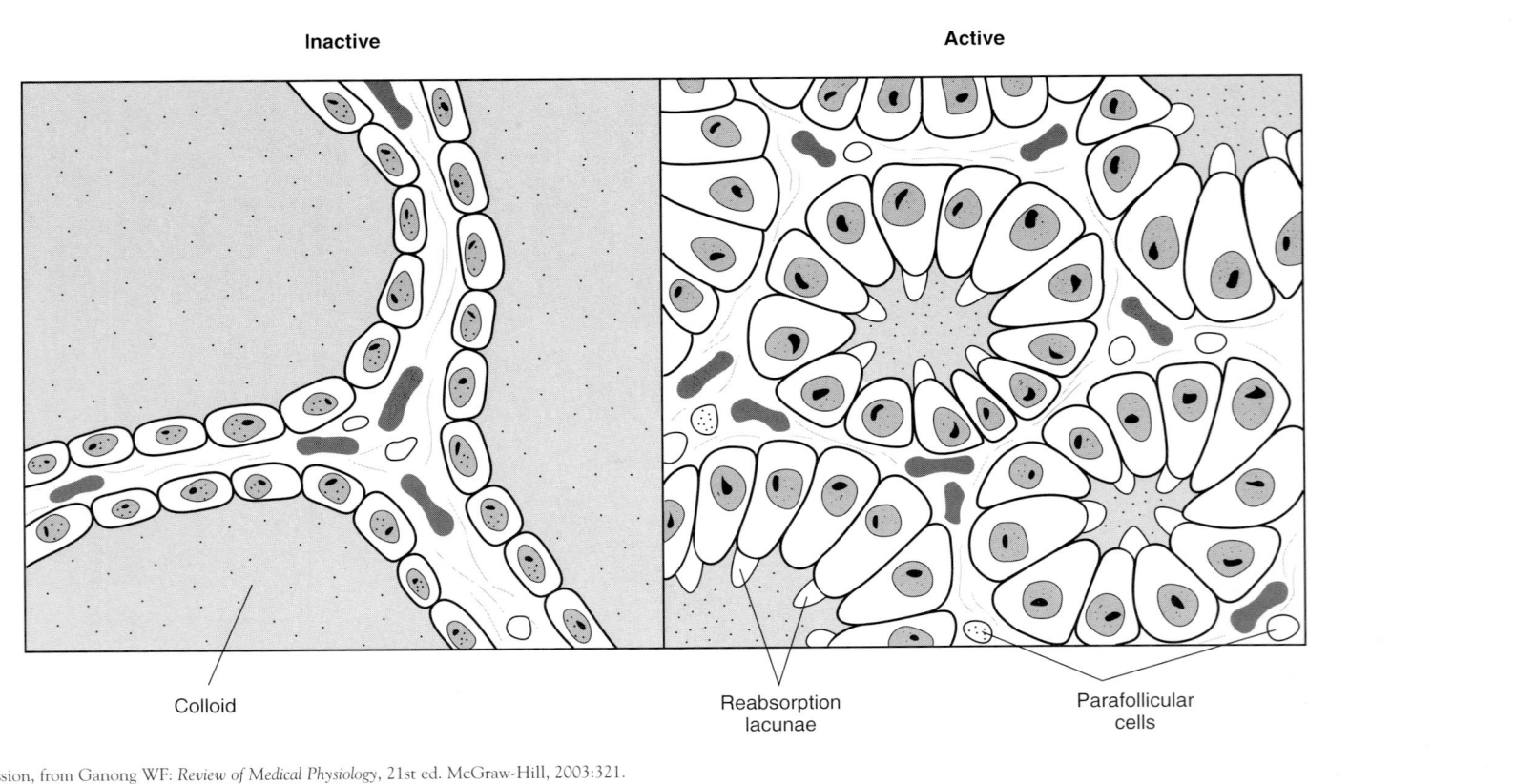

Inactive

Active

Colloid

Reabsorption lacunae

Parafollicular cells

THYROID ANATOMY

Gross Anatomy

- Located in the anterior neck, and the two lobes lie on either side of the trachea.
- Thyroglossal duct marks path of thyroid from tongue to neck (may persist into adulthood).
- Isthmus is ridge of tissue connecting two lobes.
- Pyramidal lobe arises from isthmus in front of larynx.

Microscopic Anatomy

- Acini, or *follicles*, are made up of cuboidal cells and filled with proteinaceous *colloid*.
- Inactive gland: large follicles, abundant colloid, flat lining cells
- Active gland: small follicles, minimal colloid, cuboid lining cells.
- Parafollicular cells or C cells: secrete calcitonin.

THYROID HORMONES

Hormone	Description
Thyroglobulin	• Glycoprotein made by thyroid cells and secreted in colloid by exocytosis of granules that also contain thyroid peroxidase. • Hormones remain bound by thyroglobulin until secreted.
T_4	• Major product of thyroid. • Functions as prohormone.
T_3	• Primarily formed in peripheral tissues by deiodination of T_4; some is secreted from thyroid. • Provides almost all thyroid activity in target cells (more active than T_4).
Reverse T_3	• Inactive. • Produced from deiodination of T_4 when less active thyroid needed.

SYNTHESIS AND SECRETION OF THYROID HORMONES

Synthesis	Secretion
1. Ingested iodine is converted to iodide and absorbed.	1. Iodinated thyroglobulin is stored within follicle lumen as colloid.
2. Iodide is actively transported into thyroid against electrical and chemical gradients.	2. Iodinated thyroglobulin is transferred into cell via endocytosis.
3. Iodide is incorporated into tyrosine molecules within thyroglobulin.	3. Lysosomal proteases release free T_4 and T_3 into bloodstream.
4. Thyroid peroxidase catalyzes oxidation of iodide and its substitution for hydrogen in benzene ring of tyrosine (called iodination), producing MIT and DIT.	4. Iodine liberated by deiodination of MIT and DIT is reutilized in gland.

- T_3 = MIT + DIT
- T_4 = DIT + DIT

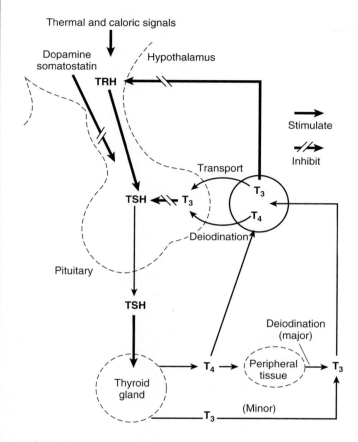

Modified, with permission, from Berne RM, Levy NM: *Principles of Physiology*, 3rd ed. Mosby, 2000:551.

- Iodide is essential for normal thyroid synthesis and function. Both iodide deficiency and excess inhibit thyroid function.
- The ratio of T_4 to T_3 is 10:1. When iodide is low or the thyroid gland is overstimulated, conditions are favorable for T_3 production.
- T_3 inhibits TSH and TRH via negative feedback.
- Cortisol, dopamine, GH, somatostatin, stress, and heat inhibit TSH.
- Excess anions, iodide, lithium, and thiouracils inhibit T_4 synthesis.

EFFECTS OF THYROID HORMONES

Type of Effect	Action
Metabolism	• Increases metabolic rate, encourages catabolic state; if food intake is not increased, weight is lost. • Stimulates O_2 consumption and substrate use. • Stimulates Na^+-K^+-ATPase pump. • Mobilizes fatty acids, increases rate of carbohydrate absorption, and lowers circulating cholesterol. • Increases need for vitamins, which may cause vitamin deficiency. • Increases heat production: resulting increase in body temperature leads to vasodilation and sweating.
Heart	• Increases number and affinity of β-adrenergic receptors in heart. • Increases sensitivity of heart to inotropic and chronotropic effects of catecholamines.
Nervous System	• Has critical effects on development of central nervous system: growth of cerebral and cerebellar cortex, protein and lipid content of myelin and neurotransmitters and receptors, effects on emotions and responses. • Sympathetic nervous system (epinephrine, norepinephrine) increase metabolic rate and produce cardiovascular effects similar to thyroid hormones. • Catecholamine levels are normal in hyperthyroidism, but cardiovascular effects, tremulousness, and sweating produced by thyroids are reduced or abolished by sympathectomy and β-blockers (β-blockers are weak inhibitors of extrathyroidal conversion of T_4 to T_3).
Growth	• Essential for normal growth and maturation. • Stimulates linear growth, development, and maturation of skeleton. • Stimulates secretion of GH and potentiates its effects. • Increases dissociation of O_2 from hemoglobin by increasing 2,3-diphosphoglycerate.
Reproduction	• Stimulates milk secretion. • Essential for normal menstrual cycles and sperm production.

HYPERTHYROIDISM VERSUS HYPOTHYROIDISM

Feature	Hyperthyroidism	Hypothyroidism
Causes	Graves disease.	Fetal thyroid dysgenesis.
	Administration of T_3 or T_4.	Inborn errors of thyroid hormone synthesis.
	Ectopic thyroid tissue.	Maternal antithyroid antibodies that cross placenta (T_4 crosses placenta; unless mother is hypothyroid, fetal development is normal until birth).
	Toxic thyroid adenoma (solitary of multinodular).	Maternal iodine deficiency.
	Thyroiditis.	Hypothalamic hypothyroidism.
	Mutations that activate TSH receptor.	Hypopituitary hypothyroidism.
Signs and Symptoms	Weight loss and increased metabolism.	Weight gain and decreased metabolism.
	Cardiovascular symptoms (eg, tachycardia, high output failure).	Cardiovascular symptoms (low cardiac output).
	Heat intolerance, increased sweating.	Cold intolerance, decreased sweating.
	Warm, soft skin.	Dry, yellowish skin (carotenemia), hair loss.
	Hyperphagia, excessive thirst.	Slow, husky voice.
	Irritability, restlessness, tremor, insomnia.	Fatigue, depression.
	Muscle weakness (thyrotoxic myopathy), atrophy.	Muscle weakness.
	Osteoporosis.	Inhibition of GH, growth retardation, skeletal immaturity.

Continued

HYPERTHYROIDISM VERSUS HYPOTHYROIDISM (Continued)

Feature	Hyperthyroidism	Hypothyroidism
	Exophthalmos, goiter.	Elevated cholesterol.
	Rapid mentation.	• Mental retardation in children, slow mentation, poor memory. • Severe mental symptoms = "myxedema madness."
Diagnosis	Decreased response of TSH to TRH caused by negative feedback of thyroid hormones on pituitary.	• Primary hypothyroidism: test dose of TSH results in no increase in thyroid hormone; TSH has increased response to TRH. • Hypothalamic hypothyroidism: TSH responds normally to TRH. • Hypopituitary hypothyroidism: TSH does not respond to TRH.

COMMON THYROID DISORDERS

Disorder	Description	Clinical Presentation	Treatment
Cretinism	• Congenital hypothyroidism. • One of most common causes of preventable mental retardation.	Protuberant abdomen and tongue, dwarfism, mental retardation.	Oral thyroid supplementation (based on weight).
Graves Disease	• Autoimmune disease. • α-TSH receptor antibodies cause thyroid gland hyperactivity, resulting in elevated thyroid hormone levels and depressed TSH secretion.	See previous table for symptoms of hyperthyroidism.	Antithyroid drugs (eg, propylthiouracil, methimazole), radioiodine, or both.
Hashimoto Thyroiditis	Autoimmune thyroiditis that causes swelling of the gland and partial or total failure of thyroid hormone secretion.	Cold intolerance, fatigue, weight gain, constipation, goiter.	Thyroid hormone replacement if needed.
Myxedema	Adult hypothyroidism.	See previous table for symptoms of hypothyroidism.	Thyroid hormone replacement.
Thyroid Storm	Severe exacerbation of hyperthyroidism.	• Sudden onset. • Tachycardia, sweating, fever, possible congestive heart failure or pulmonary edema.	• β-Blockers for thyrotoxicosis and thyroid storm. • β-Blockers inhibit extrathyroidal conversion of T_4 to T_3.

III. Calcium, Phosphate, Bone, and Parathyroid Glands

CALCIUM AND PHOSPHATE

Feature	Calcium	Phosphate
Description	• Major cation in crystalline structure of bone and teeth. • 99% is in skeleton. • Free, ionized (active) form is vital second messenger (eg, blood coagulation, muscle contraction, nerve function).	• The major intracellular anion. • 85–90% is in skeleton. • Component of many intermediates in glucose metabolism. • Part of structure of high-energy transfer compounds (eg, ATP) and cofactors.
Regulation	• PTH and vitamin D increase plasma Ca^{2+}. • Calcitonin decreases plasma Ca^{2+}. • *Plasma [Ca^{2+}] rises or falls with plasma albumin levels, with no biological consequence as long as [Ca^{2+}] remains in normal range.* • Alkalosis increases protein-bound form and decreases free form; acidosis has opposite effect.	Vitamin D increases P_i absorption in intestine, but this effect is overridden by PTH stimulation of renal P_i excretion, leading to decreased plasma P_i.
Metabolism	Vitamin D (1,25 dihydroxycholecalciferol) stimulates GI tract absorption, renal reabsorption, and bone resorption (mobilizes Ca^{2+} from bone).	Vitamin D stimulates GI tract absorption and bone resorption (mobilizes P_i from bone).
	98–99% of Ca^{2+} filtered by kidneys is reabsorbed, 60% in proximal tubules.	85–90% of filtered P_i is reabsorbed, most in proximal tubule.
	• GI tract absorption adjusts to Ca^{2+} intake to maintain steady state. • High protein diet increases GI absorption in adults and predisposes to renal stone formation.	GI absorption is relatively constant and linearly proportionate to dietary intake.
Clinical Significance	Low [Ca^{2+}] causes neuromuscular irritability (eg, numbness, paresthesias, tetanic contractions of hands and feet [carpopedal spasm] and larynx [may lead to airway obstruction or asphyxia]).	Severe P_i depletion may result in cardiac and skeletal muscle dysfunction, abnormal bone growth, and hemolysis.

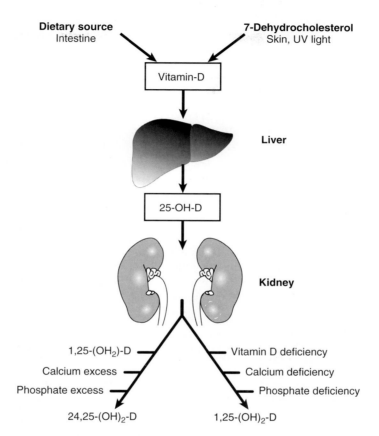

Dietary source
Intestine

7-Dehydrocholesterol
Skin, UV light

Vitamin-D

Liver

25-OH-D

Kidney

1,25-(OH₂)-D
Calcium excess
Phosphate excess

Vitamin D deficiency
Calcium deficiency
Phosphate deficiency

24,25-(OH)₂-D

1,25-(OH)₂-D

25-OH-D = 25-hydroxyvitamin D; 1,25-(OH)$_2$-D = calcitriol; 24,25-(OH)$_2$-D = 24,25-dihydroxyvitamin D; UV = ultraviolet.

COMPARISON OF HORMONES THAT REGULATE CALCIUM LEVELS

Feature	PTH	Calcitriol	Calcitonin
Description	Hormone that *increases plasma [Ca²⁺] and decreases plasma [Pᵢ]*.	Hormone (most biologically active form of vitamin D) that increases plasma [Ca²⁺] and [Pᵢ].	Hormone that decreases plasma [Ca²⁺] and [Pᵢ].
Site of Production	Parathyroid glands.	Formed from vitamin D in liver and kidneys.	Thyroid parafollicular C cells.
Stimulatory Factors	*Low serum [Ca²⁺]* and high serum [Pᵢ].	• Low serum [Ca²⁺] and [Pi] • Prolactin, estrogen, pregnancy calcitonin, and growth hormone	• High serum [Ca²⁺]. • β-agonists, CCK, dopamine, gastrin, glucagon, secretin, food ingestion, estrogen, and pregnancy stimulate calcitonin.
Inhibitory Factors	• Vitamin D deficiency. • Severe magnesium deficiency.	High serum [Pi] and [Ca²⁺] (via negative feedback on PTH).	Low serum [Ca²⁺], PTH, vitamin D.
Mechanisms	• Stimulates Ca²⁺ resorption in bone (inhibits osteoblasts and stimulates osteoclasts). • Stimulates renal Ca²⁺ resorption in thick ascending limb and distal tubule of kidney. • Stimulates calcitriol production, thereby increasing Ca²⁺ absorption by GI tract and stimulating bone resorption. • Increases urinary Pᵢ excretion.	• Increases Ca²⁺ and Pi absorption by GI tract. • Stimulates Ca²⁺ and Pi bone resorption (via osteoclast stimulation). • Stimulates renal Ca²⁺ resorption (via decreasing renal Ca²⁺ excretion).	• Stimulates deposition of Ca²⁺ in bone (via osteoclast inhibition). • Increases excretion of Ca²⁺ in urine.
Clinical Significance	Hyperparathyroidism causes hypercalcemia, hypophosphatemia, and hypercalciuria, leading to demineralization of bones and formation of renal stones.	• Poor diet, lack of sunlight, and GI disease can result in fat malabsorption, liver disease, and kidney failure; all these disorders can cause vitamin D deficiency. • Hyperthyroidism inhibits calcitriol, resulting in osteoporosis.	• Calcitonin is used to block bone resorption when it is abnormally high (eg, Paget disease and osteoporosis). • Calcitonin is elevated in medullary thyroid cancer, Zollinger-Ellison syndrome, and pernicious anemia.

BONE ANATOMY

Anatomic Perspective	Structure	Description
Microanatomy	Osteoblast.	• Cell of mesodermal origin responsible for bone formation. • Differentiates into osteocytes.
	Osteoclast.	Multinucleate cell responsible for bone resorption.
	Osteocyte.	• Osteoblast that has ceased activity and has become embedded in bone matrix. • Receives nutrients from Haversian canals via canaliculi.
	Compact, or cortical bone.	• Outer layer of bone. • Accounts for 80% of bone in body, primarily appendicular skeleton (arms, legs).
	Trabecular, or spongy bone.	• Inner layer of bone. • Accounts for 20% of bone in body (but has greater surface area than cortical bone), primarily axial skeleton (skull, ribs, vertebrae, pelvis). • Made of spicules or plates. • High metabolic activity. • Nutrients diffuse from bone ECF into trabeculae.
	Haversian system.	Haversian canals, their surrounding blood vessels, and collagen arranged in concentric layers forming cylinders called osteons or Haversian systems.
Macroanatomy	Diaphysis.	Shaft of long bone.
	Epiphysis.	Specialized area at end of long bone that is separated from shaft by epiphyseal plate.
	Epiphyseal plate.	Area of epiphyses made of actively proliferating cartilage where bone lengthens by laying down new bone on end of shaft; this process is promoted by GH and IGF-I.
	Metaphysis.	Growing part of long bone that lies between epiphysis and diaphysis.

STRUCTURE OF BONE

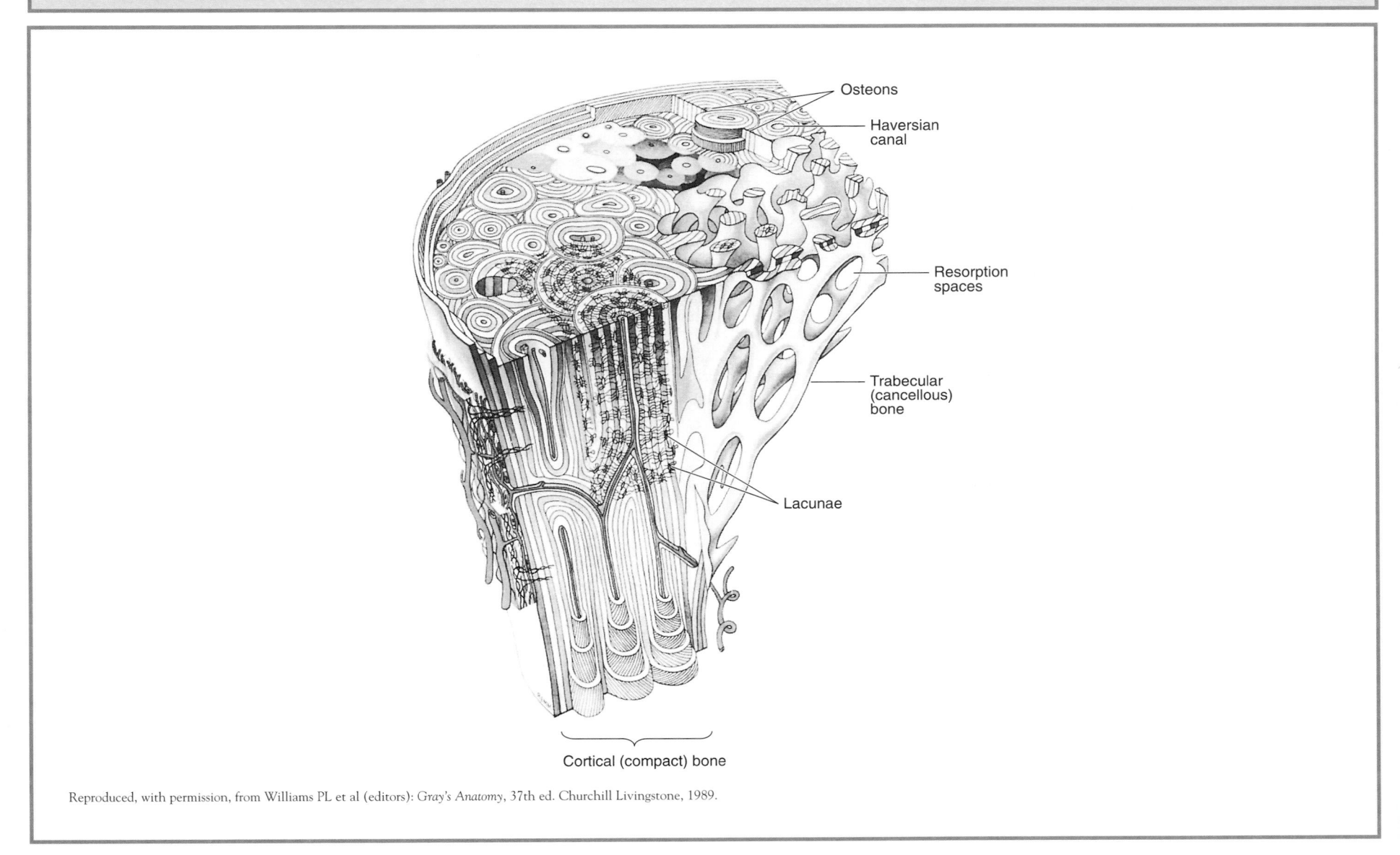

Osteons

Haversian canal

Resorption spaces

Trabecular (cancellous) bone

Lacunae

Cortical (compact) bone

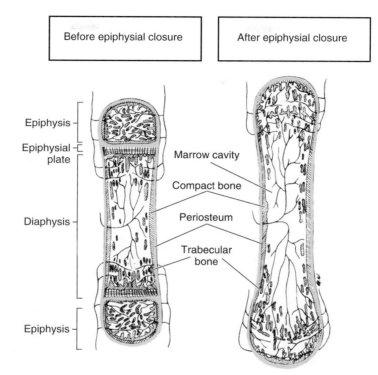

Before epiphysial closure

After epiphysial closure

Epiphysis

Epiphysial plate

Diaphysis

Epiphysis

Marrow cavity

Compact bone

Periosteum

Trabecular bone

Epiphyseal closure occurs when epiphyses unite with the shaft and growth ceases. This process is caused by estrogens and occurs in an orderly, temporal sequence. The last epiphyseal closure normally occurs after puberty. Sexually precocious individuals are often dwarfs, and castrated men with low estrogen levels tend to be tall, because epiphyses remain open past the normal age of puberty.

Reproduced, with permission, from Ganong WF: *Review of Medical Physiology*, 20th ed. McGraw-Hill, 2001:371.

BONE REMODELING

Process	Location	Mechanism	Effects of Time
Resorption initiates formation.			
Bone Resorption	Occurs on inner surface of cortical bone, diminishing bone mass by extracting Ca^{2+} and destroying organic matrix.	Osteoclasts attach to osteon and secrete collagenase and other enzymes, tunneling through mineralized bone and releasing organic products into ECF.	Rates of formation and resorption are equal until 40–50 years of age, when resorption begins to exceed formation and total bone mass slowly decreases.
Bone Formation	Occurs on outer surface of cortical bone.	• Osteoblasts secrete type I collagen and create osteoid matrix in which calcium and phosphate is deposited with aid of alkaline phosphatase. • Mineralization leads to formation of hydroxyapatite crystals. • Osteoblast loses its synthetic activity and becomes osteocyte.	Formation exceeds resorption during growth.

BONE DISEASES

Disease	Description/Causes	Clinical Presentation
Osteitis	Inflammation of bone.	• Bone pain. • Frequently occurs after radiation therapy.
Osteitis Fibrosa Cystica	• Severe hyperparathyroidism, resulting in marrow fibrosis and increased bone remodeling. • Resorption > formation.	• Bone weakness, frequent fractures. • Decalcification and large, punched-out cystic areas of bone filled with osteoclasts that appear as "tumors" on X-ray. • Increased osteoblastic activity. • Increased plasma alkaline phosphatase.
Osteogenesis Imperfecta	Brittle bone disease caused by congenital mutations in genes that code for collagen.	Frequent fractures, scoliosis.
Osteomalacia	Vitamin D deficiency in *adults*, resulting in defective calcification of bone matrix and softening of bones.	• Bone weakness, bowing of weight-bearing bones, bone pain, vertebral collapse, stress fractures, dental deficits, hypocalcemia. • Responds to treatment with vitamin D.
Osteomyelitis	Inflammation of bone marrow caused by infection.	Bone pain with localized swelling, general malaise, nausea, fever.
Osteopetrosis	• Defective osteoclasts unable to resorb bone, leading to increased bone density. • Bone formation > bone resorption.	• Brittle bones that fracture easily. • Neurologic defects caused by narrowing of foramina. • Hematologic abnormalities caused by crowding out of marrow cavities.
Osteoporosis	• Decreased bone strength and mass caused by loss of matrix and minerals. • Most common cause is involutional osteoporosis caused by advancing age. • Disuse osteoporosis occurs in patients who are immobilized. • Associated with glucocorticoid excess (Cushing syndrome), untreated hyperthyroidism, and DM.	• Fractures, especially of distal forearm (*Colles fracture*), vertebral bodies, and hip where there is high content of trabecular bone. • Associated with menopause or estrogen deficiency and andropause or testosterone deficiency. • "Widow's hump" (kyphosis), vertebral fractures, hip fractures. • Women have less bone mass than men, and after menopause they lose it initially more rapidly than men of comparable age.

Continued

BONE DISEASES (Continued)

Disease	Description/Causes	Clinical Presentation
		• Estrogen treatment arrests progress of disease, as does increased calcium intake and moderate exercise. • Bisphosphonates such as alendronate (Fosamax) and risedronate (Actonel) inhibit osteoclast bone resorption and are used to treat osteoporosis and osteopenia.
Rickets	Vitamin D deficiency in *children* resulting in defective calcification of bone matrix and softening of bones.	• Weakness and bowing of weight-bearing bones, abnormal closure of epiphyses. • Dental deficits, hypocalcemia. • Some forms respond to treatment with vitamin D, and others are resistant.

ANATOMY OF THE PARATHYROID GLANDS

Description	Components
• Four yellow-brown endocrine glands. • Lie posterior to thyroid, usually two at superior poles and two at inferior poles.	Chief cells: • Smaller cells, present throughout life. • Synthesize and secrete PTH.
	Oxyphil cells: • Less abundant, larger cells that appear at puberty and increase in number with age. • Function is unknown.

ACTIONS OF PARATHYROID HORMONE (PTH)

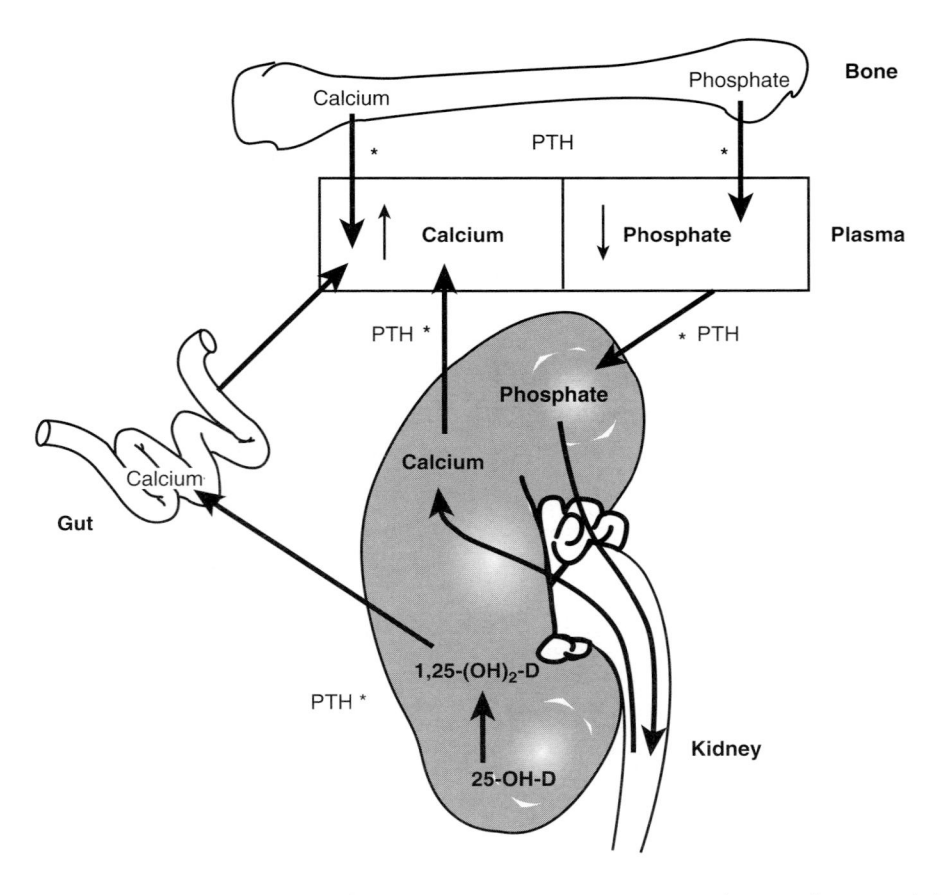

PTH acts directly on bone and kidneys and indirectly on the gut via vitamin D to increase plasma calcium and decrease plasma phosphate.

25-OH-D = 25-hydroxyvitamin D; 1,25-(OH)$_2$-D = calcitriol.

METABOLIC EFFECTS OF PARATHYROID DISORDERS

Disorder	PTH	Vitamin D	Serum Ca2+	Serum Pi	Bone Resorp-tion	Urine Ca2+	Urine Pi	Associated Clinical Conditions
Primary Hyperparathy-roidism	↑ (primary event)	↑	↑	↓	↑	↑	↑	Parathyroid gland tumor (usually benign), renal stones, osteitis fibrosa.
Secondary Hyperparathy-roidism	↑	↓	↓ (primary event)	↑	↑	↑	↑	Chronic renal disease, renal failure, rickets, bone fractures.
Pseudohyper-parathyroidism	↑ (primary event)	↑	↑	↓	↑	↑	↑	• Breast, kidney, and ovarian cancers may produce PTH-related protein. • Secondary hyperparathyroidism is also caused by exogenous PTH.
Primary Hypoparathy-roidism	↓ (primary event)	↓	↓	↑	↓	↓	↓	• Inadvertent parathyroidectomy during thyroid surgery. • Paresthesias, tetany.
Secondary Hypoparathy-roidism	↓	↑	↑ (primary event)	↓	↓	↓	↓	Hypercalcemic states.
Pseudohypo-parathyroidism	↑ or normal (primary event)	↓	↓	↑	↓	↓	↓	Familial benign hypocalciuric, hypercalcemia, mutation of Ca^{2+} receptor gene, resulting in Ca^{2+} receptors that are insensitive to PTH.

IV. Pancreas

HORMONES OF THE ENDOCRINE PANCREAS

Type of Islet Cell	Product	Action
A (25%)	Glucagon.	Regulation of metabolism of carbohydrates, proteins, and fats.
B (60%)	Insulin.	Regulation of metabolism of carbohydrates, proteins, and fats.
D	Somatostatin.	Regulation of islet cell secretion.
F	Pancreatic polypeptide.	Slows absorption of food.

☞ A Gardner **BIDS** For Pansies: **A** makes **G**lucagon

                                  B makes **I**nsulin

                                  D makes **S**omatostatin

                                  F makes **P**ancreatic polypeptide

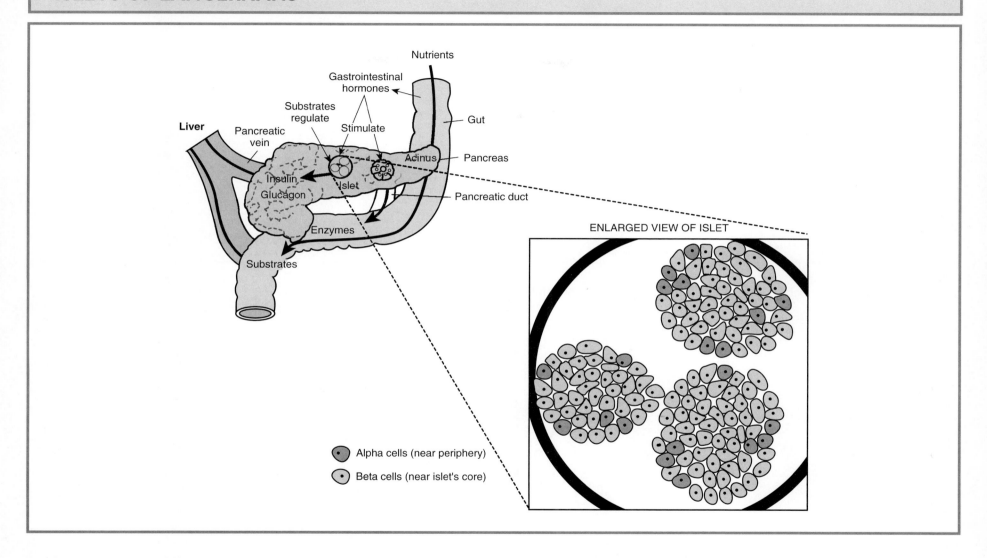

Nutrients

Gastrointestinal
hormones

Substrates
regulate

Stimulate

Liver

Pancreatic
vein

Gut

Acinus

Pancreas

Insulin

Islet

Glucagon

Pancreatic duct

Enzymes

Substrates

ENLARGED VIEW OF ISLET

Alpha cells (near periphery)

Beta cells (near islet's core)

INTERACTIONS BETWEEN HORMONES OF THE ENDOCRINE PANCREAS

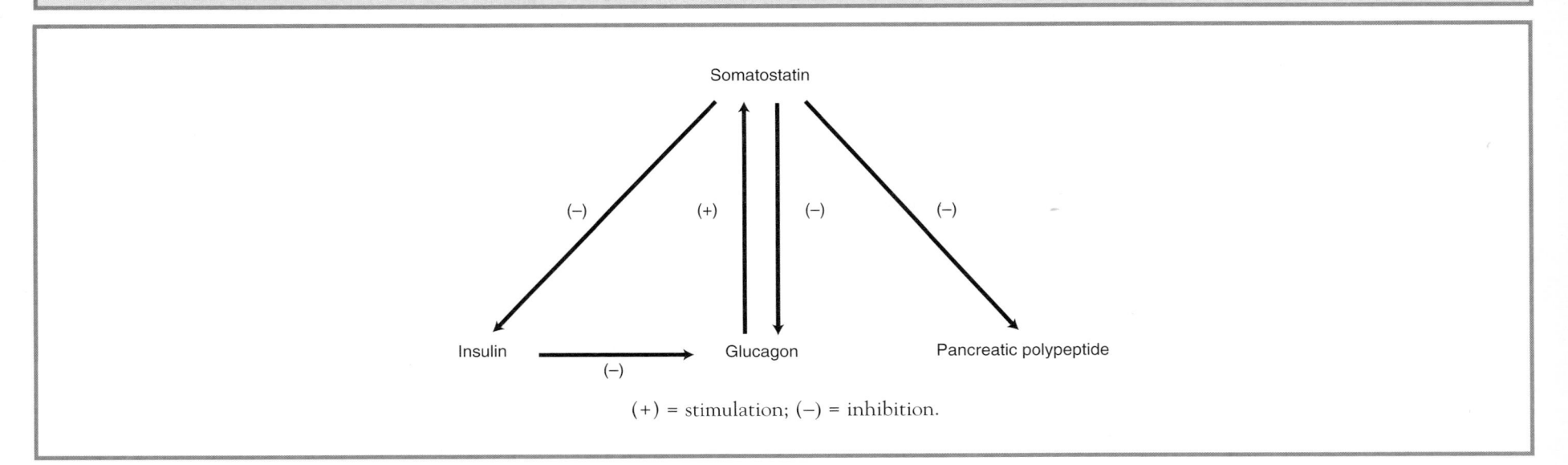

(+) = stimulation; (−) = inhibition.

INSULIN SYNTHESIS

Hormones Involved	Process
Preproinsulin	Synthesized in rough endoplasmic reticulum of B cells.
Proinsulin	• Result of folding, which is facilitated by C peptide.
	• Measurement of C peptide by radioimmunoassay provides index of B cell function in patients receiving exogenous insulin.
Insulin	• Action of proteases on proinsulin forms insulin.
	• Insulin is packaged in Golgi apparatus and expelled by exocytosis via fenestrations of capillary endothelium into bloodstream.

INSULIN REGULATION

Serum Glucose	Resulting Insulin Activity	Regulatory Process	Mechanism	Clinical Symptoms
Low	Low	*Insulin secretion suppressed via activation of glucagon, epinephrine, GH, and cortisol.*	Glucagon and epinephrine increase in hepatic glucose production (glycogenolysis).	• Hypoglycemia may cause confusion, irritability, muscular weakness, incoordination, and sweating. • *Many of these symptoms are similar to patients with DM and hyperglycemia—intracellular glucose is low in both states.*
			GH and cortisol decrease glucose utilization in peripheral tissues.	If severe (eg, insulin shock), coma may result that mimics diabetic coma, but without Kussmaul breathing or acetone breath.
High	High	Rapid transport of glucose into muscle cells.	Insulin facilitates transfer of insulin through muscle cell membrane.	• Abnormal hyperglycemia may cause polyuria, polydipsia, polyphagia, and fatigue. • For severe symptoms, see "Metabolic Changes in Diabetes Mellitus," p. 439.
		Increase in storage of glucose in liver as glycogen.	Insulin inhibits liver phosphorylase and increases glucokinase.	

EFFECT OF INSULIN ON ENERGY SUBSTRATES

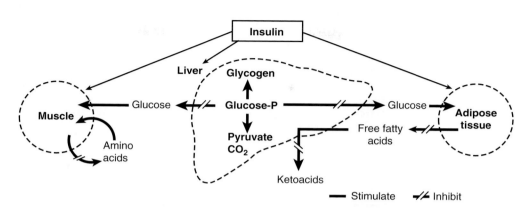

Insulin stimulates the uptake of glucose and amino acids into tissues and inhibits the release of FFAs and ketoacids from tissues.

Modified, with permission, from Berne RM, Levy MN: *Principles of Physiology*, 3rd ed. Mosby, 2000:512.

EFFECT OF GLUCAGON ON ENERGY SUBSTRATES

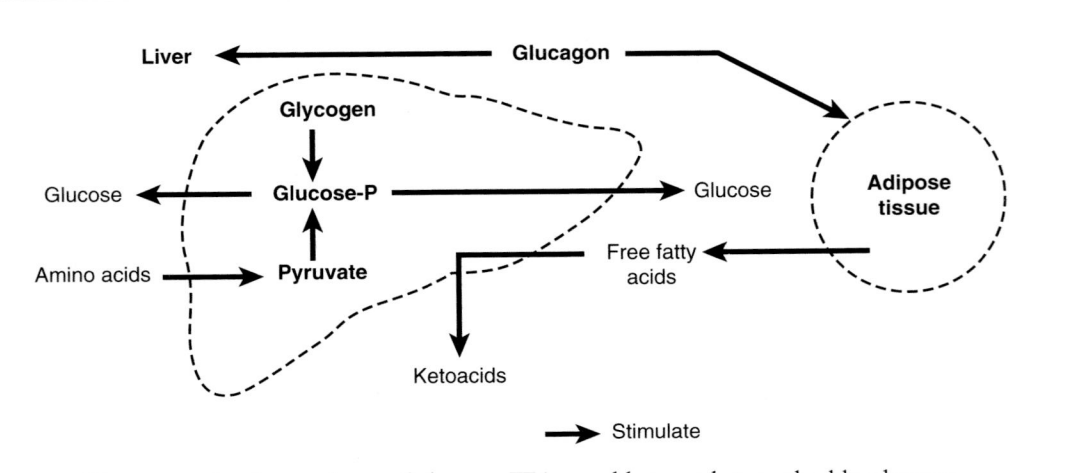

Glucagon stimulates release of glucose, FFAs, and ketoacids into the bloodstream.

Modified, with permission, from Berne RM, Levy MN: *Principles of Physiology*, 3rd ed. Mosby, 2000:516.

COMPARISON OF INSULIN WITH GLUCAGON

Feature	Insulin	Glucagon
Effects	Glucose transport: insulin facilitates glucose entry into cells by increasing number of glucose transporters in cell membrane.	Stimulates release of glucose into bloodstream.
	Anabolic.	Catabolic.
	Hormone of "energy storage."	Hormone of "energy release."
	Glycogenesis, antigluconeogenic, antilipolytic, antiketotic.	Glycogenolytic, gluconeogenic, lipolytic, ketogenic.
	Stimulates uptake of amino acids, FFAs, ketones, and K^+ into cells.	Stimulates release of amino acids, FFAs, and ketones into bloodstream.
	Stimulates synthesis of glycogen, proteins, lipids.	Stimulates glycogen, protein, and lipid degradation.
	Excess causes hypoglycemia.	Excess worsens DM.
	Deficiency causes DM.	Deficiency causes hypoglycemia.
Stimulators	Glucose.	Hypoglycemia, amino acids.
	Glucagon, secretin, CCK, gastrin, gastric inhibitory peptide.	CCK, gastrin, cortisol.
	β-Adrenergic stimulation.	β-Adrenergic stimulation.
		Exercise, infection, and other stresses.
Inhibitors	Glucagon, epinephrine, GH, cortisol.	Insulin, somatostatin, secretin.
	Hypoglycemia.	Glucose, FFAs.
	α-adrenergic stimulation.	α-Adrenergic stimulation.
	K^+ depletion, hyperaldosteronism, thiazide diuretics.	

TYPES OF DIABETES MELLITUS

Feature	Type 1	Type 2
Age of Onset	Usually < 40 years.	Usually > 40 years.
Insulin Requirement	Always.	Not in early stages of disease.
Involves Obesity	No.	Yes.
Autoimmune Destruction of B Cells in Pancreatic Islets	Yes.	No.
Involves Insulin Resistance	No.	Yes.
Ketosis as Complication	Yes.	Rarely.

DIAGNOSTIC TESTING FOR DIABETES MELLITUS

Test	Description	Results for Normal Patient	Results for Patient with DM
Hemoglobin A_{1C}	• Index of diabetic control for 4–6-week period before measurement. • When glucose is episodically elevated over time, small amounts of hemoglobin A are nonenzymatically glycosylated to form hemoglobin A_{1C}.	• < 6.5%. • Normal level also indicates well-controlled DM.	• > 6.5%. • Excellent: 6.5–7.5%. • Good: 7.5–8.5%. • Fair: 8.5–9.5%. • Poor: > 9.5%.
Fasting Blood Glucose Level	Early morning level.	80–110 mg/dL.	> 110 mg/dL.
Oral Glucose Tolerance Test	75 g glucose/300 mL H_2O (or 1 g glucose/kg body weight) administered in fasting state.	Fasting glucose < 115 mg/dL. 2-hour value < 140 mg/dL. No value > 200 mg/dL.	2-hour value and one other value > 200 mg/dL.

EFFECTS OF INSULIN DEFICIENCY

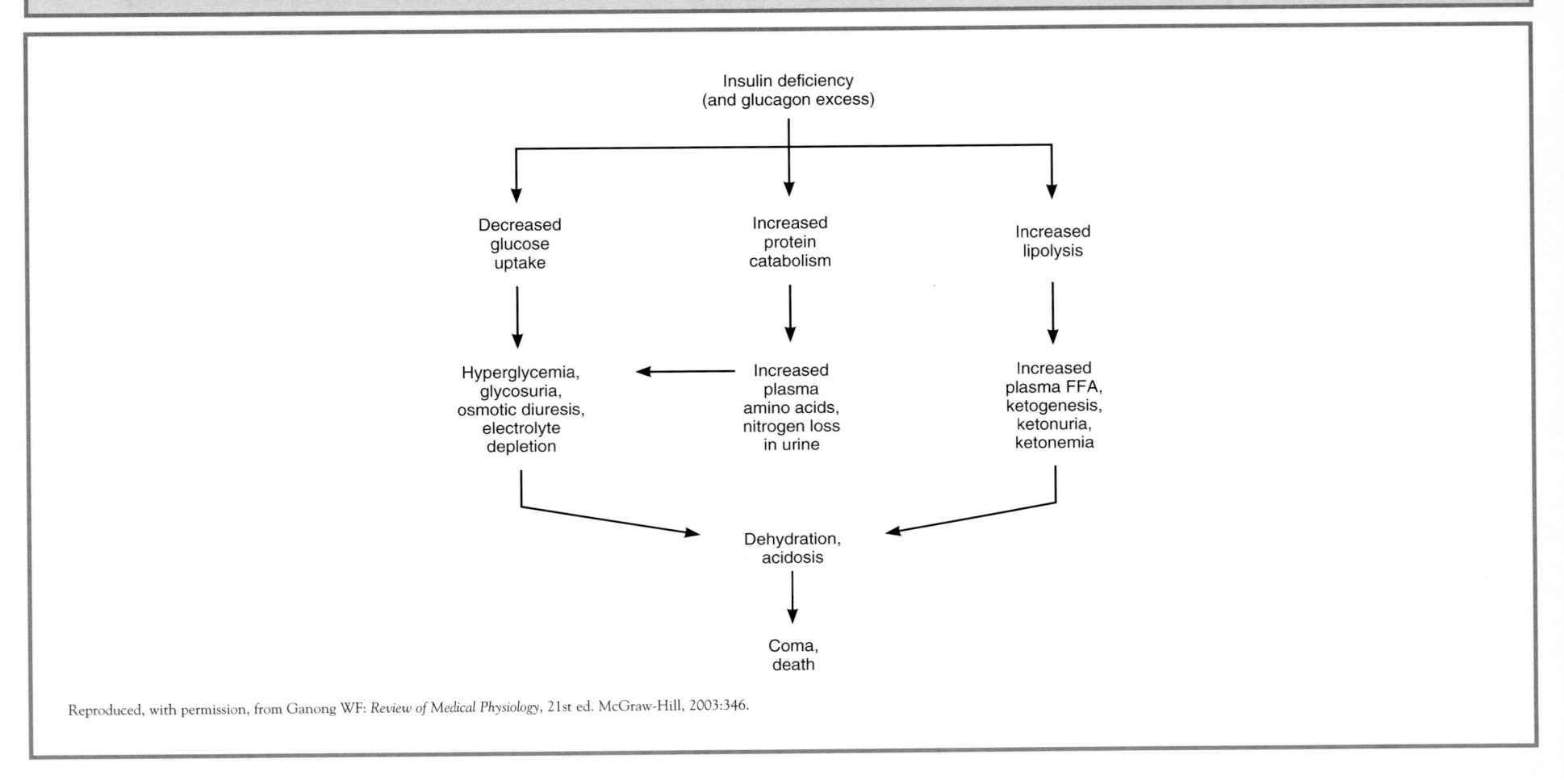

Reproduced, with permission, from Ganong WF: *Review of Medical Physiology*, 21st ed. McGraw-Hill, 2003:346.

METABOLIC CHANGES IN DIABETES MELLITUS

Metabolic Changes	Signs and Symptoms
Reduced entry of glucose and amino acids into peripheral tissues and increased liberation of glucose into circulation from liver.	Significant hyperglycemia, including during fasting and postprandial states.
Intracellular glucose deficiency forces energy requirements to be met by increasing catabolism of fat.	Weight loss.
• Hypersecretion of glucagon and glucocorticoids increases amino acid supply for gluconeogenesis. • Accelerated protein catabolism and decreased protein synthesis causes protein depletion.	• Body enters "starvation" state. • Serum albumin decreases.
Circulating FFAs are increased as result of insulin inhibition of lipase and hypersecretion of glucagon.	*Ketosis* (excess acetyl coenzyme A causes excess production of acetoacetate, acetone, and β-hydroxybutyrate to be formed in liver and enter circulation).
Excess extracellular glucose causes hyperosmolality of blood. Hyperosmolality of blood causes renal capacity for glucose reabsorption to be exceeded.	Hyperosmolar plasma, leading to total body depletion of K^+ and Na^+ and severe *metabolic or lactic acidosis*. • Glycosuria and osmotic diuresis causing *polyuria*. • Resultant dehydration leading to *polydipsia*. • *Polyphagia* occurs in attempt to cover glucose loss, leading to further mobilization of protein and fat stores and weight loss.

COMPLICATIONS OF DIABETES MELLITUS

Type	Description	Clinical Findings
Cardiovascular	Accelerated atherosclerosis caused by increased LDLs, low levels of HDLs, triglycerides, and hypertension.	Increased frequency of stroke and myocardial injury.
	Atherosclerosis in macrovasculature and extremities.	Claudication.
	Damage to microvasculature of eye.	• Diabetic retinopathy leading to cataracts, blindness. • Chronic skin ulcerations leading to gangrene (especially feet).
Neurologic	Damage to microvasculature of nerves in extremities.	Peripheral neuropathy: anesthesia and burning sensation of feet, lack of awareness of damage to feet leading to ulcers.
	Damage to microvasculature of nerves in bladder.	Neurogenic bladder: urinary retention and associated increased risk of urinary tract infections.
Renal	Damage to microvasculature of nephron.	• Diabetic nephropathy: gradual reduction of renal function, with rising creatinine.
Metabolic	Electrolyte abnormalities, acidic urinary loss of Na^+ and K^+, loss of water.	• Common cause of renal failure, requiring dialysis. • Diabetic ketoacidosis: severe metabolic acidosis. • Low plasma pH stimulates respiratory center, leading to Kussmaul breathing (rapid, deep respirations). • Other symptoms: acetone breath, vomiting, dehydration, hypotension; may progress to coma and death. • *Diabetic ketoacidosis is a medical emergency and is most common cause of early death in clinical DM.*

V. Adrenal Gland

ANATOMY OF THE ADRENAL GLAND

Structure	Description	Function
Cortex	• Outer zone. • 80% of weight. • Derived from mesoderm. • ☞ Remember the three zones using GFR.	Main source of corticosteroid hormones (all three zones secrete corticosterone).
	• Zona Glomerulosa. • Outermost layer.	• Secretes mineralocorticoid aldosterone. • ☞ "Salt" = mineralocorticoids.
	• Zona Fasciculata. • Middle layer.	• Secretes glucocorticoid cortisol. • ☞ "Sugar" = glucocorticoids.
	• Zona Reticularis. • Innermost layer.	• Secretes sex steroid precursors, androstenedione, DHEA, DHEA sulfate, and trace amounts of testosterone and estrogen. • ☞ "Sex" = sex steroids.
Medulla	• Inner zone. • 20% of weight. • Derived from neuroectoderm.	• Secretes catecholamines, epinephrine (90%), and norepinephrine (10%). • All circulating epinephrine derived from medulla. • Almost all circulating norepinephrine derived from sympathetic nerve terminals and brain.
	Chromaffin cells contain granules that release catecholamines and are innervated by cholinergic preganglionic fibers of sympathetic nervous system.	• Part sympathetic nervous system ganglion, part endocrine gland. • Acts in concert with "fight-or-flight" response.

SYNTHESIS OF ADRENAL CORTICAL HORMONES

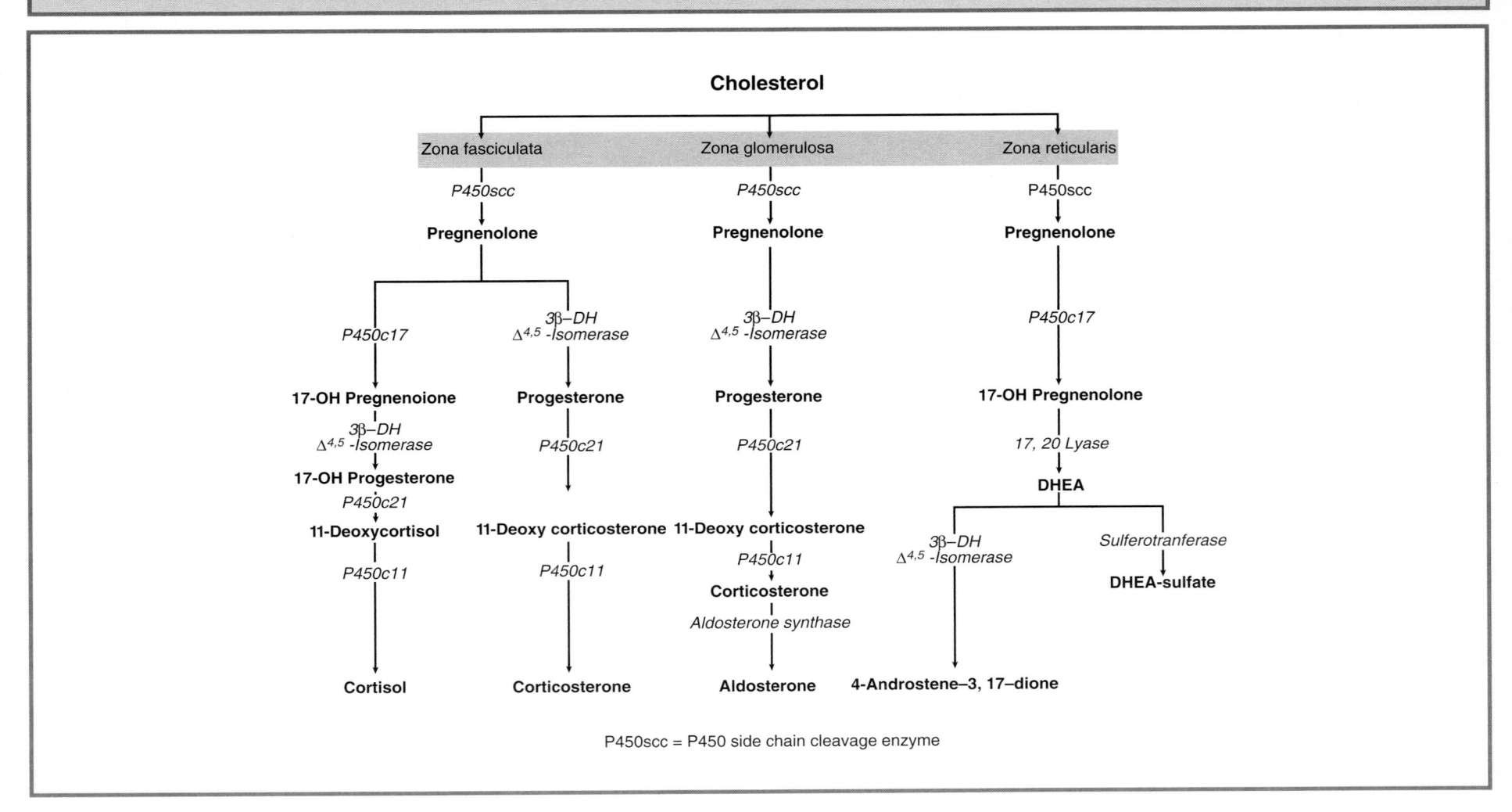

COMPARISON OF ADRENAL CORTICAL HORMONES

Feature	Aldosterone	Cortisol	Androstenedione and DHEA
Description	Mineralocorticoid secreted from zona glomerulosa.	Glucocorticoid secreted from zona fasciculata.	Sex steroid precursors to testosterone and estradiol that are secreted from zona reticularis.
	C21 steroid, also called 17-hydroxycorticosteroid due to hydroxyl group at 17 position.	C21 steroid, also called 17-hydroxycorticosteroid due to hydroxyl group at 17 position.	C19 steroids, also called 17-ketosteroid due to keto group at position 17.
Function	• *Increases renal Na⁺ reabsorption and K⁺ excretion, which leads to expanded ECF volume.* • *Acts primarily on distal tubule and collecting duct.*	• *Catabolic and diabetogenic.* • *Opposes insulin.* • *Supports glucose production from protein and storage of glucose as glycogen.* • *Essential during fasting.*	Promotes masculinization and feminization.
	Part of renin-angiotensin-aldosterone system (see Chapter 6, Renal System).	• Stimulates GH. • Inhibits gastrointestinal Ca^{2+} absorption and stimulates renal Ca^{2+} excretion, leading to hypocalcemia. • Inhibits bone formation and stimulates bone resorption.	Promotes protein anabolism and growth.
Regulation	*Stimulated by low ECF volume, hyperkalemia, hyponatremia, and stress.*	CRH → ACTH → cortisol, with negative feedback from cortisol on both CRH and ACTH.	CRH → ACTH → secretion of adrenal androgens.
	Initially stimulated by ACTH, until renin decreases and ANP increases.	Stimulated by stress (exercise, hypoglycemia, sepsis, surgery).	*Secretion of adrenal androgens is controlled by ACTH, not by gonadotropins.*
	ANP inhibits renin secretion and decreases responsiveness of zona glomerulosa to angiotensin II.	Cortisol secretion is pulsatile and diurnal. • Peak: 2 hours before waking. • Nadir: just before sleep.	

Continued

COMPARISON OF ADRENAL CORTICAL HORMONES (Continued)

Feature	Aldosterone	Cortisol	Androstenedione and DHEA
Metabolism	• Metabolized in liver and kidneys. • Excreted in urine as glucuronide conjugates.	• Metabolized in liver. • Excreted in urine as glucuronides.	• Metabolized in liver. • Excreted in urine as 17-ketosteroids (as are gonadal androgens).
Clinical Significance	• Excess aldosterone leads to K⁺ depletion, increased ECF volume, and hypertension. • When ECF reaches certain point, Na⁺ excretion is increased, and *edema does not develop* (escape phenomenon, thought to be caused by ANP). • *Mineralocorticoids do not produce edema.* • Drugs that decrease aldosterone and elevate K⁺: β-blockers (propanolol), inhibitors of prostaglandin synthesis (indomethacin), and angiotensin-converting enzyme inhibitors (eg, captopril).	• *Urinary 17-hydroxycorticoid level is used as index of cortisol secretion.* • Urinary 17-hydroxycorticoid level is elevated in Cushing syndrome, stress, oral contraceptive use, pregnancy. • Cortisol is used to treat autoimmune disease and organ transplant patients because of its anti-inflammatory and anti-immune effects. • Anti-inflammatory response of cortisol may increase patient's susceptibility to opportunistic infections, cause slow wound healing, or delay diagnosis. • Large doses of cortisol for long periods result in osteoporosis and suppress CRH/ACTH, leading to atrophy of adrenal cortex.	• Excess androstenedione and DHEA cause precocious puberty in boys, female pseudohermaphroditism, and female adrenogenital syndrome. • Conversion of androstenedione to estrogens is important source of estrogens in men and postmenopausal women. • Urinary 17-ketosteroid levels are decreased in panhypopituitarism, Addison disease, and castration. • Urinary 17-ketosteroid levels are elevated in adrenal cortex abnormalities (adrenogenital syndrome, adenoma, carcinoma, Cushing disease), pituitary and ACTH tumors, and interstitial testicular tumors.

- *To avoid complications of sudden cessation of steroid therapy, steroid dose must be decreased slowly over time.*

- Cortisol excess increases glucose, which increases insulin.

- Insufficient insulin response may result in DM.

ALDOSTERONE SECRETION

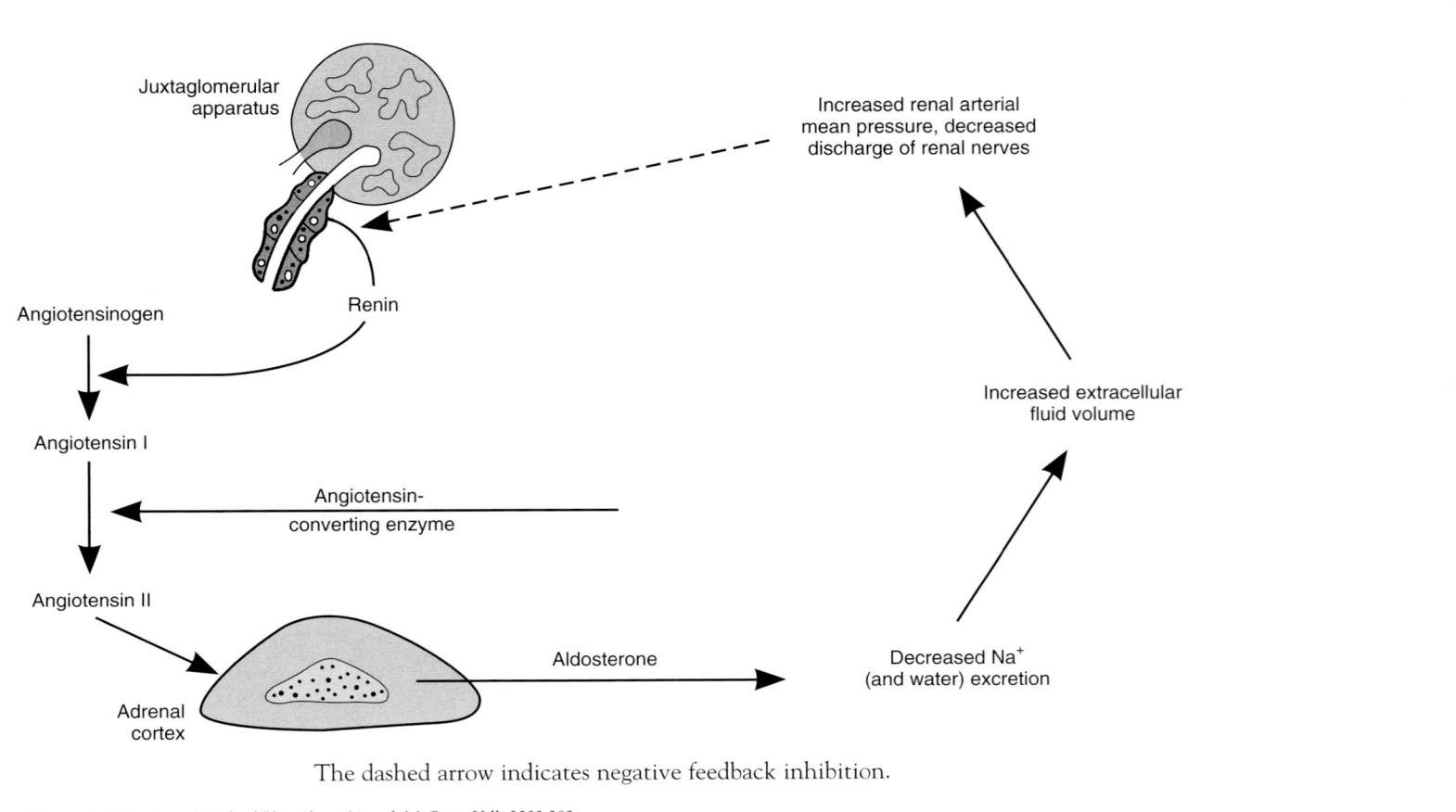

The dashed arrow indicates negative feedback inhibition.

ADRENAL DISORDERS

Disorder	Description	Types	Signs and Symptoms
Addison Disease	Deficiency of glucocorticoids and mineralocorticoids caused by destruction of adrenal cortex.	• Primary disease usually caused by autoimmune inflammation of adrenal cortex. • Secondary disease autoimmune pituitary disorder. • Tertiary disease autoimmune hypothalamic disorder.	Natriuresis, dehydration, hypotension, hyperkalemia, hyponatremia, hyperchloremic acidosis, fatigue, weight loss.
			• Elevated ACTH levels cause diffuse tanning of skin (hyperpigmentation) characteristic of chronic glucocorticoid deficiency. • *Hyperpigmentation is not present in milder secondary and tertiary forms because ACTH is low, not high.*
			• Inability to excrete water load produces *danger of water intoxication*. • Glucose infusion may cause high fever (glucose fever) followed by vascular collapse and death. • Fasting causes fatal hypoglycemia; *any stress may cause vascular collapse*.
			Deficiency of adrenal sex hormones usually has little effect in presence of normal testes or ovaries.
			Addisonian crisis occurs when mineralocorticoid and glucocorticoid deficiency cause severe hypotension, circulatory insufficiency and (fatal) shock.
Congenital Adrenal Hyperplasia	• Congenital defects in enzymes lead to deficient cortisol secretion, causing increased ACTH and hyperplasia.	*21β-hydroxylase deficiency is cause in 90-95% of cases.*	• *21β-hydroxylase deficiency causes salt-losing form.* • Mineralocorticoid deficiency and excess aldosterone-antagonizing steroids cause loss of Na^+.
	• Steroid production is shunted to androgens, causing virilization (if severe, may result in female pseudohermaphroditism).	*11β-hydroxylase deficiency is second most common cause.*	• *11β-hydroxylase deficiency causes hypertensive form.* • Excess secretion of 11-deoxycortisol and 11-deoxycorticosterone causes salt and water retention and, in two thirds of cases, hypertension.

Continued

ADRENAL DISORDERS (Continued)

Disorder	Description	Types	Signs and Symptoms
	• Enough glucocorticoids and mineralocorticoids are usually formed to sustain life.		
Pheochromocytoma	Benign tumor of chromaffin cells of adrenal medulla that secretes catecholamines.		• Hypertension, tachycardia, palpitations, headache, anxiety, chest pain, cold perspiration, hyperglycemia, glycosuria, weight loss, elevated metabolism. • *Elevated urinary excretion of catecholamines or their metabolites (metanephrines and vanillylmandelic acid).*

DISORDERS OF ALDOSTERONE

Disorder	Description	Signs and Symptoms	Important Points
Hyperaldosteronism	Primary disease caused by adrenal disorder: *adenoma of zona glomerulosa (Conn syndrome)*, adrenal hyperplasia, or adrenal cancer. *Secondary disease: congestive heart failure, cirrhosis, nephrosis.*	Fluid retention *without edema*, hypertension, hypokalemia, hypernatremia, metabolic alkalosis, weakness, tetany, polyuria.	• Primary hyperaldosteronism: low renin. • Secondary hyperaldosteronism: high renin. Treat with aldosterone antagonists such as spironolactone.
Pseudohypoaldosteronism	Resistance to action of aldosterone in patients with renal disease.	Hyperkalemia, salt wasting, hypotension.	Low renin.
Glucocorticoid-remediable Aldosteronism	Autosomal dominant disorder.	Hypertension.	• Increase in aldosterone secretion from ACTH is no longer transient. • Treatment with glucocorticoids suppresses aldosterone hypersecretion and associated hypertension.

CUSHING SYNDROME

Causes	Signs and Symptoms
Cushing syndrome—prolonged excessive increase in plasma glucocorticoids.	
ACTH-independent: • Prolonged *exogenous glucocorticoids (most common)*. • Glucocorticoid-secreting adrenal tumors (adenomas, carcinomas).	Increased mineralocorticoids cause salt and water retention that leads to hypertension and K^+ depletion.
ACTH-dependent: • ACTH-secreting pituitary adenoma (also known as Cushing *disease, most common*). • Ectopic ACTH syndrome (e.g., in lung cancer, medullary thyroid cancer). • Abnormal CRH secretion.	Increased glucocorticoid secretion causes increased adrenal androgens, which cause increased facial hair (hirsutism) and acne.
Pseudo-Cushing syndrome is caused by stress, serious infections, severe obesity, and depression.	• Excess protein catabolism, thin skin, easy bruising, poorly developed muscles, purple striae on abdomen (caused by lack of collagen and easy tearing of tissues), thin hair. • Decreased bone formation and increased bone resorption cause osteoporosis. • Fat collects in abdominal wall, face ("moon faced"), and upper back ("buffalo hump"). • Lacks progressive tissue damage associated with Cushing syndrome.

TESTS USED TO DIAGNOSE CUSHING SYNDROME

Test	Description	Indication	Results
24-Hour Urinary Free Cortisol Level	Most specific, usually first test performed.	Determine if cortisol levels are elevated.	> 50–100 µg/d suggests Cushing syndrome.
Ambulatory AM and PM Cortisol Levels	Blood cortisol levels.	Determine if normal circadian rhythm in plasma cortisol is present when 24-hour urinary level is elevated or equivocal.	Patients with Cushing syndrome lack normal diurnal variation or have higher-than-normal basal levels.
Dexamethasone Suppression	• Dexamethasone, a synthetic glucocorticoid, is given. • 24-hour urinary cortisol levels are measured.	• Determine if cortisol levels are elevated in patients with equivocal 24-hour urinary cortisol. • Helps identify pseudo-Cushing syndrome.	Normal (Cushing syndrome not present): dexamethasone signals pituitary to reduce ACTH secretion, causing blood and urine cortisol levels to decrease.
	Low-dose dexamethasone (often given first 2 days).	Determine presence of Cushing syndrome.	Cushing syndrome: cortisol is not suppressed by low-dose dexamethasone.
	High-dose dexamethasone (often given second 2 days).	Distinguishes between pituitary, adrenal, and ectopic etiology for Cushing syndrome.	Pituitary adenoma: 50% or greater suppression of patient's cortisol levels.
			Adrenal cortex: no suppression of patient's cortisol levels.
			Ectopic ACTH: cortisol levels are completely suppressed.
CRH Stimulation	Patients are injected with CRH, and blood levels of ACTH and cortisol are measured.	Distinguishes between pituitary and ectopic ACTH and cortisol-secreting adrenal tumors.	Pituitary adenoma: ACTH and cortisol levels rise.
			Adrenal tumor: baseline low ACTH and high cortisol levels are not affected by ACTH.
			Ectopic ACTH: baseline high ACTH and cortisol levels are not altered by CRH.

Dexamethasone-CRH	Combination of two tests described above.	Distinguishes between Cushing syndrome and pseudo-Cushing syndrome.	Believed to provide a more accurate diagnosis.
Imaging	Computed tomography or magnetic resonance imaging.	Detect tumors (eg, pituitary, adrenal).	
Petrosal Sinus Sampling	• Blood is drawn from petrosal sinuses, which drain pituitary, via femoral line. • ACTH levels are measured.	Distinguishes between pituitary and ectopic Cushing syndrome.	Pituitary adenoma: ACTH levels in petrosal sinuses are higher than in forearm. Ectopic ACTH: ACTH levels in petrosal sinuses and forearm are equal.

CATECHOLAMINE SYNTHESIS

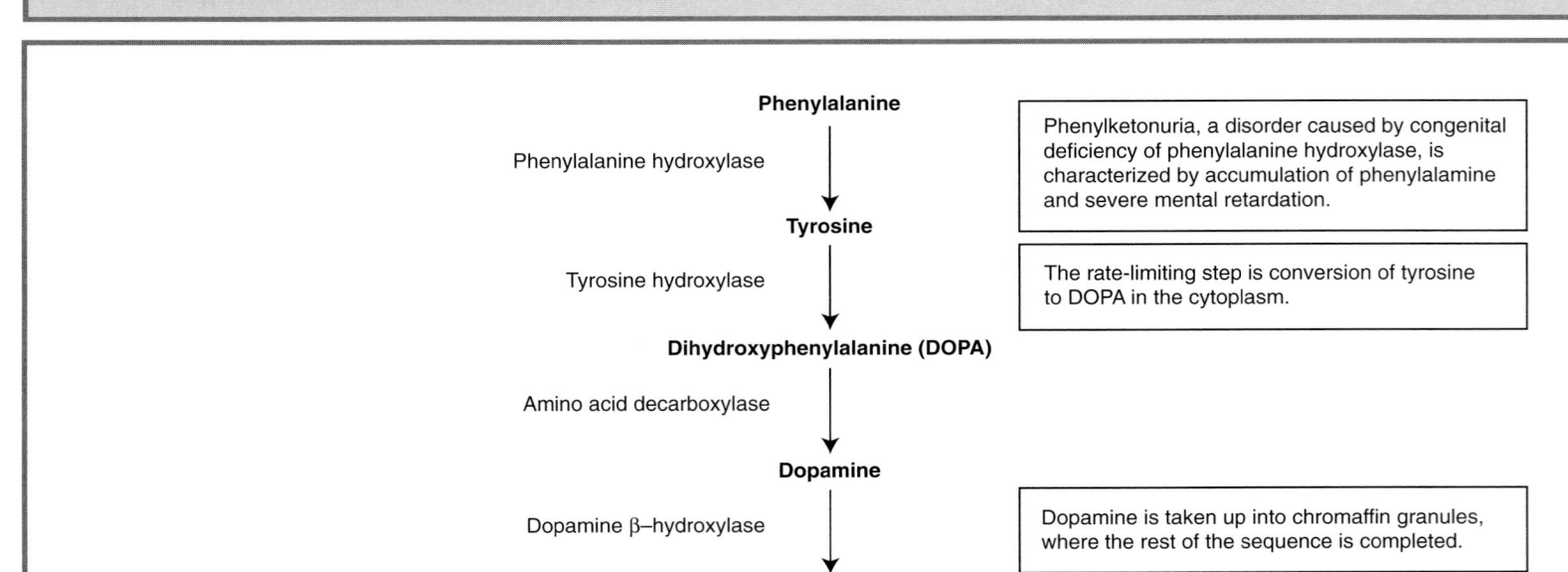

Phenylalanine

Phenylalanine hydroxylase

Phenylketonuria, a disorder caused by congenital deficiency of phenylalanine hydroxylase, is characterized by accumulation of phenylalamine and severe mental retardation.

Tyrosine

Tyrosine hydroxylase

The rate-limiting step is conversion of tyrosine to DOPA in the cytoplasm.

Dihydroxyphenylalanine (DOPA)

Amino acid decarboxylase

Dopamine

Dopamine β–hydroxylase

Dopamine is taken up into chromaffin granules, where the rest of the sequence is completed.

Norepinephrine

Phenylethanolamine–N–methyltransferase

In most granules, norepinephrine reenters the cytoplasm, where it is converted to epinephrine and taken back up into granules for storage.

Epinephrine

FUNCTIONS OF CATECHOLAMINES

Action	Mechanism
Mediate rapid fuel mobilization.	• Increase release of glucose by stimulating glycogenolysis, gluconeogenesis, and lipolysis. • Inhibit insulin secretion and stimulate glucagon secretion.
Stimulate cardiovascular system during exercise.	• Increase force and rate of cardiac contraction. • Epinephrine decreases total peripheral resistance, widens pulse pressure, and increases heart rate and cardiac output.
Increase metabolism.	Stimulate thermogenesis.

ACTIONS OF CATECHOLAMINES DURING STRESS

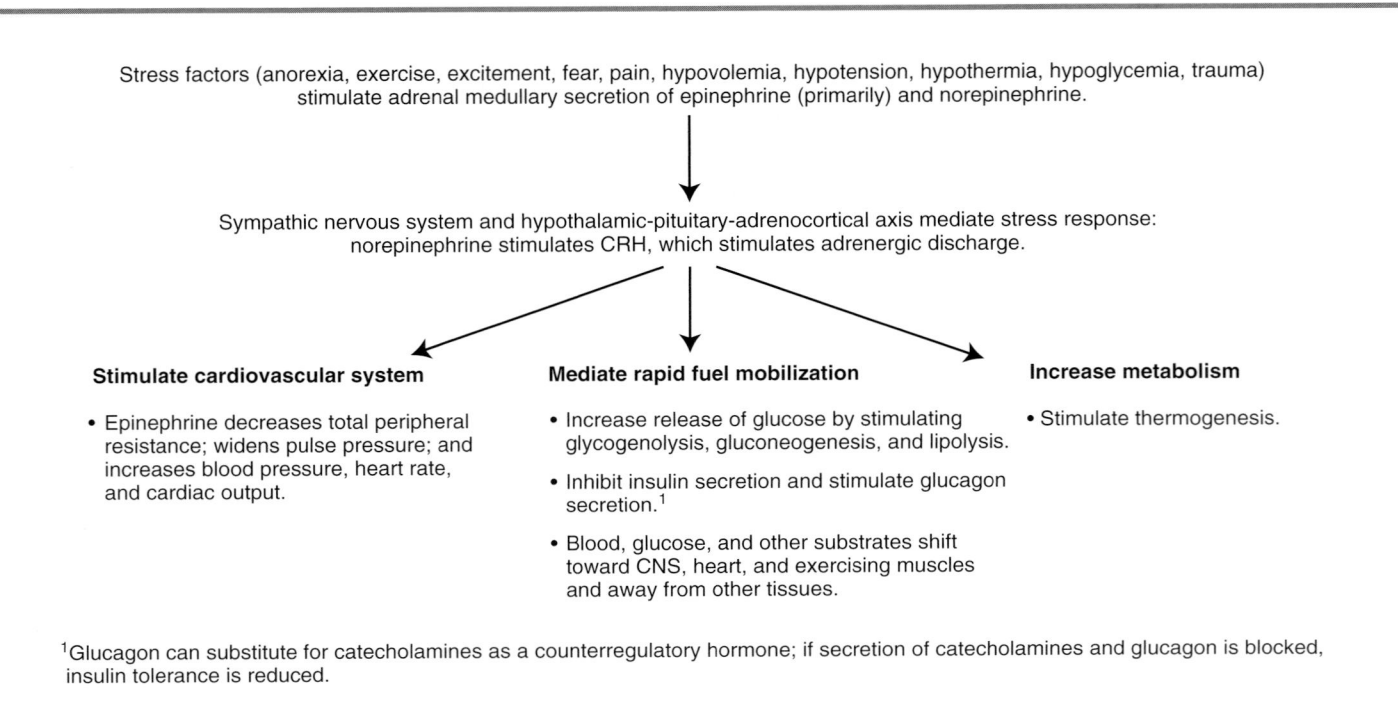

Stress factors (anorexia, exercise, excitement, fear, pain, hypovolemia, hypotension, hypothermia, hypoglycemia, trauma) stimulate adrenal medullary secretion of epinephrine (primarily) and norepinephrine.

Sympathic nervous system and hypothalamic-pituitary-adrenocortical axis mediate stress response: norepinephrine stimulates CRH, which stimulates adrenergic discharge.

Stimulate cardiovascular system

- Epinephrine decreases total peripheral resistance; widens pulse pressure; and increases blood pressure, heart rate, and cardiac output.

Mediate rapid fuel mobilization

- Increase release of glucose by stimulating glycogenolysis, gluconeogenesis, and lipolysis.

- Inhibit insulin secretion and stimulate glucagon secretion.[1]

- Blood, glucose, and other substrates shift toward CNS, heart, and exercising muscles and away from other tissues.

Increase metabolism

- Stimulate thermogenesis.

[1]Glucagon can substitute for catecholamines as a counterregulatory hormone; if secretion of catecholamines and glucagon is blocked, insulin tolerance is reduced.

VI. Pineal Gland

KEY POINTS CONCERNING THE PINEAL GLAND

Description	Action	Clinical Significance
• Arises from roof of third ventricle under posterior corpus callosum. • Connected by stalk to posterior commissure. Contains radiopaque pineal sand (calcium phosphate and calcium carbonate).	• Secretes melatonin, which is thought to play a role in sleep- wake cycle; *does not play physiologic role in regulation of skin color.* • Secretion is low during daylight and increases during dark; also higher in children and declines with age.	*Displacement of calcified pineal from its normal position indicates presence of space-occupying lesion (eg, brain tumor).* Pineal tumor associated with hypothalamic damage produces sexual precocity. Melatonin injections work like bright light. • After dark, they delay onset of sleep. • Just before dawn, they accelerate onset of the next sleep period.

CHAPTER 9

REPRODUCTIVE SYSTEM

ABBREVIATIONS

ACTH = adrenocorticotropic hormone

ATP = adenosine triphosphate

cAMP = cyclic adenine monophosphate

cGMP = guanosine adenine monophosphate

CRH = corticotropin-releasing hormone

DHEAS = dehydroepiandrosterone sulfate

DHT = dihydrotestosterone

FSH = follicle-stimulating hormone

GnRH = gonadotropin-releasing hormone

hCG = human chorionic gonadotropin

HDL = high-density lipoprotein

LH = luteinizing hormone

MIS = müllerian-inhibiting substance

PRL = prolactin

SRY = sex-determining region of the Y chromosome

SSBG = sex steroid–binding globulin

TSH = thyroid-stimulating hormone

VLDL = very low density lipoprotein

Andropause	"Male menopause," or declining sexual drive and fertility in men of middle age; associated with testosterone deficiency.
Anovulation	Failure of ovulation during menstrual cycle; occurs during first 12–18 months after menarche and again before onset of menopause.
Azoospermia	Absence of sperm in semen.
Braxton Hicks Contractions	Uncoordinated, irregular, ineffective uterine contractions that begin the last month of pregnancy; progesterone helps maintain functional quiescence of myometrium.
DHT (Dihydrotestosterone)	Metabolic product of testosterone that is necessary for normal development of male external genitalia and secondary sex characteristics at puberty.
Lactation	Secretion of milk by the mammary glands; usually begins at end of pregnancy.
Menopause	Time when ovaries become unresponsive to gonadotropins; characterized by estrogen deficiency, disappearance of menstrual cycles, hot flashes, palpitations, and vaginal dryness.
Menstruation	Periodic shedding of uterine mucosa that results in vaginal bleeding; average length of one menstrual cycle is 28 days.
Mittelschmerz	Transient lower abdominal pain and peritoneal irritation at time of ovulation; caused by minor bleeding into abdominal cavity.
Oligospermia	Inadequate number of sperm in semen (<10,000,000/mL).
Ovarian Cycle	Release of an ovum from a mature (graafian) follicle; stimulated by LH.
Parturition	Process of giving birth.
Precocious Pseudopuberty	Early development of secondary sexual characteristics without gametogenesis; caused by abnormal exposure of immature males to androgen or females to estrogen.
5α-Reductase	Enzyme that converts testosterone to DHT.
SSBG (Sex Steroid–Binding Globulin)	β-Globulin made in liver that complexes with high affinity to testosterone, DHT, and estradiol, rendering them biologically inactive; decreased by androgens and increased by estrogens.

Continued

True Precocious Puberty	Early but otherwise normal pubertal pattern of gonadotropin secretion from pituitary gland.
Uterine Cycle	Restoration of endometrium after each menstrual phase, followed by preparation of uterus for implantation of fertilized ovum.
Zona Pellucida	Protective, membranous structure surrounding ovum; made of mucopolysaccharides from granul

I. Sexual Development

HORMONAL DIFFERENCES BETWEEN MALES AND FEMALES

Feature	Male	Female
Gonadal Function	Testes produce sperm, large amounts of masculinizing androgens (testosterone), and small amounts of estrogens.	Ovaries produce oocytes, large amounts of estrogens, small amounts of androgens, and *progesterone*.
Production of Other Sex Hormones	Adrenal cortex secretes androgens.	Adrenal cortex secretes androgens.
	Androgens are converted to estrogens in adipose tissue.	Androgens are converted to estrogens in adipose tissue.
Gonadotropin Secretion	GnRH from hypothalamus → LH and FSH from pituitary → testosterone.	GnRH from hypothalamus → LH and FSH from pituitary → estradiol and progesterone.
	Noncyclic.	Cyclic (eg, menstruation, pregnancy, lactation).
Chromosomal Sex	46,XY. • *SRY (testis-determining gene) on short arm of Y results in masculinization of genital tracts and external genitalia.* • No known hormonal influences are required for differentiation of the indifferent gonad into a testis.	46,XX. • One X becomes functionally inactive in all tissues outside gonad during early embryologic development. • Absence of Y results in feminization of genital tracts and external genitalia. • Absence of Y chromosome and SRY gene results in absence of testes and androgens, resulting in female internal and external genitalia.

EMBRYOLOGY OF MALE AND FEMALE INTERNAL GENITALIA

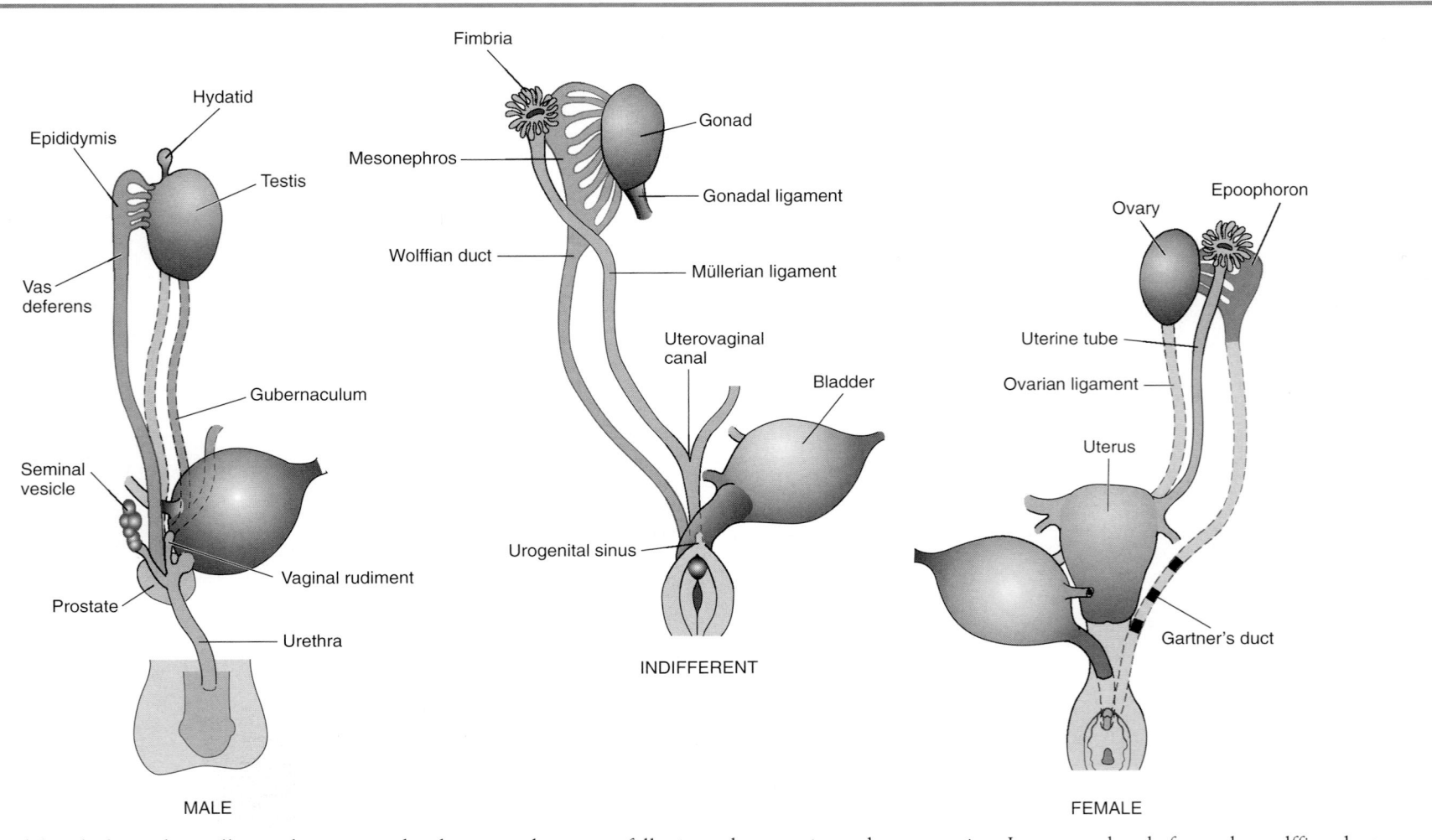

Fimbria

Hydatid

Epididymis

Testis

Mesonephros

Gonad

Gonadal ligament

Wolffian duct

Müllerian ligament

Epoophoron

Ovary

Vas
deferens

Uterovaginal
canal

Bladder

Uterine tube

Ovarian ligament

Gubernaculum

Uterus

Seminal
vesicle

Urogenital sinus

Vaginal rudiment

Prostate

Gartner's duct

Urethra

INDIFFERENT

MALE

FEMALE

In a normal female fetus, the müllerian duct system develops into the uterus, fallopian tubes, cervix, and upper vagina. In a normal male fetus, the wolffian duct system on each side develops into the epididymis, vas deferens, seminal vesicles, and ejaculatory ducts.

Modified, with permission, from Grumbach M, Conte FA: In *Williams Textbook of Endocrinology*, 7th ed. Wilson JD, Foster DW [editors]. Saunders, 1985.

DEVELOPMENT OF THE HUMAN REPRODUCTIVE SYSTEM

Period	Male	Female
Gestational Week 6	Leydig and Sertoli cells start to secrete testosterone and MIS, respectively.	Embryonic ovary does not secrete hormones.
Gestational Week 7	• Indifferent gonads start to develop into testes. • *Testosterone induces wolffian ducts to develop into epididymis, vas deferens, seminal vesicles, and ejaculatory ducts.* • Development complete at 12 weeks. • MIS causes regression of müllerian ducts.	• Indifferent gonads start to develop into ovaries. • *Müllerian ducts form uterus, fallopian tubes, cervix, and upper vagina.* • No known hormonal influences are required. • Wolffian ducts regress by 10 to 11 weeks because of absence of testosterone.
Gestational Week 8	*Induction of external genitalia by DHT.* • Genital tubercle forms glans penis. • Genital swelling forms scrotum. • Urethral and genital folds enlarge and enclose penile urethra and corpora spongiosa. • Urogenital sinus forms prostate gland.	Growth of external genitalia. • Genital tubercle forms clitoris. • Genital swelling forms labia majora. • Urethral and genital folds form labia minora. • Urogenital sinus forms lower vagina.
Gestational Week 9+	• hCG (LH-like placental hormone) stimulates early testosterone production by Leydig cells. • Continued growth of male genitalia in last 6 months gestation requires fetal pituitary LH to support testosterone production. • Testosterone burst occurs just before birth and again in neonatal period.	Later growth of female genitalia in utero may be modulated by ovarian estrogen production, which depends on fetal pituitary gonadotropins.
Puberty	Leydig cells and testes are quiescent until activated by gonadotropins in puberty.	Ovaries remain quiescent until activated by gonadotropins in puberty.
	Increased androgens suppress breast development.	Increased pubertal estrogens induce growth and differentiation of breast tissue.

HYPOTHALAMIC–ANTERIOR PITUITARY–GONADAL AXIS

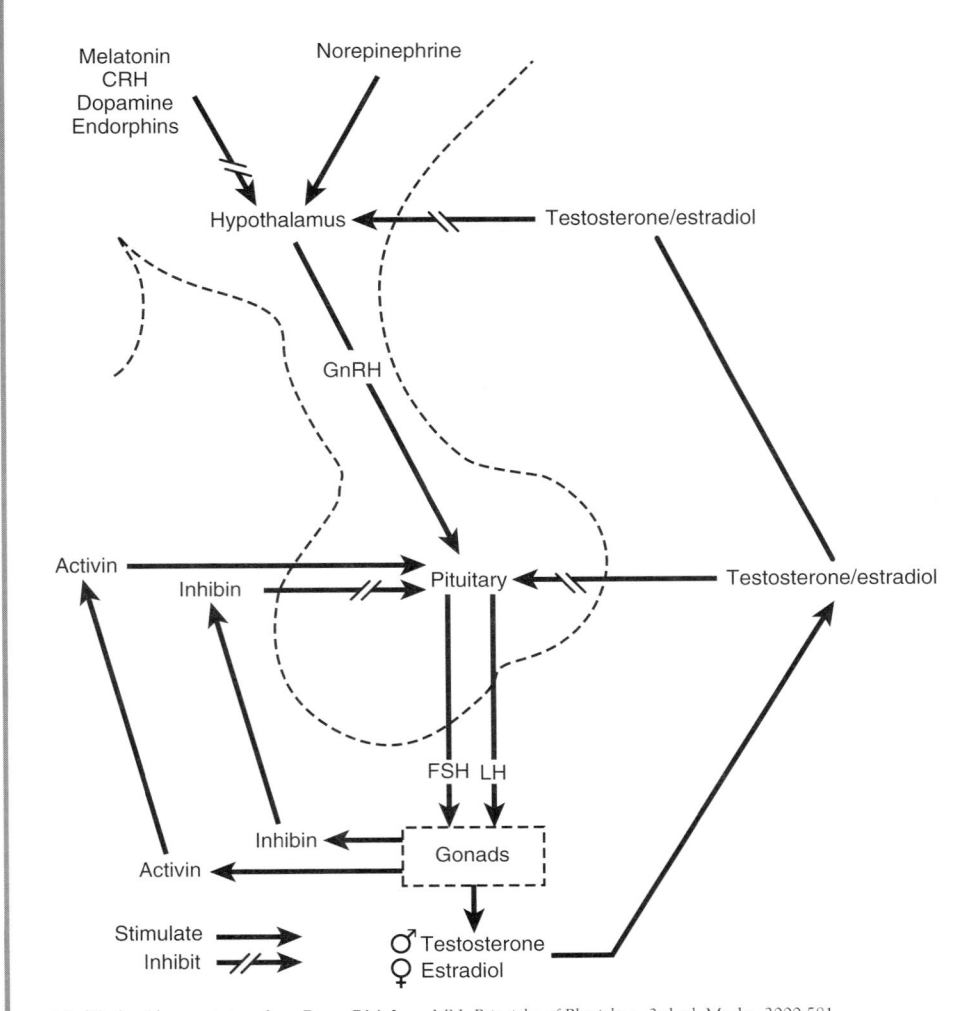

- Hypothalamic GnRH stimulates the release of LH and FSH from the pituitary.

- In turn, LH and FSH stimulate gonadal secretion—primarily testosterone in males and estradiol in females.

- LH and FSH exert negative feedback at both the pituitary and hypothalamic levels to inhibit the secretion of testosterone and estradiol.

- In addition, FSH stimulates the gonadal release of inhibin, which exerts negative feedback to preferentially block the release of FSH.

- Estradiol (in women) and the gonadal protein activin have positive feedback effects on pituitary secretion.

Modified, with permission, from Berne RM, Levy MN: *Principles of Physiology*, 3rd ed. Mosby, 2000:581.

HORMONES OF THE REPRODUCTIVE SYSTEM

Hormone	Description	Regulation	Function
GnRH	• Made in arcuate and preoptic nuclei of hypothalamus and released in *pulsatile* fashion into pituitary. • Stimulates release of gonadotropins.	• Inhibited by negative feedback from testosterone, estrogen, and progesterone. • Also inhibited by dopamine.	Stimulates LH and FSH (LH more than FSH).
	Frequency of pulsations increases late in follicular phase of menstrual cycle, causing LH surge.	*Prolonged and nonpulsatile stimulation of GnRH downregulates its receptor, leading to inhibition of gonadotropin secretion.*	Long-acting GnRH agonists are used therapeutically when gonadal androgen or estrogen production must be suppressed (eg, precocious puberty, prostate cancer, endometriosis).
LH	Gonadotropic hormone synthesized and released in *pulsatile* fashion by anterior pituitary.	Stimulated by GnRH.	Stimulates maturation of ovarian follicles and their secretion of estrogen and progesterone.
	• α Subunit is identical to TSH and FSH. • β Subunit is unique.	Inhibited by negative feedback from estrogen and testosterone.	• Stimulates ovulation, formation of corpus luteum, and progesterone secretion from corpus luteum. • *Stimulates theca and Leydig cells to secrete testosterone, and to a lesser degree, estrogens.*
FSH	Gonadotropic hormone synthesized and released by anterior pituitary.	Stimulated by GnRH.	*Stimulates granulosa and Sertoli cells to secrete estrogens and inhibin.*
	• α Subunit is identical to TSH and FSH. • β Subunit is unique.	Inhibited by inhibin.	Stimulates maturation of ovarian follicles and formation of sperm in testes.
	Injections of FSH may be used to treat patients with infertility.		• Increases sensitivity of target cells to LH by increasing number of LH receptors. • Stimulates SSBG.

Continued

HORMONES OF THE REPRODUCTIVE SYSTEM (CONTINUED)

Hormone	Description	Regulation	Function
Estrogen	• One of a group of steroid hormones including estriol, estrone, and estradiol. • Synthesized mainly by the ovaries, with small amounts made in adrenal cortex, testes, and placenta. • 98% of circulating estradiol is bound to protein; (60% to albumin and 38% to SSBG). • Metabolized in liver, secreted in bile (reabsorbed via enterohepatic circulation), and excreted in urine.	• LH promotes conversion of cholesterol to androstenedione, which is converted to estrogen. • FSH promotes estradiol secretion by increasing aromatase activity via cAMP. • Peak estrogen secretion occurs just before ovulation and during midluteal phase of menstrual cycle.	• Stimulates development of female sex organs and female secondary sexual characteristics. • See Functions of Estrogen.
Progesterone	See Hormones in Pregnancy.		
Testosterone	• Principal male sex hormone that stimulates development of male sex organs and male secondary sexual characteristics. • Synthesized mainly by testes, with small amounts made in adrenal cortex and ovaries. • 98% testosterone in plasma is bound to protein (65% to SSBG and 33% to albumin). • Only free fraction of androgens are biologically active. • Most testosterone is converted to 17-ketosteroids (eg, androsterone) and excreted in urine. • Some circulating testosterone is converted to estrogens.	LH stimulates Leydig cells to synthesize testosterone from cholesterol; cAMP increases cholesterol formation via protein kinase A.	See Functions of Testosterone, p. 469.

Activin	Gonadal protein secreted by Sertoli cells.	• Inhibited by FSH. • Stimulated by interleukin-1.	Stimulates FSH (positive feedback).
Inhibin	Gonadal protein secreted by Sertoli cells in males and granulosa cells in females.	• Stimulated by FSH. • Inhibited by interleukin-1.	• Inhibits GnRH secretion from hypothalamus. • Inhibits FSH secretion from anterior pituitary.
PRL	See "Hormones in Pregnancy", p. 470.		
MIS	Secreted by Sertoli cells in males and granulosa cells in females.	Stimulated by steroidogenic factor.	Causes regression of müllerian ducts by apoptosis and initiates testicular descent.

ESTROGEN BIOSYNTHESIS

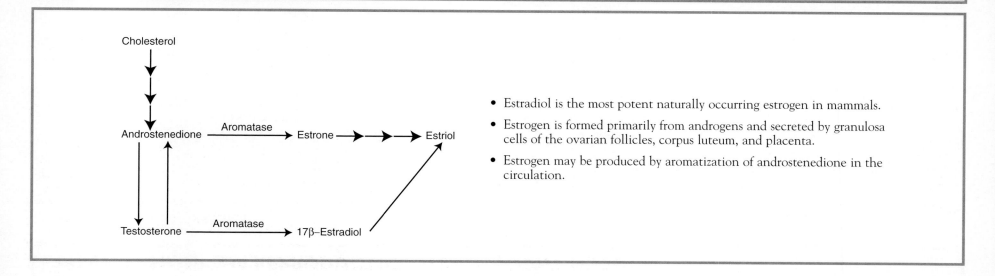

- Estradiol is the most potent naturally occurring estrogen in mammals.
- Estrogen is formed primarily from androgens and secreted by granulosa cells of the ovarian follicles, corpus luteum, and placenta.
- Estrogen may be produced by aromatization of androstenedione in the circulation.

FUNCTIONS OF ESTROGEN

Nature of Effect	Function
Reproductive	<ul><li>Causes growth of ovarian follicles.</li><li>Causes cyclic changes in endometrium, cervix, and vagina.</li><li>Increases uterine blood flow, muscle contraction, and motility of fallopian tubes.</li><li>Makes uterus more sensitive to oxytocin.</li></ul>
Puberty	<ul><li>Induces female pubertal development of secondary sex characteristics, including proliferation of mammary ducts in breasts.</li><li>*Causes epiphyseal closure.*</li></ul>
Other	<ul><li>Low levels cause negative feedback inhibition on GnRH and gonadotropins (LH and FSH), leading to decreased estrogen secretion (eg, oral contraceptives [estrogen-progesterone combinations] decrease secretion of gonadotropins to levels below those needed monthly to produce mature ovum).</li><li>High levels cause positive feedback on LH and FSH (eg, elevated estrogen causes LH and FSH surges during menstrual cycle).</li><li>*Causes increased secretion of angiotensinogen, resulting in salt and water retention, and thyroid-binding globulin.*</li></ul>

FUNCTIONS OF TESTOSTERONE

Nature of Effect	Function	Clinical Significance
Reproductive	Maintains spermatogenesis along with FSH.	Testosterone levels, and, therefore, spermatogenesis, gradually decrease (but are maintained) as men age.
	Develops and maintains male external genitalia and male secondary sex characteristics via conversion to DHT by 5α-reductase.	• 5α-Reductase inhibitors are used to treat male disorders. • Example: high-dose finasteride (Proscar) is used to treat benign prostatic hypertrophy, and low-dose finasteride (Propecia) is used to treat baldness.
Other	• Exerts protein-anabolic effect. • Promotes growth and libido.	• Testosterone creates greater bone mass in males than in females, protecting against osteoporosis. • Risk of osteoporosis increases as testosterone decreases.
	• Inhibits GnRH from hypothalamus. • Inhibits LH from anterior pituitary.	Negative feedback inhibition: • Testosterone inhibits GnRH secretion from hypothalamus → decreased testosterone. • Testosterone inhibits LH secretion from anterior pituitary → decreased testosterone.
	Serves as source of estrogen. • 80% of estradiol and 95% of estrone in males is formed from aromatization of circulating testosterone and androstenedione in adipose tissue and liver. • Remainder is derived from testes (Leydig and Sertoli cells).	Peripheral aromatization of estrogens from androgens is primary source of estrogens in men and increases with increased weight and age.
	Increases VLDL but decreases HDL.	Higher risk of coronary artery disease in men than in women.
	Stimulating erythropoietin.	Increases red blood cell mass.

HORMONES IN PREGNANCY

Hormone	Description/Regulation	Functions
Progesterone	Hormone secreted by ovarian follicles, corpus luteum, and placenta (small amounts are secreted from adrenal glands and testes). • Stimulated by LH. • Secretion increases late in follicular phase and during luteal phase.	• Serves as intermediate in steroid biosynthesis in all tissues that secrete steroid hormones. • Inhibits LH (and progesterone) secretion by negative feedback. • *Causes cyclic changes in endometrium, cervix, and vagina.* • Potentiates inhibitory effects of estrogens, preventing ovulation. • Thermogenic (believed to be responsible for increase in basal body temperature at ovulation). • In pregnancy, it stimulates secretion of nutrients for early zygote, decreases sensitivity of myometrial cells to oxytocin, and induces PRL synthesis. • Stimulates development of lobules and alveoli in breast. • Supports secretory function of breast during lactation.
hCG	• Glycoprotein produced by syncytiotrophoblast. • Composed of same α subunit as LH, FSH, and TSH with unique β subunit.	• *Maintains corpus luteum* and stimulates it to secrete hormones during pregnancy. • Its presence in urine is used to detect pregnancy within 9 days of conception.
	• Normally produced in small amounts by fetal liver and kidney. • Secreted in small amounts by gastrointestinal and other tumors in both sexes. • Its presence in urine is used to detect pregnancy within 9 days of conception.	• Stimulates early secretion of testosterone by Leydig cells. • *Critical to differentiation of male genital tract.*
Human Chorionic Somatomammotropin (human placental lactogen)	Hormone secreted by syncytiotrophoblast with structure similar to human growth hormone.	• "Maternal growth hormone of pregnancy." • Helps divert glucose to fetus.

Relaxin	• Hormone secreted from ovaries, corpus luteum, decidua, and placenta during pregnancy. • Stimulated by hCG.	Loosens ligaments of pubic symphysis, softens cervix, and decreases uterine muscle contractility, which facilitate fetal delivery.
PRL	• Anterior pituitary gland hormone. • Excess secretion causes impotence and hypogonadism in males and osteoporosis due to estrogen deficiency in females. • *Associated with chromophobe adenomas of anterior pituitary and secondary amenorrhea.* • *Secretion is increased by nipple stimulation, exercise, and stress.* • Tonically inhibited by dopamine (PRL-inhibiting hormone) from hypothalamus. • Stimulated by maternal estrogen. • Inhibits its own secretion via negative feedback.	• Inhibits effects of gonadotropins. • Stimulates production of progesterone by corpus luteum and production of milk after childbirth. • Suppresses ovulation in nursing mothers by inhibiting GnRH (thereby also inhibiting LH).
Oxytocin	• Hypothalamic hormone secreted via posterior pituitary gland. • *Secretion increased by nipple stimulation.*	• Increases contraction of womb during labor and stimulates ejection of milk from breast. • Oxytocin (Pitocin) given to induce uterine contractions and to control or prevent hemorrhage after birth.

PUBERTY

Sex	Age (y)	Hormonal Changes	Physical Changes
Males	7–10	LH and FSH levels remain low until increased synthesis and release of GnRH occurs, causing a gradual increase in androgen secretion.	Linear growth.
	10–12	*Adrenarche* is onset of increase in secretion of adrenal androgens.	
	9–17	Increases in plasma LH and FSH occur.	Enlargement of testes is first physical sign of puberty.
		Secretion of testosterone rapidly increases.	Pubarche is development of axillary and pubic hair.
		• DHT and its binding with stronger affinity to androgen receptor is required for development of prostate as well as development and maintenance of secondary sex characteristics.	• Scrotum becomes pigmented and rugose. • Muscle mass increases, and shoulders broaden. • Linear growth reaches peak velocity. • Growth ceases 1–2 years after adult testosterone levels are reached. • Larynx enlarges, vocal cords grow, and voice deepens. • Sebaceous gland secretions thicken. In one third of boys, transient stimulation of breast growth occurs, probably caused by increased production of estradiol, and as testosterone levels predominate, breast tissue regresses.
Females	7–10	• LH and FSH levels remain low until increased synthesis and release of GnRH occurs, causing a gradual increase in estrogen secretion. • *Adrenarche* is onset of increase in secretion of adrenal androgens.	Linear growth.

9–17	• Plasma LH and FSH increase. • Pulsatile pattern emerges, and ratio of LH to FSH increases. • Secretion of estrogens rapidly increases.	*Thelarche:* breast development is first event.
	Levels of adrenal DHEAS increase.	*Pubarche* is development of axillary and pubic hair (due primarily to androgens).
	Withdrawal of estrogen secretion from graafian follicles undergoing atresia induces bleeding.	• *Menarche* is start of menstruation. • *Initial periods are anovulatory, and regular ovulation starts 12–18 months later.* • Peak velocity of growth is attained earlier in girls. • Height increase usually stops 1–2 years after onset of menses.

COMPARISON OF ANDROPAUSE AND MENOPAUSE

Process	Hormonal Changes	Physical Changes
Andropause	Testes gradually lose responsiveness to gonadotropins, leading to gradual decrease in testosterone and inhibin.	Gradual testicular atrophy with decrease in number of Leydig and Sertoli cells.
	Secretion of LH and FSH increase as result of decreased negative feedback from androgens.	Decline in libido and sperm production (some spermatogenesis persists into ninth decade).
	Moderate increase in estrogen production with advancing age.	Osteoporosis.
Menopause	Decline in number of primordial follicles causes ovaries to become unresponsive to gonadotropins.	• Irregular menses that cease at 45–55 years of age. • Average age of menopause is 52.
	Ovaries no longer secrete progesterone and estradiol.	Atrophy of uterus and vagina.
	• Secretion of LH and FSH increase as result of decreased negative feedback from estrogens. • FSH > LH.	Hot flashes, night sweats.
	Small amounts of estrogen formed by aromatization of androstenedione in circulation (adrenal androgens become predominant source of estrogen).	Osteoporosis.

ABNORMAL SEXUAL DIFFERENTIATION

Type	Description	Examples
Mixed Gonadal Dysgenesis (mosaicism)	• 46,XY/45,XO. • Testis on one side and streak gonad on other side. • External genitalia usually incompletely virilized male. • Internal structures variable.	McCune-Albright syndrome: precocious puberty, amenorrhea, galactorrhea.
Pure Gonadal Dysgenesis	Nondisjunction of sex chromosomes during first meiotic division.	Turner syndrome: 45,XO; bilateral streak gonads; underdeveloped müllerian tract; webbed neck; short stature; sexual infantilism.
True Hermaphrodite (rare)	Flawed mitosis in early zygote produces a mosaic (two or more populations of cells with different chromosome complements).	• XX/XY. • Both ovaries and testes are present.
Female Pseudohermaphrodite	• 46,XX. • SRY negative. • Only ovarian tissue present. • Female internal genitalia with male external genitalia.	*Congenital adrenal hyperplasia*, Mayer-Rokitansky syndrome (müllerian agenesis), exposure to maternal androgens at 8–13 weeks gestation.
Male Pseudohermaphrodite	• 46,XY. • SRY positive. • Only testicular tissue present. • Male internal genitalia with female external genitalia.	Persistent müllerian duct syndrome: male infant with inguinal hernias containing uterus, fallopian tubes, or both. *5α-Reductase deficiency, resulting in no DHT:* • Male internal genitalia, including testes, but female external genitalia. • Affected child usually raised as girl. • At puberty, LH secretion and circulating testosterone levels are increased, and patient develops male body contours and male libido. • Patient often then "becomes" boy.

		Testicular feminization syndrome: defective androgen receptors.
		• Female infant with inguinal hernia containing normal testes.
		• Presents as primary amenorrhea.
		• Patient is phenotypically tall with normal female breasts and external genitalia.
Nondisjunction	• Pairs of homologous chromosomes fail to separate during meiosis or a chromosome fails to divide at anaphase of mitosis or meiosis. • Results in cell with abnormal number of chromosomes.	Klinefelter syndrome (*most common type*) • XXY. • High incidence of mental retardation. • Abnormal seminiferous tubules (infertility). • Normal male external genitalia.
		XXX (superfemale): no characteristic abnormalities.
		Down syndrome (trisomy 21).
Transposition of Parts of Sex Chromosomes	Short arm of father's Y chromosome is transposed to father's X chromosome during meiosis.	Genetic male with XX.
	Deletion of SRY portion of Y chromosome.	Genetic female with XY.
Hypergonadotropic Hypogonadism	• Hormonal deficiency at level of gonad. • Circulating gonadotropin levels are elevated. • Circulating testosterone in males or estrogen in females is depressed.	• Males: cryptorchism, varicocele, viral orchitis (mumps), defects of Y chromosome or androgen receptors. • Females: Turner syndrome, defects of estrogen receptors.
Hypogonadotropic Hypogonadism	• Deficiency at level of pituitary or hypothalamus. • Circulating gonadotropins, testosterone (males), and estrogen (females) are depressed.	*Kallmann syndrome:* failure of GnRH secretion resulting in secondary testicular failure, associated anosmia.

II. Male Reproduction

MALE REPRODUCTIVE SYSTEM

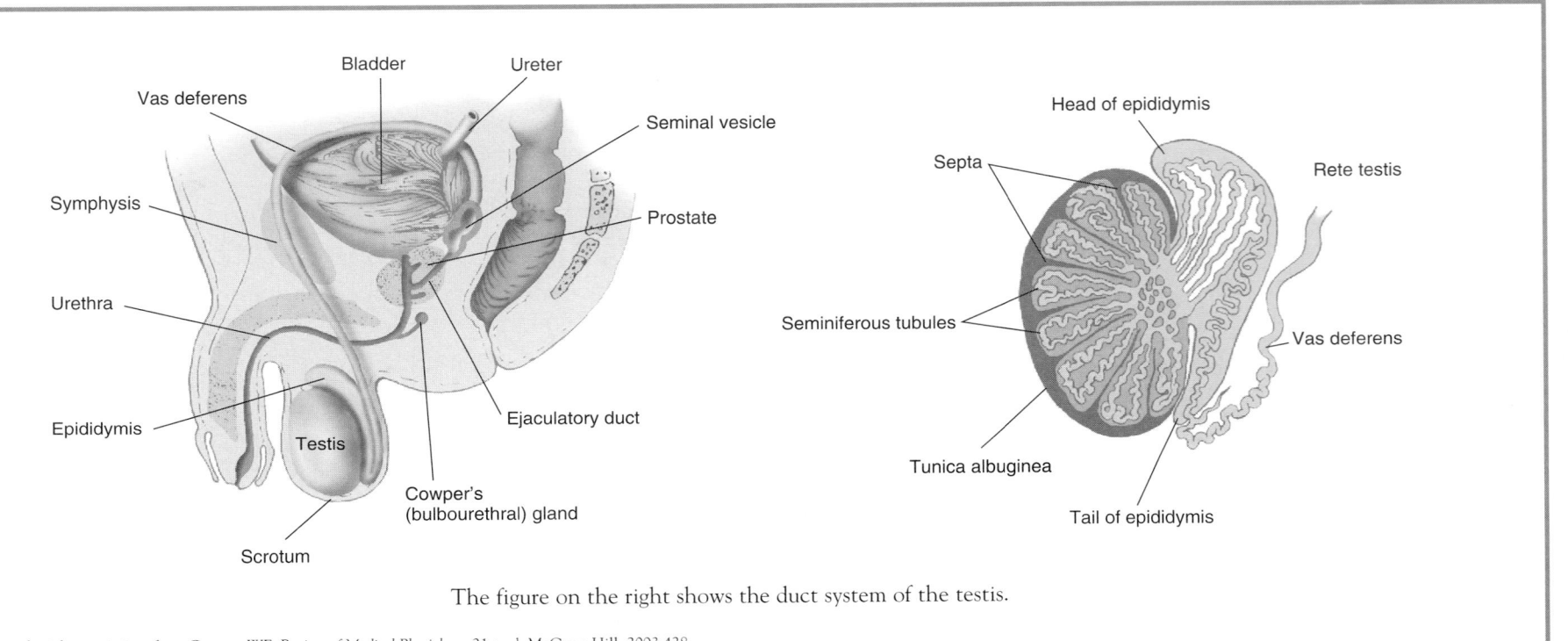

The figure on the right shows the duct system of the testis.

Reproduced, with permission, from Ganong WF: *Review of Medical Physiology*, 21st ed. McGraw-Hill, 2003:428.

MALE REPRODUCTIVE ANATOMY

Structure	Description	Function
Testes	• Male gonads. • Each adult gonad is 40 g in weight and 4.5 cm in length. • Location in scrotum allows them to be maintained 1°–2° C below core body temperature, which facilitates sperm production.	Sperm production. Cryptorchidism: undescended testes. • Occurs in 10% of newborn males. • Treatment with gonadotropic hormones or surgery. • Risk of damage to spermatogenic epithelium if not corrected early. • Associated with higher incidence of testicular cancer.
Seminiferous Tubules	• Form 80% of testis. • Coiled mass of loops that drain into head of epididymis.	Site of spermatogenesis.
Epididymis	Convoluted tube that connects testis to vas deferens.	Maturation (2–4 weeks) and storage (in tail) for spermatozoa.
Vas Deferentia	Pair of ducts with muscular wall.	• Store and carry spermatozoa from epididymis to ejaculatory duct. • Contraction aids in ejaculation.
Ejaculatory Ducts	Ducts within body of prostate.	Carries spermatozoa into urethra for emission.
Prostate	Accessory sex gland below bladder that opens into urethra.	• Secretes alkaline fluid, forming part of semen. • Helps neutralize acid pH of female genital secretions.
Seminal Vesicles	Paired accessory sex glands that open into each vas deferens before vas deferens joins urethra.	Provides largest, terminal portion of ejaculate that contains fructose (nutrition for spermatozoa) and prostaglandins.
Leydig Cells	• Interstitial cells and connective tissue of testis. • Form 20% of testis.	Stimulated by LH from pituitary to secrete testosterone.
Sertoli Cells	Large, pale cells in walls of seminiferous tubules.	• Anchor and nourish developing germ cells. • Tight junctions between them form blood-testis barrier. • *Secrete androgen-binding protein, inhibin, and MIS.* • Contain aromatase, which can convert androgens to estrogens.

Continued

MALE REPRODUCTIVE ANATOMY (Continued)

Structure	Description	Function
Blood-Testis Barrier	Components: • Basement membrane. • Peritubular cells. • Tight junctions and cytoplasm of Sertoli cells.	• Excludes harmful substances from intercellular fluid bathing maturing germ cells and from tubular fluid surrounding spermatozoa. • Products from later stages of spermatogenesis are prevented from diffusing back into bloodstream and producing antibodies. • Provides germ cells with high local concentrations of testosterone from Leydig cells and protein and other products from Sertoli cells; this is essential for spermatogenesis.

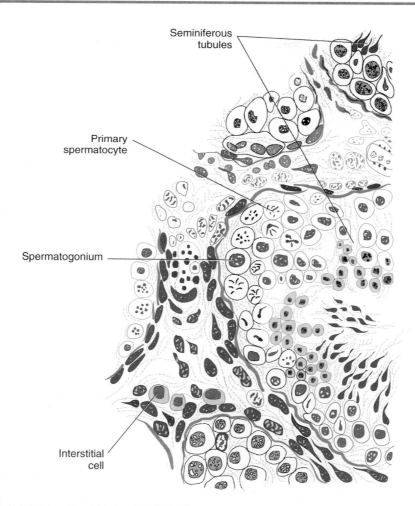

Seminiferous tubules

Primary spermatocyte

Spermatogonium

Interstitial cell

Reproduced, with permission, from Ganong WF: *Review of Medical Physiology,* 21st ed. McGraw-Hill, 2003:428.

SPERMATOGENESIS

Structure	Description	Function	Product
Spermatogonia	• Immature male germ cells near basal lamina. • Until puberty, multiplication is insignificant. • After puberty, multiplication continues throughout life.	Undergo two *mitotic* divisions within basal compartment.	Three active cells (primary spermatocytes) and one resting cell.
Primary Spermatocytes	• Products of mitosis. • Generated by spermatogonia beginning at puberty.	Enter prophase of meiosis, *first reduction division*, in which they remain for 20 days.	Two secondary spermatocytes.
Secondary Spermatocytes	Products of first meiotic division.	Undergo second meiotic division.	Four spermatids.
Spermatids	• Products of second meiotic division. • *Contain haploid number of 23 chromosomes*: 22 autosomes and either one X or one Y chromosome. • Head has nucleus and acrosomal cap, which contains hydrolytic and proteolytic enzymes that facilitate penetration of ovum. • Body (middle piece) and tail contain mitochondria and ATP that generate motile energy, and contractile microtubules aid in flagellar motion.	Undergo nuclear condensation, shrinkage of cytoplasm, formation of acrosome, and development of tail.	• Four spermatozoa (sperm). • 100–200 million sperm can be produced daily. • Sequence of spermatozoa development occurs over 50–70 days. • Groups of adjacent spermatogonia initiate cycle of development every 16 days.

ERECTION AND EJACULATION

Events	Description	Mechanism	Clinical Significance
Erection: *Parasympathetic Control*	• Simultaneous dilation of arterioles, filling of venous sinuses, and constriction of veins.	*Activation of cGMP, a vasodilator, by nitric oxide.*	• Sildenafil (Viagra) inhibits breakdown of cGMP by phosphodiesterase. • Used to treat erectile dysfunction.
		Prostaglandin E$_1$ is also a vasodilator.	• Alprostadil (Muse; prostaglandin E$_1$). • Used to treat erectile dysfunction.
Emission: *Sympathetic Control*	Semen moves into urethra.	Contraction of smooth muscle of vas deferens and seminal vesicles in response to stimuli from hypogastric nerves.	
Ejaculation: *Sympathetic Control*	• Semen is propelled from urethra at time of orgasm.	Contraction of bulbocavernosus muscle.	

☞ Parasympathetic: "Point", Sympathetic: "Shoot."

III. Female Reproduction

FEMALE REPRODUCTIVE SYSTEM

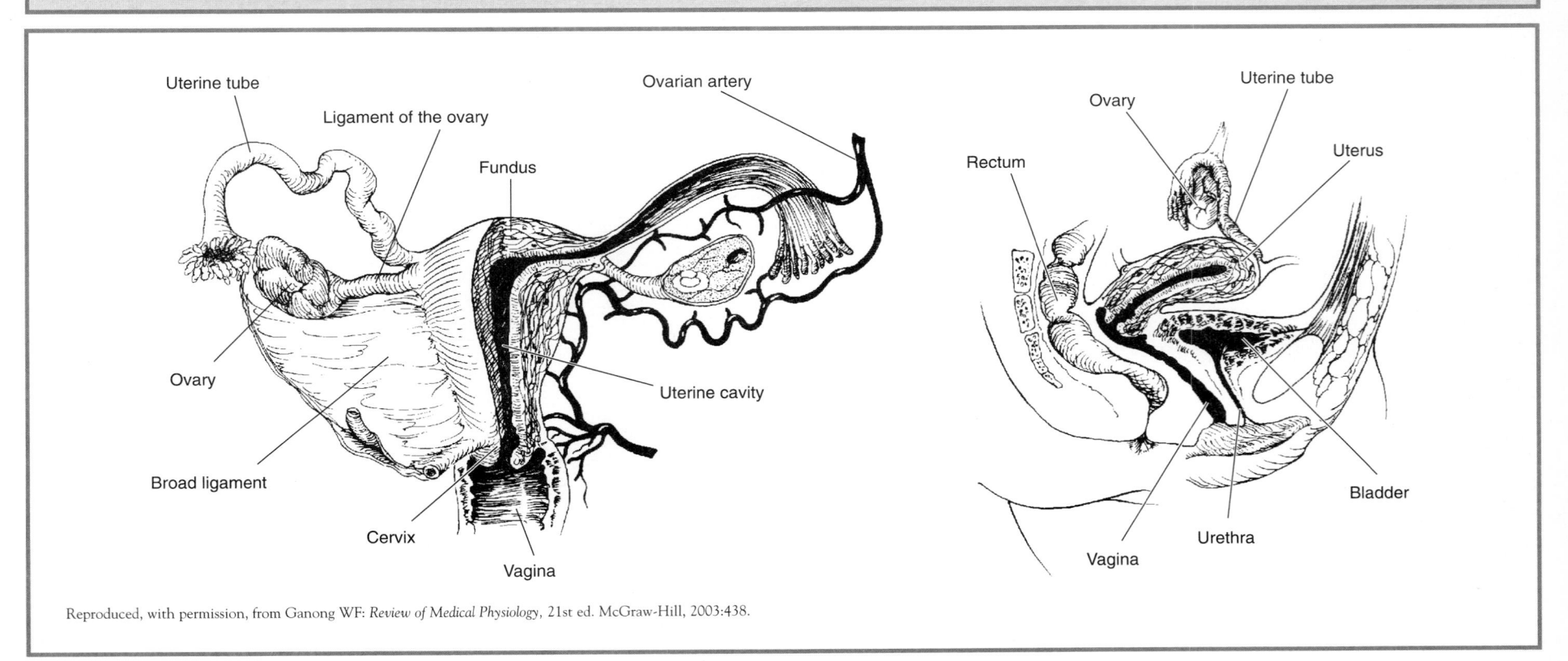

Reproduced, with permission, from Ganong WF: *Review of Medical Physiology*, 21st ed. McGraw-Hill, 2003:438.

Structure	Description	Function
Ovaries	• Female gonads. • Have three zones: cortex, medulla, and hilum. • Cortex: lined by germinal epithelium and contains oocytes enclosed in follicles in various stages of development as well as surrounding stroma of connective tissue and interstitial cells. • Medulla and hilum: contain scattered steroid-producing cells.	Produces ova and steroid hormones in response to gonadotropins in cyclic fashion. ☞ :**RIPE** (ovarian hormones)—**R**elaxin, **I**nhibin, **P**rogesterone, **E**strogen
Granulosa Cells	• Surround oocyte. • Form corona radiata. • Analogous to Sertoli cells in male.	Secrete estrogens.
Theca (Interstitial Cells)	• Form vascular theca interna and theca externa (made of loose connective tissue and smooth muscle) that surround oocyte. • Analogous to Leydig cells in male.	Secrete androgens.
Luteal Cells	Transformed granulosa and theca cells.	Secrete progesterone.
Uterus	• Muscular pelvic organ suspended by ligaments. • Inner mucous lining is endometrium (decidua is endometrium of pregnancy). • Outer muscular lining is myometrium. • Connected to fallopian tubes proximally and cervix distally.	Houses, nurtures, and eventually evacuates mature fetus.
Fallopian Tubes (Oviducts, Uterine Tubes)	• Tubes that extend from uterus and open into abdominal cavity. • Ovarian end has fimbriated ends that help guide ovum.	• Conduct ova from ovary to womb. • Serve as site for fertilization of ovum and sperm.

Continued

FEMALE REPRODUCTIVE ANATOMY (Continued)

Structure	Description	Function
Vagina	Muscular tube lined with mucous membrane that connects cervix to exterior of body.	Estradiol increases cornification of epithelium and vaginal secretion, enhancing conditions for fertilization.
Cervix	• Neck of uterus. • Located at distal end of uterus.	Helps maintain competency of fetus.
Breasts	• Mammary glands. • Made of glandular lobules embedded in fatty tissue. • Milk passes from lobules into ducts that discharge into nipple.	Secrete milk to provide nutrition for infant.

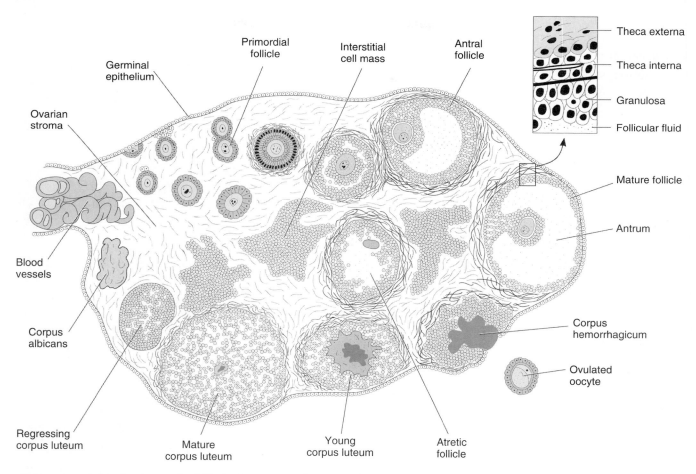

This diagram shows the sequential development of a follicle, formation of a corpus luteum, and follicular atresia. A section of the wall of a mature follicle is enlarged at the upper right.

Reproduced, with permission, from Gorbman A, Bern H: *Textbook of Comparative Endocrinology*. Wiley, 1962.

OOGENESIS

Cell	Description	Function	Product
Oogonium	• Primordial female germ cell. • Earliest stage in formation of an ovum. • Oocyte and surrounding granulosa and theca cells.	Enters prophase of meiosis after mitotic proliferation.	• 6–7 million oogonia by 20th week of gestation. • Some oogonia degenerate, leaving 2 million primordial follicles at birth, 50% of which are atretic. • Normally, about 1 million undergo first part of first meiosis. • Combination of primary oocytes and spindle cells yields primordial follicle.
Primary Oocyte	• Product of oogonium. • Arrested in prophase of meiosis. • Throughout life, undergoes either atresia (caused by apoptosis) or ovulation.<hr>• *No new ova formed after birth.* • Attrition or ovulation continues until reproductive capacity ends (unlike males, whose supply of spermatogonia is continually renewed).<hr>• Number of ova in both ovaries at puberty is < 300,000. • Only one per cycle normally reaches maturity, and the rest degenerate.	*Completes first meiotic division at ovulation.*	One secondary oocyte and the first polar body, each with 46 chromosomes.<hr>At 5 to 6 months gestation, spindle cells are transformed into cuboidal granulosa cells, forming a primary follicle.<hr>• Granulosa and theca cells make several layers around oocyte, producing secondary follicle, which is contained within mature ovarian (graafian) follicle. • Mature ovarian follicle undergoes ovulation.
Secondary Oocyte	• Product of primary oocyte as result of ovulation. • Receives most of cytoplasm, while second polar body fragments and disappears.	• Begins second meiotic division and stops at metaphase. • *Division completed only when sperm penetrates oocyte.*	Mature ovum and second polar body, each with 23 chromosomes (haploid).

MENSTRUAL CYCLE

Uterine Cycle	Ovarian Cycle	Associated Hormonal Changes
Follicular Phase (preovulatory phase): days 1–13		
• Under influence of estrogens from developing follicle, endometrium increases rapidly in thickness. • Uterine glands lengthen.	• Menstrual bleeding begins. • Several *primordial follicles* enlarge. • *Antral follicles* form.	• Before follicular phase, FSH and LH are at their lowest, with LH:FSH ratio slightly > 1. • One day before onset of menses, FSH begins gradual increase that continues through the first half of follicular phase. • LH increases slightly later (see "Hormones and Changes in the Endometrium During the Menstrual Cycle").
	• FSH supports early maturation of ovarian follicles. • LH is kept low because of negative feedback from estrogen (inhibin is low and FSH is elevated).	• Second half of follicular phase, FSH falls slightly and LH continues to increase. • LH:FSH ratio approaches 2.
	• Day 6: one follicle in one ovary starts to grow rapidly and becomes *dominant follicle*. • Other follicles regress and become *atretic follicles*.	• Day 6: estradiol begins gradual increase, stimulated by FSH. • Later in follicular phase, estradiol increases more sharply (caused by increased granulosa cell secretion of inhibin, which decreases FSH) and peaks just before ovulatory phase.
	36–48 hours before ovulation, estrogen feedback becomes positive and initiates LH surge.	• LH continues to rise until it peaks. • FSH also peaks with smaller spike.
Ovulation: day 14 (may last 1–3 days)		
No significant changes.	• *LH surge triggers ovulation 9 hours later* and is responsible for initial formation of corpus luteum • Mature (graafian) follicle ruptures, and ovum is extruded into abdominal cavity. • Fimbriated ends of fallopian tubes pick up ovum and transport it to uterus.	LH and FSH spike.

Continued

MENSTRUAL CYCLE (CONTINUED)

Uterine Cycle	Ovarian Cycle	Associated Hormonal Changes
Ovulation: day 14 (may last 1–3 days) (Continued)		
	• Ovum lives 72 hours after it is extruded from follicle. • *Most fertile time is 48 hours before ovulation.* • If ovum is not fertilized, it leaves through vagina (endometrium is shed and menstruation occurs).	
	Ovulation is associated with increase in basal body temperature.	Progesterone increases.
Luteal Phase (secretory phase): days 15–28		
• After ovulation, endometrium becomes more vascularized and edematous under influence of estrogen and progesterone from corpus luteum. • Uterine glands become coiled and tortuous and secrete clear fluid.	• Ruptured follicle fills with blood (corpus hemorrhagicum). • Granulosa and theca cells lining follicle proliferate. • Clotted blood replaced with yellow, lipid-rich luteal cells, forming *corpus luteum*.	*Tenfold increase in plasma progesterone from corpus luteum.*
Late in luteal phase endometrium makes PRL (function unknown).	If fertilization occurs, corpus luteum persists and menstruation ceases until after delivery of infant.	• *Placenta secretes hCG, which supports corpus luteum.* • Luteal cells secrete estrogens and progesterone. • LH and FSH secretion is low because of elevated estrogens, progesterone, and inhibin.

- If no fertilization occurs, corpus luteum regresses, resulting in withdrawal of hormonal support.
- Endometrium becomes thinner, spinal arteries spasm, and necrosis occurs (aided by prostaglandins).
- Endometrium is shed, leading to menstrual flow, and new cycle starts.

- Stratum functionale is superficial two thirds of endometrium, supplied by spiral arteries and shed during menstruation.
- Stratum basale is deep layer supplied by basilar arteries that is not shed during menstruation.

If no fertilization occurs, corpus luteum begins to degenerate due to prostaglandins (luteolysis) 4 days before next menses and is replaced by scar tissue, forming corpus albicans.

- If no fertilization occurs, corpus luteum degenerates.
- Progesterone, estradiol, and inhibin decrease to baseline at end of luteal phase.
- FSH and LH increase.
- Menstrual bleeding starts.

HORMONES AND CHANGES IN THE ENDOMETRIUM DURING THE MENSTRUAL CYCLE

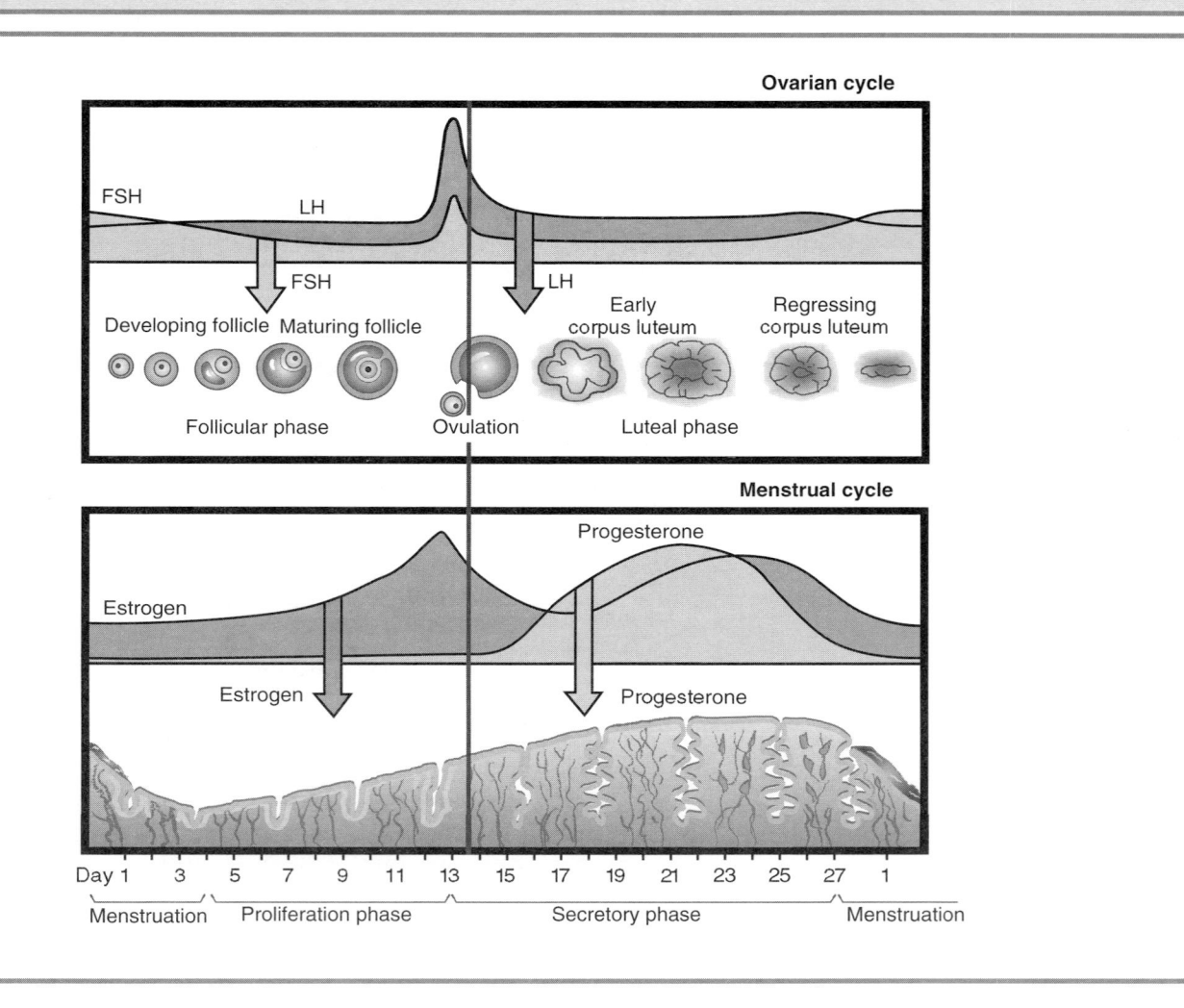

MENSTRUAL ABNORMALITIES

Disorder	Description
Amenorrhea	Absence of menses.
Primary Amenorrhea	Menstrual bleeding has never occurred.
Secondary Amenorrhea	Cessation of menses in females with previously normal periodic bleeding (caused by pregnancy until proved otherwise).
Hypomenorrhea	Scanty flow during regular menses.
Menorrhagia	Abnormally profuse flow during regular menses.
Metrorrhagia	Uterine bleeding between menses.
Menometrorrhagia	Irregular periodicity, amount, or duration of menses.
Oligomenorrhea	Reduced frequency of menses.
Dysmenorrhea	• Painful menstruation, often caused by accumulation of prostaglandins in uterus. • Inhibitors of prostaglandin synthesis provide relief..
Premenstrual Syndrome	• Irritability, bloating, edema, emotional lability, decreased ability to concentrate, depression, headache, and constipation during last 7–10 days of menstrual cycle. • Also known as premenstrual tension or luteal phase dysphoric disorder.
Polycystic Ovary Syndrome (Stein-Leventhal Syndrome)	• Incomplete development of graafian follicles resulting from inadequate LH. • Follicles fail to ovulate and remain as multiple cysts, distending ovary. • Further hormone imbalance (eg, excessive theca production of androgens) leads to obesity, infertility, and hirsutism.

IV. Pregnancy

FERTILIZATION

Millions of sperm are deposited into vagina during sexual intercourse.

- Approximately 50–100 sperm reach the ovum and bind to the zona pellucida.
- Ovum must encounter sperm within 12–24 hours of ovulation for fertilization to occur.
- Sperm must reach ovum within 48 hours after entering vagina.
- Capitation is the process by which sperm contact the female reproductive tract for several hours, increasing their motility and enhancing their ability to penetrate the ovum.

Acrosomal reaction:

- Acrosome breaks down, releasing enzymes, including acrosin.
- These enzymes disperse the cumulus oophorus and facilitate sperm penetration through the zona pellucida.

Fertilization of ovum by sperm occurs in the midfallopian tube.

- Fusion to ovum membrane is mediated by the protein fertilin on sperm head.
- Fusion initiates development and reduces membrane potential of the ovum, preventing polyspermy.
- Structural change in zona pellucida provides long-term protection against polyspermy.
- Breakdown of fusion area leads to release of sperm nucleus into cytoplasm of ovum.

IMPLANTATION

Step	Event
1	Blastocyst moves down fallopian tube into uterus over 3 days, during which time it reaches 8- or 16-cell stage.
2	Implantation in uterus begins within another 2–3 days.
3	• Once blastocyst contacts endometrium, it becomes surrounded by syncytiotrophoblast (outer layer) and cytotrophoblast (inner layer). • Implantation usually occurs on dorsal uterine wall.
4	Fetus and placenta develop.

HORMONAL CHANGES AFTER IMPLANTATION

Step	Change
1	Placenta secretes hCG and stimulates corpus luteum to grow and secrete estrogen, progesterone, and relaxin.
2	After sixth week of pregnancy, placenta produces sufficient hormones to take over function of corpus luteum.
3	Corpus luteum function begins to decline after 8 weeks of pregnancy (but persists throughout).
4	hCG decreases after an initial rise, but estrogen and progesterone increase until just before parturition. • Placenta synthesizes pregnenolone and progesterone from cholesterol. • Some pregnenolone and progesterone enters fetal circulation where is used as substrate for synthesis of fetal adrenal steroids.

STAGES OF LABOR

Stage	Description	Maternal Changes	Fetal Changes
1	• Gradual dilation and effacement of cervix, with uterine contractions. • Duration: 10–25 hours.	• Latent phase: cervix dilates 0–4 cm, membranes spontaneously rupture, and contractions become more regular. • Active phase: cervix dilates 4–8 cm. • Transition phase: cervix dilates 8–10 cm (full dilation). Positive feedback loop: uterine contractions dilate cervix, leading to secretion of oxytocin and prostaglandin that stimulates uterine contractions.	• Placental CRH increases at term, leading to increased fetal DHEAS, which causes increased placental estrogens. • Placental and fetal hypothalamic CRH increases fetal ACTH and cortisol, which stimulates fetal lung maturation and promotes closure of ductus arteriosus.
2	• Full cervical dilation to delivery. • Duration: 30–120 minutes	• Once fully dilated, uterine contractions can expel fetus through cervix and vaginal opening. • Episiotomy may prevent uncontrolled tearing of perineum.	• Fetal-placental circulation ceases. • Ductus arteriosis closes because of decreased prostaglandins. • Decrease in pulmonary vascular resistance allows aeration of fetal lungs.
3	• Delivery of placenta. • Duration: 5–30 minutes.	• Myometrial contractions constrict uterine vessels and prevent excessive bleeding. • Removed placenta must be examined for tears, because retained placental tissue may result in prolonged bleeding.	

FUNCTION OF HORMONES DURING LACTATION

Estrogen	Oxytocin	Prolactin
During pregnancy, high PRL, estrogens, and progesterone promote full lobuloalveolar development of breasts Drop in circulating estrogen after delivery initiates lactation (estrogen antagonizes the milk-producing effect of prolactin).	• Stimulated by nursing. • Causes contraction of myoepithelial cells of alveoli, promoting flow of milk into areola.	• Stimulated by nursing. • Stimulates milk production after childbirth. • Inhibits GnRH, which inhibits ovulation. • Women who nurse regularly have amenorrhea for 25–30 weeks. • Women who do not nurse have first menstrual period 6 weeks after delivery. • 50% of cycles first 6 months after resumption of menses are anovulatory. • Risk of pregnancy while nursing is 5–10% due to resulting low estrogen and progesterone levels

INDEX

baroreceptor(s), 127
    cardiovascular regulation by, 127, 196
    maintenance of ECF volume by, 332
baroreceptor reflex, 197, 198
basal ganglia, 95
basal ganglia lesions, movement disorders due to, 105
basal metabolic rate, 369
basilar artery, 201
basilar membrane, 88, 89, 102
basophils, 129
BBB (bundle branch block), 190, 192
B cells, 129, 134, 135
Becker muscular dystrophy, 45
"bend, the," 312
beriberi, 392
beta cells, 429
ß neuron, 97
ß-oxidation, 370, 371, 386
ß-receptors, cardiovascular regulation by, 195, 202
beta waves, 113
Bezold-Jarisch reflex, 197
bicarbonate (HCO$_3^-$)
    absorption of, 293
    CO$_2$ transport in blood via, 238
    formation from NH$_4^+$ of, 357–58
    and H$^+$ secretion, 359
    measurement of, 362
    resorption of filtered, 358
bicarbonate (HCO$_3^-$) buffer system, 354, 355
bile, components of, 285
bile acids, 285
    conjugated, 259, 285
bile canaliculi, 283
bile duct, 283, 287
    ampulla of, 287
bile pathway, 286
bile pigment(s), 285
bile pigment gallstones, 285

bile salts, 259, 285
binasal heteronymous hemianopsia, 83
Biot breathing, 254, 255
biotin, 393
bipolar limb leads, 178
bitemporal heteronymous hemianopsia, 83
black widow spider bite, 34
bladder
    anatomy of, 306
    innervation of, 317
    neurogenic, in diabetes mellitus, 440
blastocyst, 493
blind loop syndrome, 273
blindness, unilateral, 83
blind spot, 75
blood-brain barrier, 56, 201
blood cells
    disorders of, 143–45
    types of, 129–30
blood coagulation, 137
blood components, structure and function of, 129–30
blood flow
    dynamics of, 146–54
    factors that influence, 149–50
blood groups, 133
blood pressure, 149
    high, 154
blood-testis barrier, 478
blood vessels
    parallel and series arrangement of, 150, 151
    radius of, 149
    structure and function of, 146–47
blood viscosity, 150
body fluid(s), 46–52
body fluid compartments, 46
body fluid volume, 328–45
body water, characteristics of, 328
Bohn effect, 235

bone(s)
    anatomy of, 419–21
    compact (cortical), 419–21
    trabecular (spongy, cancellous), 419–21
bone conduction, 90
bone diseases, 423–24
bone formation, 422
bone remodeling, 422
bone resorption, 422
    parathyroid disorders and, 427
botulism, 34
Bowman capsule, 307, 310, 312
Bowman space, 311
    hydrostatic pressure in, 322
    oncotic pressure in, 322
Boyle law, 214
bradycardia, sinus, 181, 182
bradykinesia, 105
bradykinin
    cardiovascular regulation by, 194
    and glomerular filtration, 326
brain, 59–62
brain death, 117
brainstem, 59
    in motor system, 95
Braxton Hicks contractions, 459
breasts, 484
breathing
    accessory muscles of, 219
    Biot, 254, 255
    chemical control of, 248
    CNS control of, 249–50
    Kussmaul, 255, 400
    mechanics of, 215–31
    periodic, 254
    regulation of, 247
    work of, 216
broad ligament, 482
bronchial artery, 221

E

ear
- anatomy of, 84
- inner, 87–89
- middle, 86
- outer, 85

eardrum, 84, 86

ECF. *See* extracellular fluid (ECF)

ECG. *See* electrocardiogram (ECG)

edema, pulmonary, 213

Edinger-Westphal nucleus, 109

EEG. *See* electroencephalogram (EEG)

EF (ejection fraction), 159, 160

effectors, in intracellular communication, 15

efferent nerves, 56, 58

eicosanoids, 369, 382

ejaculation, 481

ejaculatory ducts
- anatomy of, 476, 477
- development of, 463
- function of, 477

ejection fraction (EF), 159, 160

elastance, 210

elastic recoil, 146, 210

electrocardiogram (ECG)
- with abnormal K⁺ concentration, 179
- of atrial rhythms, 182–84
- axis deviation on, 179
- of conduction disturbances, 188–92
- lead placements for, 178
- normal, 175–77
- of sinus rhythms, 180, 181
- of ventricular rhythms, 185–87

electrochemical potential difference, 51

electroencephalogram (EEG)
- during brain death, 117
- during seizures, 116
- during sleep, 114

electrolytes, absorption of, 293, 295

elliptocytosis, hereditary, cytoskeleton in, 7

Embden-Meyerhof pathway, 375

embryology, of reproductive system, 462, 463

emmetropia, 80

emphysema, 212
- compliance curve in, 228
- diffusing capacity in, 232
- lung compliance in, 224

endocrine, defined, 400

endocrine communication, 12, 14

endocrine pancreas, 259

endocrine system, 397–455
- adrenal gland in, 441–54
- calcium, phosphate, bone, and parathyroid gland in, 416–27
- hypothalamus and pituitary gland in, 402–7
- pancreas in, 428–40
- pineal gland in, 455
- thyroid gland in, 408–15

endocytosis, 49

endolymph, 87, 101

endometrium, in menstrual cycle, 488, 489

endoplasmic reticulum (ER), 6, 8

ß-endorphin, 31

endothelin, and glomerular filtration, 326

endothelin-1, cardiovascular regulation by, 193

endothelium-derived relaxing factor, cardiovascular regulation by, 193

end-plate potential, 40

energy balance, 372

energy metabolism, 371–72

energy storage, 372

energy transfer, between organs, 373

enkephalin, 31

enteric nervous system (ENS), 58, 107, 263, 268, 269

enterochromaffin cells, 261

enterochromaffin-like cells, 261, 288

enterogastric reflex, 271

enterohepatic circulation, 286

enterokinase, 282

entero-oxyntin, 288

enteropeptidase, 282

enuresis, nocturnal, 115

enzymes, in fatty acid metabolism, 384

eosinophils, 129

ependymal cells, 19

epididymis
- anatomy of, 476, 477
- development of, 462, 463
- function of, 477

epilepsy, 116

epinephrine, 30
- cardiovascular regulation by, 194
- and glomerular filtration, 326
- and insulin, 432
- and pulmonary resistance, 225
- synthesis of, 452

epiphyseal closure, 421, 468

epiphyseal plate, 419, 421

epiphysis, 419, 421

episodic memory, 119

epithelium, of intestinal walls, 263, 264

epoophoron, 462

equilibrium potential, for ion, 51

ER (endoplasmic reticulum), 6, 8

erection, 481

ERV (expiratory reserve volume), 215, 216

erythroblastosis fetalis, 127

erythrocytes, 129
- disorders of, 143–44

erythropoietin, 127, 304

escape phenomenon, 444

esophageal sphincter, lower, 265

esophagus, gross anatomy of, 265, 267

essential fatty acids, 369

essential hypertension, 154

essential thrombocythemia, 143

paradoxical splitting, 165
parafollicular cells, of thyroid gland, 408, 409
paralysis
   flaccid, 35
   periodic, 45
paralytic ileus, 273
parasympathetic nervous system (PNS), 58, 107,
     109–11
   cardiovascular regulation by, 195
   gastrointestinal regulation by, 268, 269, 276
parathyroid disorders, metabolic effects of, 427
parathyroid gland, anatomy of, 425
parathyroid hormone (PTH)
   actions of, 426
   and calcium metabolism, 297, 418, 426
   and H^+ secretion, 359
parietal cells, 261
   in digestion, 288
   HCl secretion by, 262
parietal lobe, 60, 62
parietal pleura, 219
parietal-temporal-occipital association area, 62
Parkinson disease, 30, 105
paroxysmal atrial tachycardia, 182
paroxysmal ventricular tachycardia, 185
pars compacta, lesions of, 105
pars reticulata, lesions of, 105
partial pressure(s), 210
   and pulmonary blood flow, 243
partial pressure of carbon dioxide (PCO_2),
     measurement of, 362
partial thromboplastin time (PTT), 138
parturition, 459
parvicellular pathway, 68
pavor nocturnes, 115
PCO_2 (partial pressure of carbon dioxide),
     measurement of, 362
PCW (transthoracic pressure), 223
peak flow, 229

PEEP (positive end-expiratory pressure), 210
pellagra, 392
pelvic nerves, 317
   and gastrointestinal motility, 268
pelvic space, 309
penis, development of, 463
pentose phosphate pathway, 375
pepsin(s), 291, 296
pepsinogens, 291
peptic cells, 261
peptic ulcer disease, 279
perfusion-limited gas exchange, 232
perfusion pressure, and renin secretion, 348
perfusion zones, 241
pericardium, 157
perilymph, 87, 101
periodic block, 189
periodic breathing, 254
periodic paralysis, 45
periosteum, 421
peripheral nervous system, 58
peristalsis, 266, 270
peritubular capillaries
   hydrostatic pressure in, 323
   oncotic pressure in, 323
   Starling forces between intercellular space and,
     323
pernicious anemia, 296, 393
peroxisomes, 7
persistent müllerian duct syndrome, 474
petrosal sinus sampling, for Cushing syndrome, 451
Peyer patches, 261
pH
   abnormalities in, 249
   cardiovascular regulation by, 193
   compensatory responses of ECF to changes in, 354
   measurement of, 362
   normal, 353
   and potassium homeostasis, 343

phagocytosis, 49
phantom limb sensation, 94
phasic stretch reflex, 100
phenylalanine, 452
phenylketonuria, 452
pheochromocytoma, 448
phosphate, 416
   clinical significance of, 416
   description of, 416
   metabolism of, 416
   parathyroid disorders and, 427
   PTH and, 426
   regulation of, 416
   renal processing of, 345
phospholipase A_2, in pancreatic juice, 282, 292
phospholipids, in bile, 285
phosphorylcreatine, 379
photopic vision, 77
physiologic dead space (VDS), 217
physiologic shunt, 245
pigment epithelium, of retina, 74
"pill rolling" movement, 105
pineal gland, 455
pinna, 85
pinocytosis, 49
pituitary adenoma, 450, 451
pituitary gland
   disorders of, 406–7
   and hypothalamus, 405
pituitary hormones, 403–4
PL (transpulmonary pressure), 223
   and distribution of ventilation, 244
placenta
   delivery of, 494
   hormones secreted by, 488, 493, 494
plasma, 46, 131
plasma cells, disorders of, 144
plasma creatinine, 325
plasma membrane, 5

respiratory alkalosis, 364
  compensatory mechanism in, 249, 363, 364
  conditions associated with, 364
  nomogram of, 365
  and ventilatory rate, 354
respiratory bronchiole, 221
respiratory compensation, 363
respiratory defense, 222
respiratory disease. *See* lung disease
respiratory distress syndrome
  adult, 212
  of premature infants, 224
respiratory epithelia, defense function of, 222
respiratory exchange ratio, 210
respiratory gas diffusion, 232–33
respiratory minute volume, 216
respiratory passages, defense function of, 222
respiratory quotient, 211
respiratory response, to stress, 251–55
respiratory system, 207–55
resting expiratory level, 216
restrictive airway disease, 211, 231
  compliance curves in, 227
  lung compliance in, 224
rete testis, 476
reticular activating system, 57
  control of breathing by, 250
reticular lamina, 89
reticulospinal tract
  medullary (lateral), 71
  pontine (medial), 71
retina, 74–75
retrograde amnesia, 119
reverse T_3, 409
RFI (renal failure index), 325
rheumatoid arthritis, mitochondria in, 6
Rh-incompatibility, 127
rhodopsin, 74, 77
riboflavin, 392

rickets, 297, 393, 424
right atrium, 155
right bundle branch, 158
right bundle branch block (RBBB), 190, 192
right hepatic duct, 287
right-sided heart failure, 174
right ventricle, 156
rigidity
  cogwheel, 105
  decerebrate, 56
  decorticate, 56
  lead pipe, 105
Rinne test, 90
risus sardonicus, 33
rods, 74, 77
rofecoxib (Vioxx), 383
rough endoplasmic reticulum (RER), 6, 8
round window, 84, 87
RR interval, 176
rubrospinal tract, 72
Ruffini corpuscle, 93
RV (residual volume), 159, 215, 216, 229
R wave, 175

S

saccades, 79
saccule, 100
sacculus, 102
sacral parasympathetic nucleus, 109
SA (sinoatrial) exit block, 188
saliva, 276
salivary amylase, 276, 289
salivary glands, in digestion and absorption of
    carbohydrates, 289
salivatory nuclei, 109
SA (sinoatrial) node, 155, 158
  blocks at, 188
sarcolemma, 36, 37

sarcomere, 36, 37–38, 39
sarcoplasmic reticulum (SR), 36, 37
sarcotubular system, 37
satiety center, 402
scala media, 87, 89
scala tympani, 87, 89
scala vestibuli, 87, 89
Schwann cell, 19, 21
sclera, 73
scorpion sting, 34
scotoma, 83
scotopic vision, 77
scrotum, 476
  development of, 463, 472
scurvy, 393
secondary active transport, 48
secondary hypertension, 154
second-degree block, 189, 191
second messengers, 15, 16
secretin, 32, 275
  in digestion, 288
  and gastric emptying, 277, 278
secretion, 305
secretory granules, 8
secretory phase, 490
segmentation, in gastrointestinal motility, 270
seizures, 116
semantic memory, 119
semicircular canals, 84, 101, 102
semilunar valves, 156
  closure of, 162, 165
seminal vesicles
  anatomy of, 476, 477
  development of, 462, 463
  function of, 477
seminiferous tubules, 476, 477, 479
senile dementia of Alzheimer type, 56
sensitization, 118
sensory association cortex, 60